Research Methods in Physical Activity and Health

D1610751

Physical activity is vital for good health. It has an established strong evidence base for its positive effects on functional capacity, reducing the risk of many chronic diseases, and promoting physical, mental and social well-being. Furthermore, these benefits are evident across a diversity of ages, groups and populations. The need for these benefits in current societies means that exercise practitioners, professional bodies, institutions, health authorities and governments require high quality evidence to establish appropriate exercise guidelines, implementation strategies and effective exercise prescription at individual, group and population levels. *Research Methods in Physical Activity and Health* is the first book to comprehensively present the issues associated with physical activity and health research and outline methods available along with considerations of the issues associated with these methods and working with particular groups.

The book outlines the historical and scientific context of physical activity and health research before working through the full research process, from generating literature reviews and devising a research proposal, through selecting a research methodology and quantifying physical activity and outcome measures, to disseminating findings. Including a full section on conducting research studies with special populations, the book includes chapters on:

- Observational and cross-sectional studies;
- Interviews, questionnaires and focus groups;
- Qualitative and quantitative research methods;
- Epidemiological research methods;
- Physical activity interventions and sedentary behaviour; and
- Working with children, older people, indigenous groups, LGBTI groups, and those physical and mental health issues.

Research Methods in Physical Activity and Health is the only book to approach the full range of physical activity research methods from a health perspective. It is essential reading for any undergraduate student conducting a research project or taking applied research modules in physical activity and health, graduate students of epidemiology, public health, exercise psychology or exercise physiology with a physical activity and health focus, or practicing researchers in the area.

Stephen R. Bird is a Research Group Leader at RMIT University, Australia. He has over 30 years of experience working in the University and Hospital sectors in the field of

Health and Exercise. He has authored five books in the field, as well as numerous book chapters and over 100 articles on the subject. He is an active member of numerous professional associations, including being a former Chair of the Physiology Section of the British Association of Sport and Exercise Sciences. His current research interests include physical activity for older people, the prevention of chronic diseases, and the use of exercise in rehabilitation programs.

Research Methods in Physical Activity and Health

Edited by Stephen R. Bird

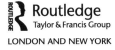

LONDON AND NEW YORK

First published 2019
by Routledge
2 Park Square, Milton Park, Abingdon, Oxon OX14 4RN

and by Routledge
52 Vanderbilt Avenue, New York, NY 10017

Routledge is an imprint of the Taylor & Francis Group, an informa business

British Library Cataloguing-in-Publication Data
A catalogue record for this book is available from the British Library

Library of Congress Cataloging-in-Publication Data
Names: Bird, Stephen R., 1959– editor.
Title: Research methods in physical activity and health / edited
  by Stephen R. Bird.
Description: Abingdon, Oxon ; New York, NY : Routledge, 2018. |
  Includes bibliographical references and index.
Identifiers: LCCN 2018037817 | ISBN 9781138067677 (hardback) |
  ISBN 9781138067684 (pbk.) | ISBN 9781315158501 (ebk.)
Subjects: LCSH: Exercise—Health aspects—Research—Methodology. |
  Health behavior—Research—Methodology. | Physical
  fitness—Research—Methodology.
Classification: LCC RA781 .R366 2018 | DDC 613.7072—dc23
LC record available at https://lccn.loc.gov/2018037817

ISBN: 978-1-138-06767-7 (hbk)
ISBN: 978-1-138-06768-4 (pbk)
ISBN: 978-1-315-15850-1 (ebk)

Typeset in NewBaskerville
by Apex CoVantage, LLC

Contents

Figures

Tables

Boxes

Contributors

Ross Arena
Department of Physical Therapy, College of Applied Health Sciences
University of Illinois at Chicago, Chicago, USA

Stephen R. Bird
School of Health and Biomedical Sciences
Royal Melbourne Institute of Technology University, Melbourne, Victoria, Australia

David R. Broom
Academy of Sport and Physical Activity
Sheffield Hallam University, Sheffield, UK

Lucy K. Byrne
School of Health Sciences
University of Tasmania, Launceston, Australia

Damian A. Coleman
Canterbury Christ Church University
Canterbury, Kent, UK

Valerie Cox
School of Life Sciences
Coventry University, Coventry, UK

Diane Crone
Cardiff Metropolitan University, Cardiff, UK

R.C. Richard Davison
School of Health and Life Sciences
University of the West of Scotland, Paisley, UK

Joshua Denham
School of Health and Biomedical Sciences
Royal Melbourne Institute of Technology University, Melbourne, Victoria, Australia

Alan E. Donnelly
Centre for Physical Activity and Health Research, Health Research Institute
Department of Physical Education and Sport Sciences
University of Limerick, Limerick, Ireland

Kieran P. Dowd
Department of Sport and Health
Athlone Institute of Technology, Westmeath, Ireland

Aunty Kerrie Doyle
School of Health and Biomedical Sciences
RMIT University, Melbourne, Australia

Kathryn Duncan
Library
Australian Catholic University, Melbourne, Australia

Michael J. Duncan
Coventry University, Coventry, UK

Panteleimon Ekkekakis
Department of Kinesiology
Iowa State University, Ames, Iowa, USA

Nir Eynon
Institute for Health and Sport, Victoria University, Australia,
and Murdoch Children's Research Institute
The Royal Children's Hospital, Melbourne, Australia

Kass Gibson
Plymouth Marjon University, Plymouth, UK

Christopher Gidlow
Centre for Health and Development
Staffordshire University, Stoke-on-Trent, UK

Paul Gorczynski
University of Portsmouth, Portsmouth, UK

Brett Gordon
La Trobe Rural Health School
La Trobe University, Bendigo, Australia

Lucy Hackshaw-McGeagh
National Institute for Health Research Bristol Biomedical Research Centre
University of Bristol, Bristol, UK

Mark E. Hartman
Department of Kinesiology
Iowa State University, Ames, Iowa, USA

Philip Hurst
Canterbury Christ Church University, Canterbury, Kent, UK

Macsue Jacques
Institute for Health and Sport, Victoria University, Melbourne, Australia

David V.B. James
School of Sport and Exercise
University of Gloucestershire, Cheltenham, UK

Damon Kendrick
Department of Health Science
Australian College of Physical Education, Sydney, Australia

Matthew A. Ladwig
Department of Kinesiology
Iowa State University, Ames, Iowa, USA

Séverine Lamon
Institute for Physical Activity and Nutrition (IPAN), School of Exercise and Nutrition
    Sciences
Deakin University, Geelong, Australia

Shanie Landen
Institute for Health and Sport
Victoria University, Melbourne, Australia

Christof A. Leicht
The Peter Harrison Centre for Disability Sport
National Centre for Sport and Exercise Medicine
School of Sport, Exercise and Health Sciences
Loughborough University, Loughborough, UK

Lorena Lozano-Sufrategui
School of Sport
Leeds Beckett University, Leeds, UK

Brigid M. Lynch
Cancer Epidemiology and Intelligence Division, Cancer Council Victoria, Melbourne,
    Australia
Centre for Epidemiology and Biostatistics, Melbourne School of Population and
    Global Health
The University of Melbourne, Australia

Noel Lythgo
School of Health and Biomedical Sciences
RMIT University, Melbourne, Australia

Nirav Maniar
School of Exercise Science
Australian Catholic University, Melbourne, Australia

Barry Mason
The Peter Harrison Centre for Disability Sport
National Centre for Sport and Exercise Medicine
School of Sport, Exercise and Health Sciences
Loughborough University, Loughborough, UK

Trine Moholdt
Department of Circulation and Medical Imaging
Norwegian University of Science and Technology, Norway

Ashleigh Moreland
School of Health and Biomedical Sciences
Royal Melbourne Institute of Technology University, Melbourne, Victoria, Australia

Marie Murphy
Dean of Postgraduate Research, Ulster University, Newtownabbey, UK

Bjarne M. Nes
Department of Circulation and Medical Imaging
Norwegian University of Science and Technology, Trondheim, Norway

Nathalie Noret
York St John University, York, UK

David Opar
School of Exercise Science
Australian Catholic University, Melbourne, Australia

Christopher S. Owens
Coventry University, Coventry, UK

Cassandra Phoenix
Department of Health
University of Bath, Bath, UK

Elizabeth Pressick
School of Health and Biomedical Sciences
RMIT University, Melbourne, Australia

Harriet Radermacher
School of Primary Health Care
Monash University, Melbourne, Australia

Shanaya Rathod
Southern Health NHS Foundation Trust
and University of Portsmouth, Portsmouth, UK

Isaac Selva Raj
School of Health and Biomedical Sciences
RMIT University, Melbourne, Australia

Nicola D. Ridgers
Institute for Physical Activity and Nutrition (IPAN)
School of Exercise and Nutrition Sciences
Deakin University, Geelong, Australia

Julian Sacre
Metabolic and Vascular Physiology
Baker Heart and Diabetes Institute, Melbourne, Australia

Anthony Shield
School of Exercise and Nutrition Sciences
Queensland University of Technology, Brisbane, Australia

Jane Sims
School of Primary Health Care
Monash University, Australia
and Department of General Practice
University of Melbourne, Melbourne, Australia

Andy Smith
York St John University, York, UK

Brett Smith
School of Sport, Exercise and Rehabilitation Sciences
University of Birmingham, Birmingham, UK

Paul M. Smith
Cardiff Metropolitan University
Cardiff, UK

Lindsey B. Strieter
Department of Physical Therapy, College of Applied Health Sciences
University of Illinois at Chicago, Chicago, USA

Keith Tolfrey
School of Sport, Exercise and Health Sciences, Paediatric Exercise Physiology Group
Loughborough University, Loughborough, UK

Jan W. van der Scheer
The Peter Harrison Centre for Disability Sport
National Centre for Sport and Exercise Medicine
School of Sport, Exercise and Health Sciences
Loughborough University, Loughborough, UK

Simone J.J.M. Verswijveren
Institute for Physical Activity and Nutrition (IPAN), School of Exercise and Nutrition
    Sciences
Deakin University, Geelong, Australia

Sarah Voisin
Institute for Health and Sport
Victoria University, Melbourne, Australia

Greig Watson
School of Health Sciences
University of Tasmania, Launceston, Australia

Jonathan D. Wiles
Canterbury Christ Church University
Canterbury, Kent, UK

Andrew D. Williams
School of Health Sciences
University of Tasmania, Launceston, Australia

Catherine Woods
Centre for Physical Activity and Health Research, Health Research Institute
Department of Physical Education and Sport Sciences
University of Limerick, Limerick, Ireland

1 Why research into health and physical activity?

Stephen R. Bird

In developed countries the prevalence of non-communicable diseases such as cardio-vascular disease (CVD) and type 2 diabetes (T2D) has increased substantially during the past 50 years.[1,2] A recognized factor contributing to the increase in these diseases is the reduction in the amount of physical activity undertaken on a daily basis by many people today compared with previous generations.[3] The proposed reasons for this include but are not limited to: (i) the mechanization of many jobs, which has resulted in a reduction in occupational physical activity and a shift towards more desk-based, sedentary occupations;[4] (ii) a reduction in incidental physical activity, where again mechanization has reduced the physical demands of household tasks and garden-ing; (iii) a reduction in active transport, with fewer people walking or cycling to work and other locations, but tending to use motorized transport; and (iv) an increase in sedentary leisure pastimes, such as television and other 'screen time' pursuits, over hobbies and interests that involve more physical activity. Hence whereas in previous generations physical activity was inherent within the lifestyle of most people, it is no longer the case. This trend towards less activity and the associated increase in the aforementioned chronic diseases has led them to be termed as 'hypokinetic diseases'. The incidence of many of these conditions is further exacerbated by changes in the availability of high-caloric foods and refined sugars that result in food intakes that exceed daily caloric expenditure (hyper-caloric). This combination of hypo-activity and hyper-caloric intakes contributes to the prevalence of obesity and many of the other risk factors associated with the chronic diseases that are now so prevalent.[5–7]

Other factors that have contributed to the recent increased prevalence of chronic diseases include improvements in surgery and the medical treatment of infectious diseases. As these have increased survival rates for trauma and infections that were previously fatal, and as a consequence, people are now living longer and becoming more susceptible to the aforementioned hypokinetic diseases and conditions that develop over a prolonged period of time. An additional consequence of more people living to an older age is an increase in the prevalence of conditions that are associ-ated with ageing, such as dementia, osteoporosis and sarcopenia. The prevalences of which are exacerbated by lifestyles that lack the physical activity known to ameliorate the development of these diseases.[8–10] Hence, whilst there are many factors contribut-ing to the increased prevalence of the aforementioned chronic diseases and condi-tions, insufficient physical activity is a consistent factor throughout.

These chronic conditions have adverse effects upon the health, functional capacity and quality of life of the individual sufferers as well as affecting their families and plac-ing a considerable burden upon the healthcare services that support them. Critically, it has been suggested that if we don't improve the health of the population, we face the prospect of an ageing society with a high prevalence of people with chronic disease and a shortage in the healthcare workforce that will be needed to look after them. Consequently, strategies and interventions that can prevent and alleviate these conditions have significant physical, mental, social and economic benefits.

The role of physical activity in reducing the risk of these diseases began to gain prominence in the research literature over 50 years ago, through the seminal research of Jerry Morris and Ralf Paffenbarger amongst others.[11–14] Building on this early scientific evidence, the case for the benefits of physical activity has continually been strengthened and broadened through the results of thousands of subsequent studies. Accordingly, physical activity is now recognized as an important factor that can benefit many aspects of physical and mental health, whilst inactivity and sedentary behaviour are recognized as significant health risks. Since as previously indicated, physical activity is no longer inherent within the lifestyles of many people, it now needs to be purposely added through the inclusion of deliberate exercise of some form. This has led to governments and health authorities promoting physical activity as a preventative measure against many diseases, as a means of recovery from many diseases and for secondary prevention (the treatment of the disease to reverse its effects and/or prevent or minimise its exacerbation). Although at this point it is worth acknowledging that whilst physical activity guidelines tend to focus on meeting physical activity targets in terms of minutes and sessions per week, there is some debate about whether it is the amount of physical activity that's undertaken on a regular basis, or physical fitness, that's quintessential to the attainment of good health and reduction of disease risk.[15] Inevitably there is a link between physical activity and fitness, but the distinction should be remembered.

The physical activity guidelines produced by governments and august bodies have been founded upon the knowledge gained from high-quality research that has endeavoured to identify: the physical, mental and social benefits of physical activity; the key risk factors associated with inactivity; the details for optimal exercise prescription; the factors that can facilitate participation in physical activity; and how to achieve effective lifestyle change. This research needs to continue, since whilst it is well established that 'exercise is good for you', determining the optimal type, frequency, duration, intensity and timing of the physical activity for each individual, as well as how it interacts with other lifestyle components such as nutrition, requires further elucidation, as do the precise mental, metabolic and physical responses and adaptations to physical activity. Furthermore, despite the overwhelming acceptance of the importance of physical activity, the majority of adults in many countries fail to achieve the minimum requirements for good health,[16] and hence research that can guide and inform effective behaviour change continues to be of vital importance. The need for ongoing, current research into physical activity and health will always be necessary as the society in which people live is subject to continual change. For example, some of the current impediments to being physically active were not an issue or even in existence a generation ago. Including the aforementioned decline in occupations that require physical activity, the reduction in active transport, and the increase in sedentary leisure pursuits (television and other screen time). Similarly, some of the current means for encouraging and promoting physical activity, such as social media, GPS watches and computer-interfaced software support programmes, were also not in existence a few years ago, and have therefore warranted the attention of current researchers. Future developments in information and communication technologies will thereby continue to present new challenges and opportunities for future generations of researchers. In parallel with this, there have been extraordinary developments in techniques and equipment for measuring physiological, metabolic, molecular and other aspects of the body, which have increased our knowledge of how the body works. This means that health and physical activity studies can now measure adaptations and responses in ways that were previously inconceivable, thereby presenting the opportunity for research studies to investigate in greater detail the issues of health and physical activity. Nevertheless, these ground-breaking techniques will only produce valid data if the basic principles behind physical activity research are adhered to. This means that even in studies where the latest equipment and techniques are being used, components of the study design, such as the process for participant recruitment, screening, compliance, control of confounding factors and many other aspects, must be considered carefully.

Furthermore, ongoing technological developments provide opportunities for researchers in other ways as they enable sophisticated data analyses on personal devices that previously would have had to have been undertaken by hand, which in many cases was not feasible. This has thereby enabled the design and analysis of studies with larger data sets and more factors to be assessed in ways that were not previously possible, as illustrated by the interest in interrogating 'Big Data'. Even at a much more basic level it is interesting to compare the lack of mention of checks for statistical violations, normality, sphericity and power analyses in many of the research papers published 40 years ago, whereas these are now a common expectation of undergraduate projects. Likewise in the fields of qualitative research, technological developments have facilitated new, innovative and effective ways to collect, analyse and interpret data. Additionally, access to these technologies and sophisticated analysis programmes has enabled the findings of previous studies to be re-evaluated, the data interrogated in greater depth and for the interaction between, and influence of, many more factors to be included in ways that were not previously possible.

For the researcher the ultimate goal must be to have an impact that in some way benefits the health of individuals and society. Measures of this impact and benefit are recognized through their inclusion in the assessment of research grant applications, reviews for publication and research ratings. If we are successful and our findings are translated into policy and action, the impact on society will be dramatic. Indeed, the established benefits of physical activity are plentiful and as former American College of Sports Medicine president Robert Sallis stated at the launch of the 'Exercise is Medicine' initiative on 5 November 2007: "*if we had a pill that conferred all the proven health benefits of exercise, physicians would widely prescribe it to their patients and our healthcare system would see to it that every patient had access to this wonder drug*".[17] a point concurred upon by Jerry Morris in the context of cardiovascular disease when he described exercise as public health's 'best buy'.[18]

Another challenge facing current and future generations of researchers is that the general public are continually bombarded with a plethora of unfounded claims and the marketing of diets and interventions that have no evidence for their health benefits or effectiveness. The nature of these are often attractive to those seeking a quick fix without the need for commitment and effort. Something that is exemplified by regular features in the media on progress towards the 'exercise pill'. However, given the breadth of health benefits conveyed by physical activity it is difficult to envisage how a pill could deliver all the positive responses and adaptations. Furthermore, as discussed by Hawley and Holloszy, "why search for a pill when exercise with all its diverse beneficial health benefits is so readily available".[19] Hence our current and future generations of physical activity researchers need to continue to present unbiased evidence from high-quality research studies, and those involved in the promotion of health and physical activity need to have the skills to identify high-quality evidence from that which is flawed and biased. They will also need to interpret potentially complex issues and disseminate the key health messages to the general public in a clear and informative manner. This is a real challenge given the nature of science as illustrated in the quote attributed to Carl Sagan:

> *Finding the occasional straw of truth awash in a great ocean of confusion and bamboozle requires intelligence, vigilance, dedication, and courage. But if we don't practice these tough habits of thought, we cannot hope to solve the truly serious problems that face us – and we risk becoming a nation of suckers, up for grabs by the next charlatan who comes along.*[20]

This nicely encapsulates the issues facing the researcher and the context in which research needs to be undertaken to identify what physical activity is beneficial to health and to refute claims that have no scientific basis. Furthermore, whilst much research has tended to focus on the benefits of physical activity for the prevention of 'ill-health', researchers also need to consider the role of physical activity in promoting good health, beyond 'being just simply free from disease', as emphasized in the WHO definition.[21]

The popularity of university programmes in this field of exercise and health, as well as the inclusion of physical activity modules in the studies of other allied health professionals, reflects the current recognition of the importance of physical activity. Likewise the inclusion of research methods in the undergraduate and post-graduate curricula of many health-related degree programmes reflects the recognized needs of the future health workforce. A physical activity and health workforce and the research students who will become the elite researchers of the future, who can understand, participate in and contribute to high-quality research in this field is of vital importance. Beyond undergraduate programmes and in the wider context, 'Physical Activity and Health Research' is conducted by health researchers and their colleagues based in hospitals, research institutes and universities. The nature of such research, involving human participants, means that the design of studies that utilize the most appropriate research methods is paramount for the production of high-quality research, and must withstand the rigorous scrutiny of ethics committees and funding bodies. Hence a strong knowledge and understanding of research methods is essential for both established researchers and those early in their research career who will need to collaborate and undertake multi-disciplinary research that may require extending their existing expertise into related but less familiar methods and paradigms. The purpose of this text is therefore to provide researchers of all levels with an insight into research techniques, processes and the issues of working with different groups. For those who are early in their research careers it seeks to provide a broad coverage of and introduction to research methods in our field, whilst for more experienced researchers it may provide a new awareness of methods that they may not have used previously and specific considerations that are pertinent when working with different groups, who they may not previously be familiar with. The text has been written to enable readers to dip into specific chapters and then pursue the topic in greater depth or breadth if required, by referring to the referenced literature. To conclude, this text aims to contribute to the pursuit of high-quality research studies that will inform future policy and exercise prescription for the improvement of health. I'm sure that I can speak on behalf of all the authors by wishing you all the best with your research as you strive to achieve this objective.

References

1 World Health Organization. Available 05/2018, from: www.who.int/news-room/fact-sheets/detail/diabetes
2 World Health Organization. Available 05/2018, from: www.who.int/cardiovascular_diseases/en/
3 Griffith R, Lluberas R, Lührmann M. Gluttony and sloth? Calories, labor market activity and the rise of obesity. *J Eur Econ Assoc.* 2016; **14**:1253–86.
4 Church TS, Thomas DM, Tudor-Locke C, Katzmarzyk PT, Earnest CP, et al. Trends over 5 Decades in U.S. Occupation-Related Physical Activity and Their Associations with Obesity. *PLoS One.* 2011; **6**(5):e19657. DOI: 10.1371/journal.pone.0019657
5 Lee IM, Shiroma EJ, Lobelo F, Puska P, Blair SN, Katzmarzyk PT. Effect of physical inactivity on major non-communicable diseases worldwide: an analysis of burden of disease and life expectancy. *Lancet.* 2012; **380**(9838):219–29.
6 Barry VW, Baruth M, Beets MW, Durstine JL, Liu J, Blair SN. Fitness vs. fatness on all-cause mortality: a meta-analysis. *Prog Cardiovasc Diseases.* 2013; **56**(4):382–90.
7 Gupta S, Rohatgi A, Ayers CR, Willis BL, Haskell WL, Khera A, et al. Cardiorespiratory fitness and classification of risk of cardiovascular disease mortality. *Circulation.* 2011; **123**(13):1377–83.
8 Kohrt WM, Bloomfield SA, Little KD, Nelson ME, Yingling VR; American College of Sports Medicine. American College of Sports Medicine Position Stand: physical activity and bone health. *Med Sci Sports Exerc.* 2004; **36**:1985–96.
9 Ahlskog JE, Geda YE, Graff-Radford NR, Petersen RC. Physical exercise as a preventive or disease-modifying treatment of dementia and brain aging. *Mayo Clin Proc.* 2011; **86**(9):876–84.
10 Denison HJ, Cooper C, Sayer AA, Robinson SM. Prevention and optimal management of sarcopenia: a review of combined exercise and nutrition interventions to improve muscle outcomes in older people. *Clin Interv Aging.* 2015; **10**:859–69.
11 Morris JN, Heady JA, Raffle PA, et al. Coronary heart-disease and physical activity of work. *Lancet,*1953; **265**:1111–20.
12 Morris JN, Heady JA. Mortality in relation to the physical activity of work: a preliminary note on experience in middle age. *Br J Ind Med.* 1953; **10**:245–54.
13 Paffenbarger RS Jr, Brand RJ, Sholtz RI, et al. Energy expenditure, cigarette smoking, and blood pressure level as related to death from specific diseases. *Am J Epidemiol.* 1978; **108**:12–8.
14 Paffenbarger RS, Hale WE. Work activity and coronary heart mortality. *N Engl J Med.* 1975; **292**:545–50.
15 Blair SN, Cheng Y, Holder JS. Is physical activity or physical fitness more important in defining health benefits? *Med Sci Sports Exerc.* 2001; **33**(6 Suppl):S379–99; discussion S419–20.
16 World Health Organisation. Prevalence of insufficient physical activity. Geneva, Switzerland: World Health Organization Press; 2010, viewed June 22, 2015. Available from: www.who.int/gho/ncd/risk_factors/physical_activity_text/en/#
17 Exercise is Medicine. Video of news conference. Available from: www.exerciseismedicine.org
18 Morris JN. Exercise in the prevention of coronary heart disease: today's best buy in public health. *Med Sci Sports Exerc.* 1994; **26**:807–14.
19 Hawley JA, Holloszy JO. Exercise: it's the real thing! *Nutr Rev.* 2009; **67**(3):172–8.
20 Available from: www.azquotes.com/quote/412007?ref=charlatans
21 World Health Organization. Available from: www.who.int/about/mission/en/

2 The historical and current context for research into health and physical activity

Stephen R. Bird and David R. Broom

Historical beliefs in the benefits of physical activity

"All parts of the body which have a function, if used in moderation and exercised in labors in which each is accustomed, become thereby healthy, well developed and age more slowly, but if unused they become liable to disease, defective in growth and age quickly".[1] This well-known quote by the Greek physician Hippocrates (~470–375 BCE) highlights the historical belief that regular physical activity was an essential part of a healthy lifestyle. There is evidence to suggest that modern-day homo sapiens have evolved from hunter gatherers where physical activity was a daily occurrence. At that time, much greater levels of incidental physical activity were demanded than in the present day through the hunting and gathering of food, the requirement to walk everywhere as well as the hand-made production of tools, clothing and cooking items. Whilst life expectancy in these times was considerably shorter than it is now, premature deaths were not due to a lack of physical activity, but were caused by injury, illness, disease and poor nutrition.

With the onset of farming and the establishment of cities, physical activity remained a major part of the lives of most people throughout history. However, affluence for some may have reduced their physical activity to levels below that for optimal heath, as suggested by the quote attributed once again to Hippocrates (~470–375 BCE): *"If we could give every individual the right amount of nourishment and exercise, not too little and not too much, we would have found the safest way to health".*[1] Likewise, the quote attributed to Plato (427–347 BCE): *"Lack of activity destroys the good condition of every human being, while movement and methodological physical exercise save it and preserve it",*[2] conveys the same sentiments. Indeed, the importance of exercise for health appears in the practises of many early civilizations, including Yoga in India and Tai Chi chuan in China.

As we move closer to modern times, the message of the need to be physically active for the attainment of good health continued to have its advocates, including John Dryden (1631–1700) who said: *"Better to hunt in fields, for health unbought, than fee the doctor for a nauseous draught, the wise, for cure, on exercise depend; God never made his work for man to mend".*[3] Also, Thomas Jefferson (1762–1826) stated: *"Leave all the afternoon for exercise and recreation, which are as necessary as reading. I will rather say more necessary because health is worth more than learning".*[4] Of course, at this point in history, most people were physically active, through agricultural and manufacturing jobs that involved physical labour, and usually having to walk to get from one place to another during a typical day. Hence most people would have been considered very active by today's standards, with the exceptions to this again being those who had the affluence to be able to choose to refrain from physical labour and had the means to overindulge. However, with the advent of the Industrial Revolution (~1760–1840) there was a rapid increase in the mechanization of jobs and transport: which perhaps provided an even stronger context for exercise advocates continuing to promote their belief in the importance of exercise, as illustrated by the quote from Edward Stanley (1799–1869): "*Those who think they have not time for bodily exercise will sooner or later have to find time for illness*".[5]

Central to the decline in physical activity and increase in sedentary behaviour is the abundance of labour-saving devices, reducing the need for physical labour in factories; the growth of office-based jobs that involve sitting at a desk for 8 hours plus a day; the growth of seated leisure-time pursuits, such as watching television and playing computer games; and people using motorized transport for even the shortest journeys. Consequently, physical activity has been engineered out of everyday life and therefore our obesogenic environment promotes weight gain. Indeed, even the design of buildings favours less physical activity, thereby reducing energy expenditure, as can be attested by anyone who has used the motorized walkway at the airport or the lifts (elevators) in a hotel or office rather than climbing or descending the stairs. Typically, the lifts are well appointed and highly visible, providing an easy and welcoming route to other floors in the hotel, whereas the stairs tend to be hidden and often decorated in a utilitarian rather than opulent style, making them a far less attractive and accessible option. Using historical data on time spent on travel, leisure activities, occupational and domestic work, Ng and Popkin estimated that between 1961 and 2005 physical activity levels dropped by around 20% in the UK.[6] Although voluntary, active leisure and recreational activities have increased slightly, occupational and domestic activity has fallen to a large extent. Worryingly, they predict that by 2030, time spent in sedentary behaviour will exceed 50 hours per week.

The establishment of scientific evidence for the benefits of physical activity

Thus far, this chapter has included numerous quotes from eminent, learned scholars and whilst we may believe them word for word, they are essentially providing personal opinions based on observations, which is often referred to as anecdotal evidence i.e. based on casual observations or indications rather than rigorous or scientific analysis. In such, there is a high risk of bias and this level of evidence lacks the level of 'scientific' rigour that we as exercise scientists would expect today through our quantitative and qualitative research methodologies. Indeed even in the preceding opening section of this chapter, we as authors are ourselves guilty of such biases as we have chosen to include only quotes in favour of physical activity, rather than systematically evaluating and presenting quotes both in favour and against. Hence the opening section must be viewed as a narrative, rather than an unbiased systematic review undertaken using the protocols described in Chapter 5.

Unlike the historical advocates of physical activity, researchers in the second half of the 20th century and those of today have the tools and techniques to investigate these concerns in a scientific manner. The ability for which has been facilitated by the widespread adoption of the scientific method and the later availability of computers that have enabled the interrogation of large data sets and complex analyses, which means that the sentiments of these earlier quotes are now supported by what we may deem to be 'hard scientific evidence'. Ironically, the development of research methods in health and physical activity has coincided with many 'developed' countries experiencing the 'inactivity revolution'. Through the scientific method, quantitative analyses, epidemiology and qualitative studies have provided support for the importance of physical activity and the findings largely concur with the opinions of its historical advocates including those we quoted earlier. This evidence generated by scientific studies extends beyond 'personal opinion' and has superior credence, since such studies can account for the risk of personal prejudices, bias and confounders.

One of the earliest examples of a scientific study into the potential benefits of physical activity on health was the ground-breaking work of Jerry Morris and his co-researchers who studied the cardiovascular disease (CVD) risk of people with active occupations compared with those with more sedentary occupations. Most renowned of which was their work in comparing the conductors and drivers of London buses. The premise of this comparison was that the job of the conductors required them to spend many hours a day walking up and down the double-decker bus, climbing and descending the stairs to collect the fares from passengers. Whereas by comparison the bus drivers were seated for much of their working day and hence had very little physical activity built into their job. These studies provided a strong statistical association between the nature of the job and the prevalence of CVD, with the conductors exhibiting far lower risk of coronary heart disease.[7] For a review of the work of Professor Morris and his contribution to the field of physical activity and health research see Paffenbarger et al.[8] Such findings were supported by other studies, including those of Paffenbarger and colleagues who compared the CVD risk of longshore workers whose job required manual labour, with those who worked in an office.[9,10] They found that the most active group of cargo handlers, who expended over 1,000 kcal more than other longshoremen, had coronary heart disease (CHD) death rates significantly lower than their sedentary colleagues and these differences remained when smoking, body mass index and blood pressure were considered.

With the increased prevalence of sedentary jobs in the 20th century and having identified health issues associated with a sedentary occupation, a key physical activity and health research question became whether those who had a sedentary occupation could alleviate health risks through the pursuit of active leisure, such as sport or walking. Here again, the scientific evidence demonstrated that active leisure did indeed reduce risk as demonstrated by the studies of Morris et al.,[11,12] and the classic 'Harvard Alumni' study by Paffenbarger and colleagues.[13,14] Interestingly, these later studies also revealed that whilst it was preferable to be active throughout life, commencing activity in middle adulthood could still reduce health risk, even if someone had been inactive in their younger years. Furthermore, the studies also demonstrated that if someone had been active when young, but then became inactive, then their earlier years of activity did not provide ongoing protection and risk reduction throughout their life. Hence for optimal health, physical activity needed to be continued throughout life. So, the association between regular physical activity (whether through work or leisure) and a reduced risk of certain diseases had become well established by the late 1980s.

From the pioneering work of Morris and colleagues and Paffenbarger and colleagues' studies, there was a clear association between an active occupation or leisure-time physical activity and a reduced risk of certain diseases. However, whilst the association is strong, 'cause and effect' cannot be proven, since it was possible that individuals may have 'self-selected' the nature of their job based on their health or other factors. For example, it could be that less healthy and overweight individuals would opt for more sedentary occupations such as driving and desk work rather than more active and physically demanding jobs. There could be other confounders also e.g. being a bus driver may be more stressful than being a conductor which could have resulted in greater incidence of CVD. In recent decades, to establish 'cause and effect', intervention studies using a Randomized Controlled Trial (RCT) design have been instrumental in providing evidence for the health benefits of undertaking regular physical activity.[15,16] Details of the features of RCTs are presented in Chapter 13, but in the summary, the people participating in the trial are randomly allocated to either the group receiving the treatment being investigated, which in this case may be a particular form of exercise or exercise psychology intervention (there may be more than one of these intervention groups if more than one intervention is being assessed) or to a control group that may receive no treatment, continue with their usual lifestyle, or in some cases continue to receive the established current standard treatment or usual care. Changes in the intervention group(s) can then be compared with the control group, and each other if there's more than one intervention. Randomization minimizes selection bias and the different comparison groups allow the researchers to determine any effects of the treatment when compared with the no-treatment group, while other variables are kept constant (see Chapter 13 for details). The RCT is often considered the gold standard for a clinical trial, although it should still be noted that even intervention studies may not fully remove all bias, since those who volunteer to participate are likely to have an interest in their health and undertaking physical activity.

Nevertheless, the combined research evidence from multiple RCTs synthesized into systematic reviews and meta-analyses that show cause and effect, as well as large epidemiological, observational studies that show association, strongly advocates the health benefits of physical activity. This has resulted in clear messages and guidelines from national expert authorities such as the American College of Sports Medicine,[17] the British Association of Sport and Exercise Sciences[18] and Exercise and Sport Science Australia.[19] Organizations such as the World Health Organization and the International Society of Physical Activity and Health run global physical activity campaigns and initiatives to encourage people to meet the recommended levels of physical activity, which for many people must be deliberately added to their daily routine, given the sedentary nature inherent in the lifestyles of many people today – seated work, motorized transport, television watching, etc.

Current research issues

With a lack of physical activity being a major health issue, the need for more research that can inform, and guide policy and strategies has become imperative. Support for physical activity and health-related messages now come from tens of thousands of studies and the general concept that exercise is good for your health is widely accepted and promoted by national campaigns. Those new to the field may be surprised to learn that this was not always the case. By way of illustration, in the 19th century there was a belief that vigorous exercise could be harmful to health, which stimulated investigations into the longevity of the Oxford and Cambridge rowing crews from 1829 to 1869.[20] The findings of which indicated that their life expectancy was a couple of years longer than would be predicted from life tables, suggesting no ill effect from their vigorous rowing activity whilst at University. Yet the concern about the potential ill effects of exercise persisted in that a common belief was that exercise and vigorous sport was for the young, and that vigorous exercise 'wore out' the body, with a belief that as a person aged it was time to rest and conserve the body: and it was only 40–50 years ago that this belief was effectively questioned.

The best way to promote participation in physical activity in a sustainable manner, what exercise and how much, are questions that researchers in the physical activity and health field continuously strive to provide answers to, but we need to know more. In part this is due to the fact that as society continues to evolve, so the answers and strategies need to evolve with it, as evidenced by the relatively recent introduction of digital technologies to support exercise programmes. Additionally, with the advent of new technologies and techniques we are now able to investigate and collect data on topics and in detail that was not possible just a few years ago. Furthermore, much of the focus of early studies was on physical health and the reduction in the risk of CVD: with a later broadening focus to include type 2 diabetes, osteoporosis and cancers. In more recent years, the research field has further expanded to consider the benefits of physical activity on mental health, cognitive performance and improved physical function with age, all of which are areas of increasing concern in societies today. Hence many questions remain unanswered, and the optimal 'dose' continues to be debated. Consequently, issues still being pursued by researchers are: what exercise, how much, how vigorous, and how often? Some researchers are working at the level of population responses, others on selected groups and individuals and yet others delve into the molecular basis for adaptations that convey good health. At a practical level, for the health advocates who simply say, 'do some exercise' is somewhat akin to a physician saying 'take some medicine'. There are so many variables to be considered if the optimal exercise prescription for that person is to be recommended. Hence the answers to the aforementioned questions will continue to help inform and guide effective exercise prescription for optimal health.

Of current interest is the suggestion that vigorous exercise could be more beneficial in reducing all-cause mortality risk. A suggestion that has been evident for many years since it was reported as a factor in the studies by Morris and colleagues,[11,12] as well as the 'Harvard Alumni studies',[14] with more recent epidemiological evidence being provided by numerous studies.[18,21] Other research questions of current concern include whether we can accumulate the health benefits of exercise in short bursts,[22–24] and the issue of whether any amount of physical activity can counteract the ill effects of prolonged sitting for many hours a day.[25,26] Also, of ongoing interest is whether short bouts of activity known as High Intensity Interval Training (HIT) are efficacious and should be included in the public health message.[27]

Research continues to identify the healthiest exercise prescription for each individual and importantly seeks to find the best way to increase physical activity participation and compliance with any prescribed exercise programme, which is an important issue since even the very best possible exercise programme is of no benefit if no one does it. A view that's reflected in the quote from Oscar Wilde (1854–1900): "*To get back my youth I would do anything in the world, except take exercise, get up early or be respectable*".[28] Indeed the reluctance to find time to exercise and the perceived preference for medicine to solve the ills of inactivity remain, despite no medication to date having the breadth and extensive health benefits that's provided by exercise, with relatively few adverse effects if undertaken at sensibly prescribed volumes and intensities. As stated by Lessard and Hawley: "*Even though the case for a causal link between the rise in physical inactivity and the increase in insulin resistance is compelling, the use of anti-diabetic drugs continues to rise. It seems ironic that significant effort is expended in the search for drugs that mimic exercise training when exercise itself is a readily available, practical and economical therapeutic option with many beneficial effects and few, if any, adverse side effects*".[29]

In presenting this brief historical context, the authors fully acknowledge that the 'inactivity epidemic' as a major cause of premature death is primarily located in the more 'developed' countries. Nevertheless, it is a growing problem, affecting more countries and becoming of greater concern in those where it is already evident. Furthermore, despite the establishment of the scientific method, the general public are continually bombarded by a plethora of unfounded claims. This includes the marketing of diets and interventions that have no evidence for their health benefits or effectiveness but are attractive to those seeking a quick fix without the need for commitment and effort. The popular media misinforming the public is becoming a public health problem in its own right. A scenario that would appear to be comparable to the quackery and sale of unfounded elixirs in previous centuries, but with the advent of the world wide web providing greater marketing possibilities for such potions or techniques. Hence, our current and future generations of physical activity researchers need to continue to present unbiased evidence from high-quality research studies, and those involved in the promotion of health and physical activity need to have the skills to identify high-quality evidence from that which is flawed and biased. It is important for research to be undertaken to identify what physical activity is beneficial to health and to refute claims that have no scientific basis. In doing this, researchers today and into the future will need to continue to develop new research methods, tools and techniques, as old and fresh challenges are presented and the field evolves within the context of ever-changing societies.

References

1   Hippocrates. *Hippocrates: with an English translation by WHS Jones.* London: William Heineman; 1953.

2   Ashiedu B. *365 Quotes By Plato.* London: Insignia Expressions Ltd; 2016. ISBN 1530341388

3   Gaither CC, Cavazos-Gaither AE, editors. *Gaither's dictionary of scientific quotations.* Springer Science and Business Media: LLC; 2008. ISBN 978-0-387-4957-0

4   Thomas Jefferson. *Quotations of thomas jefferson.* Bedford, MA: Applewood Books; 2003. ISBN 1-55709-940-5

5   Available from: www.goodreads.com/quotes/173133-those-who-think-they-have-not-time-for-bodily-exercise

6   Ng SW, Popkin BM. Time use and physical activity: a shift away from movement across the globe. *Obes Rev.* 2012; **13**(8):659–680.

7   Morris JN, Heady JA, Raffle PAB, Roberts CG, Parks JN. Coronary heart disease and physical activity of work. *Lancet.* 1953; **ii**:1053–7, 1111–20.

8   Paffenbarger RS, Blair SN, Lee IM. A history of physical activity, cardiovascular health and longevity: the scientific contributions of Jeremy N Morris, DSc, DPH, FRCP. *Int J Epidemiol.* 2001; **30**:1184–92.

9   Paffenbarger RS Jr, Laughlin ME, Gima AS, Black RA. Work activity of longshoremen as related to death from coronary heart disease and stroke. *N Engl J Med.* 1970; **282**(20):1109–14.

10   Paffenbarger RS, Gima AS, Laughlin E, Black RA. Characteristics of longshoremen related fatal coronary heart disease and stroke. *Am J Public Health.* 1971; **61**(7):1362–70.

11   Morris JN, Chave SP, Adam C, Sirey C, Epstein I, Sheehan DJ. Vigorous exercise in leisure-time and the incidence of coronary heart disease. *Lancet.* 1973; **i**:333–9.

12   Morris JN, Everitt MG, Pollard R, Chave SP, Semmence AM. Vigorous exercise in leisure-time: protection against coronary heart disease. *Lancet.* 1980; **ii**: 1207–10.

13   Paffenbarger RS Jr, Wing AL, Hyde RT. Physical activity as an index of heart attack risk in college alumni. *Am J Epidemiol.* 1978; **108**(3):161–75.

14   Paffenbarger RS, Lee IM. A natural history of athleticism, health and longevity. *J Sports Sci.* 1998; **16**:331–45.

15 Swift DL, Lavie CJ, Johannsen NM, Arena R, Earnest CP, O'Keefe JH, et al. Physical activity, cardiorespiratory fitness, and exercise training in primary and secondary coronary prevention. *Circ J.* 2013; **77**(2):281–92.

16 Harber MP, Kaminsky LA, Arena R, Blair SN, Franklin BA, Myers J, Ross R. Impact of cardiorespiratory fitness on all-cause and disease-specific mortality: advances since 2009. *Prog Cardiovasc Dis.* 2017; **60**(1):11–20.

17 Garber CE, Blissmer B, Deschenes MR, Franklin BA, Lamonte MJ, Lee IM, Nieman DC, Swain DP. American College of Sports Medicine. American College of Sports Medicine position stand. Quantity and quality of exercise for developing and maintaining cardiorespiratory, musculoskeletal, and neuromotor fitness in apparently healthy adults: guidance for prescribing exercise. *Med Sci Sports Exerc.* 2011; **43**:1334–59.

18 O'Donovan G, Blazevich AJ, Boreham C, Cooper AR, Crank H, Ekelund U, et al. The ABC of Physical Activity for Health: a consensus statement from the British association of sport and exercise sciences. *J Sports Sci.* 2010; **28**(6):573–91.

19 Available from: www.essa.org.au

20 Morgan JE. *University oars.* London: Palgrave MacMillan; 1873.

21 O'Donovan G, Kearney EM, Owen A, Nevill AM, Woolf-May K, Bird SR. The effects of 24 weeks of moderate- or high-intensity exercise on insulin resistance. *Eur J Appl Physiol.* 2005; **95**: 522–8.

22 Murphy MH, Nevill AM, Hardman AE. Different patterns of brisk walking are equally effective in decreasing postprandial lipaemia. *Int J Obes Relat Metab Disord.* 2000; **24**(10):1303–9.

23 Woolf-May K, Kearney EM, Jones DW, Davison RCR, Coleman D, Bird SR. The effect of two 18-week walking programmes on aerobic fitness, selected blood lipids and factor XIIa. *J Sports Sci.* 1998; **16**(8):701–10.

24 Woolf-May K, Bird SR, Owen A. Effects of an 18 week walking programme on cardiac function in previously sedentary or relatively inactive adults. *Brit J Sp Med.* 1997; **31**(1):48–53.

25 Ekelund U, Steene-Johannessen J, Brown WJ, Fagerland MW, Owen N, Powell K, et al. Does physical activity attenuate, or even eliminate, the detrimental association of sitting time with mortality? A harmonised meta-analysis of data from more than 1 million men and women. *Lancet.* 2016; **388**(10051):1302–10.

26 Greer AE, Sui X, Maslow AL, Greer BK, Blair SN. The effects of sedentary behavior on metabolic syndrome independent of physical activity and cardiorespiratory fitness. *J Phys Act Health.* 2015; **12**:68–73.

27 Biddle SJH, Batterham AM. High-intensity interval exercise training for public health: a big HIT or shall we HIT it on the head? *Int J Behav Nutr Phys Act.* 2015; **12**:95.

28 Leach M. *The wicked wit of Oscar Wilde.* London: Michael O'Mara Books Ltd; 2000.

29 Lessard SJ, JA Hawley. Evidence for prescribing exercise as therapy for treating patients with type 2 diabetes. In: Hawley JA, Zierath JR, editors. Physical activity and type 2 diabetes. Champaign, IL: Human Kinetics Publishers; 2008. pp. 203–13. ISBN: 9780736064798

3 Health concepts

David R. Broom

Summary

This chapter introduces terms used in physical activity and health research to provide clarity in the reading of subsequent chapters. Definitions for commonly used metrics in health research, such as: prevalence, incidence, relative risk and odds ratios, will be provided. Hypothetical examples will be used to further understanding.

Chapter aim

By engaging with this chapter, you will be able to:

- Define health and public health;
- Define exercise, physical activity, sedentary behaviour and inactivity;
- Understand prevalence, incidence, relative risk, population attributable risk and odds ratios.

What is health?

The World Health Organization defined health in its broadest sense as:

> *a state of complete physical, mental and social wellbeing and not merely the absence of disease and infirmity.*[1]

WHO revised its definition of health as:

> *the extent to which an individual or group is able to realize aspirations and satisfy needs and to change or cope with the environment. Health is a resource for everyday life, not the objective of living; it is a positive concept emphasizing social and personal resources, as well as physical capacities.*[2]

Regardless of the definition, health describes an ability to function and the ability of individuals or populations to adapt and self-manage when facing physical, mental or social changes. It refers to the ability to maintain homeostasis and recover from injury, illness or disease. Mental, intellectual, social and emotional health is the ability to handle stress, acquire skills and maintain relationships, all of which form resources for resiliency and independent living. Activities to prevent or treat health problems and promote good health in humans is the role of public health.

What is public health?

Public health was defined by Winslow as:

> *the science and art of preventing disease, prolonging life and promoting health through the organized efforts and informed choices of society, organizations, public and private communities and individuals.*[3]

Public health interventions prevent and manage diseases, injuries and other health conditions through the promotion of healthy behaviour in populations and surveillance of cases. Public health aims to prevent health problems from happening or reoccurring by developing policy, implementing interventions, administering services and conducting research.

   Achieving and maintaining good health is an ongoing process that is influenced by personal strategies. Undertaking physical activity is a key personal strategy to achieving good health and its promotion is an integral part of public health. The epidemiologist Jeremy Morris, who was highlighted in Chapter 2, described physical activity as the 'best buy' in public health because undertaking moderate intensity physical activity has multiple health benefits.[4] This includes (but is not restricted to) the prevention and treatment of non-communicable diseases (i.e. diseases that cannot be passed from person to person) including cardiovascular disease, type 2 diabetes, obesity and some cancers.[5] Physical activity can reduce the risk of premature death, improves mental health and quality of life.[5]

What is physical activity?

Physical activity is defined by Caspersen et al. as:

> *any bodily movement produced by skeletal muscles that results in energy expenditure.*[6]

It is a broad term that describes bodily movement, posture and balance, all require energy. Physical activity includes physical education, dance activities, different types of sports, as well as indoor and outdoor play and work-related activity. It also includes active travel (e.g. walking, cycling, rollerblading and scooting) and routine, habitual activities such as using the stairs, doing housework and gardening.

What is exercise?

Exercise is defined by Caspersen et al. as:

> *a subset of physical activity that is planned, structured, and repetitive and has as a final or an intermediate objective the improvement or maintenance of physical fitness.*[6]

It is therefore assumed that exercise only involves movement represented by activities such as running, jumping, walking and swimming.[7] However, exercise can also involve movement assisted by machines or devices such as a bicycle, rower or wheelchair. There are also activities that require substantial expenditures of energy but little or no movement takes place e.g. tug of war or a rugby scrum. Clearly, exercise does not always require or involve movement so a more accurate definition of exercise is offered by Winter and Fowler as:

> *a potential disruption to homeostasis by muscle activity that is either exclusively, or in combination, concentric, eccentric or isometric.*[7]

This definition applies to exercise and physical activity that encompasses elite-standard competitive sport, activities of daily living and clinical applications in rehabilitation and public health.

What is sedentary behaviour and physical inactivity?

On the opposite end of the physical activity continuum is sedentary behaviour. There has been a substantial increase in the prominence of sedentary behaviour research because of the increasing evidence of the link between excessive sedentary behaviour and adverse health outcomes.[8] Sedentary behaviour is defined by Tremblay et al. as:

> *any waking behaviour characterized by an energy expenditure ≤1.5 metabolic equivalents while in a sitting, reclining or lying posture.*[9]

The term 'sedentary' should not be used synonymously with 'inactive' because the two behaviours are completely different. Tremblay et al. define physical inactivity as:

> *an insufficient physical activity level to meet present physical activity recommendations.*[9]

Physical activity and sedentary behaviour epidemiology

Epidemiology has been defined by Last as:

> *the study of the distribution and determinants of health related states or events in specified populations, and the application of this study to the control of health problems.*[10]

Measures of the occurrence of health-related outcomes are basic tools of epidemiology. They allow you to show the frequency of the outcome between populations and individuals.

Example – the doctor's dilemma

A doctor diagnosed 100 cases of coronary heart disease (CHD) in patients from the local population in the last year. Is this a dilemma?

Only having information on the number of cases with no information on the number of people at risk in the local population, it is impossible to conclude if this is a problem. To determine if this was a dilemma you would need to know how many people visited the doctor's surgery over the course of the year. If the doctor had only seen 100 patients then the interpretation would have been very different than if they had seen 10,000 patients.

What is prevalence?

Distribution relates to the frequency of the disease, which is typically measured as the prevalence. Prevalence quantifies the proportion of individuals in a population that exhibit the outcome of interest at a specified time. This could be a health outcome such as high blood pressure (hypertension) or a risk factor which is an exposure that has been found to be a determinant of health such as physical inactivity.

The formula for calculating prevalence as a percentage (%) =

(number of people with the health-related outcome at a specified time/number of people in the population at risk at the specified time) × 100.

Worked (hypothetical) example 1

What is the prevalence of physical activity in Sheffield if 350,000 people meet the physical activity recommendations out of a population of 551,800?

350,000 / 551,800 × 100 = 63%

Knowing the prevalence is helpful in assessing the need for health or preventive strategies. For example, the Health and Social Care Information Centre published data from the 2016 Health Survey for England which highlights 66% of men and 58% of women aged 16 years and over met the aerobic guidelines of at least 150 minutes of moderate intensity physical activity or 75 minutes of vigorous intensity physical activity per week or an equivalent combination of both, in bouts of 10 minutes or more.[11] There is clearly still a large proportion of the population that are not accruing the health benefits of an active lifestyle so physical activity interventions are needed to get more people active.

What is incidence?

Incidence quantifies the number of new occurrences of an outcome that develops during a specified time interval in an at-risk population. It is often expressed as the number of cases / 100 person years but there are variations.

The formula for calculating person-time incidence =

(number of people who develop the health-related outcome in a specified period/ sum of the periods of time for which each person in the population is at risk).

Worked (hypothetical) example 2

The following table shows four people who were observed during an epidemiological study. Each subject's person year contribution ends when that person develops a disease or the follow-up period ends.

Subject	*Developed Disease*	*Time Developed*	*Years At Risk*
A	Yes	1 year	1
B	No	N/A	5
C	Yes	4 years	4
D	No	N/A	5

Two people developed the disease which gives a total of 2 cases. When totalling the number of years at risk, this gives 15 person years. Incidence = 2 cases / 15 person years; however, it has been stated that incidence is often expressed as the number of cases / 100 person years so in this example (100 / 15) * 2 = 13 cases / 100 person years.

What is absolute risk?

The risk of something is the odds of it taking place. Absolute risk (AR) is the probability or chance of an event happening over a stated time period. Hypothetically, a woman living in England might have an absolute risk of developing breast cancer in her lifetime of 13.3%. That means out of every 100 women, about 13 will develop the disease at some point in their life if they lived in England. Absolute risk is always presented as a percentage. It is the ratio of people who have a medical event compared to all of the people who could have that medical event.

What is relative risk?

Relative risk (RR) is different from absolute risk because two groups of people are compared using incidence.

Worked (hypothetical) example 3

What is the relative risk of a heart attack in smokers compared to non-smokers if:

   The incidence of a heart attack is 17.7 per 100,000 person years among non-smokers.
   The incidence of a heart attack is 49.6 per 100,000 person years among smokers.
   The relative risk of a heart attack in smokers compared with non-smokers is (49.6 / 17.7) = 2.8. Smokers are therefore 2.8 times more likely to have a heart attack than non-smokers.

When dealing with exposures that are associated with a *decreased* risk of disease (as is often the case for physical activity), researchers take the unexposed group (the inactive group) as the reference category. The relative risk in the group exposed to physical activity is thus less than 1.

Worked (hypothetical) example 4

What is the relative risk of a heart attack in vigorous exercisers versus non-vigorous exercisers if:
   The incidence of a heart attack is 2.1 per 100 person years in vigorous exercisers.
   The incidence of a heart attack is 5.8 per 100 person years in non-vigorous exercisers.
   The relative risk of a heart attack in vigorous exercisers compared to non-vigorous exercisers is 2.1 / 5.8 = 0.36. Vigorous exercisers have a risk of a heart attack that is one third of that experienced by non-vigorous exercisers.

What is population attributable risk?

Population attributable risk (PAR) is a theoretical concept that reflects both the prevalence and the relative risk. It is beyond the scope of this chapter to present in detail the complicated equation for calculating population attributable risk, but its importance should be highlighted for informing policy and the allocation of public health resources should be highlighted.

Worked (hypothetical) example 5

The table below (adapted from Paffenbarger et al., 1986)[12] presents three different risk factors as well as a calculated relative risk of all-cause mortality (i.e. death from any cause) and the prevalence of each risk factor in a population.

Risk Factor	RR	Prevalence (%)	PAR (%)
Physical Inactivity	1.31	62.0	16.1
Hypertension	1.73	9.4	6.4
Smoking	11.76	38.2	22.5

If policy makers were to make decisions on risk factors based on the relative risk alone, it is likely that smoking cessation programmes would be the leading priority because of the highest relative risk with physical activity interventions the least important due to the lowest relative risk. However, when taking into account the prevalence, since 62% of this population is inactive which is much greater than the 38.2% that smoke, when the PAR is calculated, 16.1% of all-cause mortality is attributable to physical inactivity and 22.5% for smoking. Resources should be provided for both physical activity interventions as well as smoking cessation programmes in this population because the population attributable risk is similar. Hypertension has a higher relative risk than physical activity but a lower prevalence and therefore the lowest population attributable risk in this example.

What is an odds ratio?

An odds ratio (OR) is a measure of association between an exposure and an outcome. The OR represents the odds that an outcome will occur given a particular exposure, compared to the odds of the outcome occurring in the absence of that exposure. Similar to the relative risk, values greater than 1 indicate increased risk with less than 1 highlighting reduced risk.

Worked (hypothetical) example 6

An epidemiological study examined all-cause and cardiovascular mortality in monozygotic (same sex) twins with different levels of physical activity. If all-cause mortality odds ratio was calculated as 0.80 (95% confidence interval: 0.65, 0.99) and cardiovascular disease mortality odds ratio was calculated as 0.68 (95% confidence interval: 0.49, 0.95). Within-pair comparisons of monozygotic twins shows that, compared with their less active co-twin, the more active twin had a 20% reduced risk of all-cause mortality and a 32% reduced risk of cardiovascular disease mortality. In the all-cause mortality example we can be 95% confident that the reduced risk is between 35% and 1%.

Summary

In summary, we have defined key terms and concepts that will be used throughout this textbook. Epidemiology is the study of the distribution and determinants of health-related states and research in this area uses a number of different approaches including the calculation of prevalence, incidence, relative risk, population attributable risk and odds ratios to allow policy makers to allocate resources to tackle health problems.

Review questions

- Define health.
- Give three examples of physical activities.
- What metabolic equivalent would be classed as sedentary behaviour if in a sitting, reclining or lying posture?
- What is the prevalence of inactivity in UK females if 8 million are not meeting the physical activity guidelines out of a population of 32 million?
- Calculate the relative risk of type 2 diabetes in active compared to inactive men when type 2 diabetes incidence in active men is 35.3 per 10,000 person years and type 2 diabetes incidence in inactive men is 57.9 per 10,000 person years.
- Referring to worked hypothetical example 6, we can be 95% confident that the reduced risk of cardiovascular disease mortality is between _% and _%.

Further Reading

Caspersen CJ. Physical activity epidemiology: concepts, methods, and applications to exercise science. *Exerc Sport Sci Rev.* 1989; **17**:423–73.

References

1 World Health Organization. *Constitution of the world health organization.* Geneva, Switzerland: Author; 1948.
2 World Health Organization. *Health promotion a discussion document on the concept and principles: summary report of the working group on concept and principles of health promotion.* Copenhagen: WHO Regional Office for Europe; 1984.
3 Winslow CE. The untitled fields of public health. *Science.* 1920; **51**:23–33.
4 Morris JN. Exercise in the prevention of coronary heart disease: today's best buy in public health. *Med Sci Sports Exerc.* 1994; **26**:807–14.
5 Lancet Physical Activity Series. Physical activity 2016: progress and challenges. Available 2018 Jan 14from: www.thelancet.com/series/physical-activity-2016
6 Caspersen CJ, Powell KE, Christenson GM. Physical activity, exercise and physical fitness: definitions and distinctions for health-related research. *Public Health Rep.* 1985; **100**:126–31.
7 Winter E, Fowler N. Exercise defined and quantified according to the Systeme International d'Unites. *J Sports Sci.* 2009; **25**:447–60.
8 Thorp AA, Owen N, Neuhaus M, Dunstan DW. Sedentary behaviors and subsequent health outcomes in adults: a systematic review of longitudinal studies, 1996–2011. *Am J Prev Med.* 2011; **41**:207–15.

9   Tremblay MS, Aubert S, Barnes JD, Saunders TJ, Carson V, Latimer-Cheung AE, Chastin SF, Altenburg TM, Chinapaw MJ. Sedentary behavior research network (SBRN) – terminology consensus project process and outcome. *Int J Behav Nutr Phys Act.* 2017; **14**:75.
10 Last JM. *A dictionary of epidemiology.* New York: Oxford University Press; 1988.
11 Health and Social Care Information Centre. *Health survey for England 2016: physical activity in adults.* London: Author; 2017.
12 Paffenbarger RS Jr, Hyde RT, Wing A, Hsieh CC. Physical activity, all-cause mortality, and longevity of college alumni. *New England J Med.* 1986; **314**:605–13.

4 Nurture vs. nature

The genetics and epigenetics of exercise

Macsue Jacques, Shanie Landen, Sarah Voisin, Séverine Lamon and Nir Eynon

Aims of the chapter

The aims of this chapter are to provide a brief overview and introduction to the molecular aspects of how the body responds to exercise and why there may be variations in the magnitude of adaptation seen in individuals following similar exercise regimens. It considers the interaction between genotype, physical activity and epigenetics, and provides direction for those wishing to read the topic in more depth.

Introduction

In October 2011, *The Scientist Daily* published an article referring to discussions aroused in the past years regarding the concept of 'nature' vs. 'nurture' in human development. *The article began with an excerpt from an interview with behavioural psychologist Donald Hebb:*

> A journalist once asked the behavioural psychologist Donald Hebb whether a person's genes or environment mattered most to the development of personality. Hebb replied that the question was akin to asking which feature of a rectangle – length or width – made the most important contribution to its area.
>
> 'Nature' vs. 'nurture' is a paradigm that has been known for a long period of time, but was reinforced when it was found that patterns of heritability determined our genes. *Heritability* is defined as the proportion of variance in a trait that can be explained by genetic factors, for a particular population at a particular moment in time. With the human genome project completed in 2001,[1] scientists expected that the information contained in our genes would demystify the concept of 'nature' vs. 'nurture'. However, the scientific community soon found out that sequencing the human genome had generated more questions than it had answered.

The search for genetic variants associated with exercise responses

> At the completion of the human genome project,[1] scientists concluded that humans are ~99.9% identical in their DNA sequence. The remaining 0.1% difference is often referred to as genetic variants. Genetic variants are common in nature and are the opposite of 'rare' mutations. Those variants partly explain the heterogeneity between individuals in a variety of visible (i.e. eye colour) or invisible (i.e. blood type) traits, termed *phenotypes*. Just as specific variants can be associated with disease conditions, some variants may also cause changes in the

function of genes and proteins that are beneficial for athletic performance and adaptations to exercise training.

Despite the proven health benefits of exercise training, the type and magnitude of physiological adaptations to exercise training stimuli are highly variable between individuals.[2-4] This means that while some people show minimal improvements in specific phenotypes following exercise training ('low-responders'), others respond well ('responders') or very well ('high-responders') to similar training programmes. While various environmental factors, such as training status and nutrition, contribute to this variability ('nurture'), it is widely accepted that genetic variants also play a role in determining trainability ('nature').[5] Early studies conducted on twin pairs (monozygotic and dizygotic) and family members suggested that the heritability of exercise-related traits may vary between 81% and 86% and may be as high as 93% for some outcome variables,[6] demonstrating that genetics play an important role in exercise trainability. Such studies significantly contributed to our early understanding of the heritability of exercise-related phenotypes. However, owing to small sample sizes and poor statistical methods, these findings were often overestimated.[7] Furthermore, those studies focused on heritability only and did not investigate specific genetic variants that contribute to complex phenotypes such as exercise trainability.

In the late 90's, hypothesis-driven candidate gene studies have emerged to determine the specific genetic variants that influence exercise-related phenotypes. This approach requires a prior assumption that specific gene variants are associated with exercise-related phenotypes. Initially, this method was thought to be effective and therefore to be appropriate to complex traits (i.e. traits influenced by many genes working together), such as those underlying adaptations to exercise training.[8] To date, more than 200 genetic variants have been associated with exercise performance.[9] However, only two variants (ACE I/D and ACTN3 R577X) have shown consistent associations in various populations and conditions.[10-15]

Complex polygenic traits

Adaptations to exercise training result from a combination of complex polygenic traits, meaning that these traits are influenced by more than one gene. The identification of genetic variants that affect exercise-related genes has recently emerged as an important research focus.[16] In the last decade, new sequencing techniques, such as the Genome Wide Association Studies (GWAS), Whole-Genome Sequencing (WGS) and Exon Sequencing emerged to investigate complex polygenic traits. These approaches have made it possible to analyse up to several million different genetic variants simultaneously and are efficient in identifying novel genetic variants related to complex phenotypes, such as ageing muscle degeneration and type 2 diabetes.[17,18] However, only a handful of studies utilized these genome-wide comprehensive approaches in the field of exercise sciences. One seminal study, the HERITAGE study, performed a GWAS on 720 participants and identified a set of potential genetic variants associated with gains in maximal oxygen uptake ($\dot{V}O_{2max}$) following 20 weeks of standardized exercise training.[19] Rankinen et al.[20] identified 45 gene variants that may potentially predict elite athletic performance in a cohort of endurance athletes (The GAMES Consortium). The authors attempted to validate these markers in seven additional cohorts of endurance athletes and controls, including world-class athletes from Australia, Ethiopia,

Japan, Kenya, Poland, Russia and Spain (total of $n = 1,520$ athletes and $n = 2,760$ controls). However, these validation studies were not able to identify a panel of genes correlated with performance, with the exception of one marker, the Single Nucleotide Polymorphism (SNP) rs558129, which was associated with performance across all of the cohorts (20). A recent large-scale ($n = 195,180$) GWAS study found 16 novel *loci* (fixed position on a chromosome e.g. the position of a gene or a marker) associated with handgrip strength, a strong indicator of muscle function.[21] A number of these loci contained genes involved in skeletal muscle fibre structure and function (actg1), neuronal maintenance and signal transduction (pex14, tgfa, syt1) and psychomotor impairment (pex14, lrpprc and kansl1).[21] Although the field of exercise genomics has greatly advanced, available training studies are often limited by small sample number and lack of tightly controlled study design. As a consequence, Genomic, Transcriptomic, Proteomic, and Metabolomic (OMICS) profile of response to exercise training remains poorly characterized.[4] A recent, multi-centred cohort called the Gene SMART (Skeletal Muscle Adaptive Response to Training) study aims at recruiting 200 moderately trained, healthy Caucasians participants (all males 18–45 y, BMI < 30) in order to identify the genes that are responsible for muscle adaptions to a training regime in a tightly controlled manner. Studies such as the Gene SMART with tight control over training intervention and participants are paramount in order to further untangle the role of genetic variants in exercise response.[4]

Epigenetics – above our genes

Our genetic makeup explains some of the inter-individual variability of exercise training responses; however, attempts to identify reliable genetic markers of exercise response have delivered limited results to date. Environmental stimuli can also significantly affect exercise-related phenotype and modify the genome regulation. *Epigenetics* (in Greek 'epi' means 'on top') refers to a level of gene regulation that is sensitive to environmental stimuli. It allows cells to remember their past activity and primes them to respond to future environmental stresses. Epigenetics can be defined as the structural adaptation of chromosomal regions so as to register, signal or perpetuate altered activity states.[22] For example, exposure to heavy metals and pesticides, regular exercise, diet, smoking and obesity can all remodel the epigenome in a tissue-specific manner.[23–25] One interesting feature of epigenetic modifications is that they are not confined to the initial cells that have been affected, meaning that they can be passed on to daughter cells during mitosis and meiosis.[23] Contrary to genetic variations, epigenetic changes can be influenced by environmental factors, and many are likely to be reversible. Importantly, epigenetics can mediate compensatory responses to rapid environmental change in humans, such as those occurring during demanding physical activity. It is therefore essential to understand the mechanisms underlying these processes. Epigenetic modifications often involve the addition of chemical groups to the DNA or to the histone proteins that DNA coils around, such as methylation, acetylation, phosphorylation, ubiquitylation and sumoylation.[23] Since Waddington first coined the term 'epigenetics' in 1956,[26] the definition of epigenetics has considerably evolved and there are ongoing discussions regarding which marks should be considered 'epigenetic' since some marks are not heritable through cell divisions or quickly disappear once the initial stimulus is gone.[27–31] However, it is generally accepted that epigenetic modifications fall broadly into three categories: (1) DNA methylation, (2) histone modification and (3) microRNAs (miRNAs). In this chapter we will only briefly discuss DNA methylation, and histone modifications (for detailed review on those terms see Weinhold,[23] Felsenfeld[32] and Denham[33]).

DNA methylation and exercise

Research on exercise training and epigenetics is still in its infancy, and only a few studies have looked at DNA methylation changes after chronic exercise training.[34–39] There is however growing evidence corroborating the influence of exercise on the methylome. Exercise training may induce changes in the methylation status of important genes involved in muscle structure and function, and thus possibly model long-lasting expression patterns that are advantageous to respond to exercise.[40–43] In 2012, a seminal study demonstrated that the promoter regions of key genes involved in exercise response are strongly hypomethylated immediately after strenuous exercise and re-methylated at 3 hours post exercise.[44] In addition, in a recent study by Bajpeyi et al.,[45] participants performed a single bout of exercise, and were divided into responders and non-responders based on their levels of methylation at an important regulatory region of PGC1α, a master regulator of mitochondrial function in the cell and a critical determinant of cardiovascular disease and obesity.[45,46] High-responders showed *nucleosome repositioning* (where nucleosomes are located with respect to the genomic DNA sequence) after the exercise bout, along with a significant decrease in intra-myocellular lipid content, suggesting an increase in PGC1α activity. Other studies have observed changes in DNA methylation after chronic exercise training. For example, six months of exercise training (spinning and aerobics) led to genome-wide methylation changes in human adipose tissue, which may reflect a change in lipid metabolism.[35] Nitert et al. also observed changes in methylation and gene expression patterns in skeletal muscle after a six-month endurance exercise intervention.[36] In another study, three months of sprint interval training was associated with DNA methylation changes in sperm. Intriguingly, those modifications occurred in genes that were correlated with neurological diseases such as schizophrenia and Parkinson's disease.[34] Suggestions have also been made that muscle memory is influenced by epigenetic patterns: for a detailed review see Sharples et al.[47]

Histones modifications and exercise

A limited number of studies have researched histone modification after exercise. Skeletal muscle contraction induces phosphorylation of histone deacetylases (HDAC), which allows for the relaxation of regulatory regions of chromatin in exercise-related genes.[48,49] Acute exercise enhances signal transduction via signalling cascades that are associated with phosphorylation of specific HDAC isoforms.[50,51] In skeletal muscle, the class II HDACs 4, 5, 7 and 9 are pivotal in muscle development and adaptation. For example, exercise training initiates the nuclear export of HDACs 4 and 5, secondary to their phosphorylation by CaMKII and AMPK. These kinases (CaMKII and AMPK) in turn respond to changes in sarcoplasmic calcium levels and energy consumption.[52] Liu et al. also found that slow fibre type electrical stimulation of cultured adult skeletal muscle fibres induced HDAC translocation out of the nucleus, alleviating transcriptional repression.[53] These findings suggest that histone acetylation is regulating part of the response to acute exercise. Perhaps due to the dynamic nature of histone modification, studies have primarily looked into the effect of acute, rather than long-term (chronic), exercise on histone modifications.[54] Further research on the effect of both types of exercise on histone modifications is required as current assumptions suggest that histone modifications could be playing a large role in the response to exercise. Uncovering the role of the 'histone code' and its function following exercise training will lead to a broader understanding of how muscle activity regulates gene expression and pinpoint the importance of skeletal muscle plasticity in health and disease.[52] For more detailed reviews on histone modifications and exercise refer to McGee and Hargreaves,[52] Howlett[55] and Hargreaves.[56]

Summary

A significant body of work in the area of genetics, epigenetics and exercise suggests to the scientific community that the paradigm of 'nature' vs. 'nurture' can only be resolved by a combination of both factors. With recent advances in the field, the focus is shifting from quantifying the relative importance of 'nature' vs. 'nurture' to understanding the mechanisms that underlie adaptations to exercise training and the cross-talk between the genome and the environment. The concept of nature vs. nurture is therefore fading, and the present-day research redirects scientists to the study of the dynamic interplay between our genomes and our daily experiences.

References

1 Venter JC, Adams MD, Myers EW, Li PW, Mural RJ, Sutton GG, et al. The sequence of the human genome. *Science.* 2001; **291**(5507):1304–51.

2 Bouchard C, Rankinen T. Individual differences in response to regular physical activity. *Med Sci Sports Exerc.* 2001; **33**(6):S446–51.

3 Timmons JA, Jansson E, Fischer H, Gustafsson T, Greenhaff PL, Ridden J, et al. Modulation of extracellular matrix genes reflects the magnitude of physiological adaptation to aerobic exercise training in humans. *BMC Biol.* 2005; **3**:19. DOI: 10.1186/1741-7007-3-19

4 Yan X, Eynon N, Papadimitriou ID, Kuang J, Munson F, Tirosh O, et al. The gene SMART study: method, study design, and preliminary findings. *BMC Genomics.* 2017; **18**(Suppl 8):821. DOI: 10.1186/s12864-017-4186-4

5 Gibson WT. Core concepts in human genetics: understanding the complex phenotype of sport performance and susceptibility to sport injury. *Med Sport Sci.* 2016; **61**:1–14.

6 Klissouras V. Heritability of adaptive variation. *J Appl Physiol.* 1971; **31**(3):338–44.

7 Bouchard C. Genomic predictors of trainability (Genomics & Exercise). *Exp Physiol.* 2011; **3**(3):347–52.

8 Wang G, Padmanabhan S, Wolfarth B, Fuku N, Lucia A, Ahmetov II, et al. Genomics of elite sporting performance: what little we know and necessary advances. *Adv Genet.* 2013; **84**:123–49.

9 Loos RJF, Hagberg JM, Pérusse L, Roth SM, Sarzynski MA, Wolfarth B, et al. Advances in exercise, fitness, and performance genomics in 2014. *Med Sci Sports Exerc.* 2015; **47**:1105–12.

10 Bhagi S, Srivastava S, Sarkar S, Singh SB. Distribution of performance-related gene polymorphisms (ACTN3 R577X and ACE ID) in different ethnic groups of the Indian Army. *J Basic Clin Physiol Pharmacol.* 2013; **24**(4):225–34.

11 Wang G, Mikami E, Chiu LL, De Perini A, Deason M, Fuku N, et al. Association analysis of ACE and ACTN3 in elite Caucasian and East Asian swimmers. *Med Sci Sports Exerc.* 2013; **45**(5):892–900.

12 Amir O, Amir R, Yamin C, Attias E, Eynon N, Sagiv M, et al. The ACE deletion allele is associated with Israeli elite endurance athletes. *Exp Physiol.* 2007; **92**(5):881–6.

13 Scott RA, Irving R, Irwin L, Morrison E, Charlton V, Austin K, et al. ACTN3 and ACE Genotypes in Elite Jamaican and US Sprinters. *Med Sci Sport Exerc.* 2010; **42**(1):107–12.

14 Gayagay G, Yu B, Hambly B, Boston T, Hahn A, Celermajer DS, et al. Elite endurance athletes and the ACE I allele – the role of genes in athletic performance. *Hum Genet.* 1998;**103**(1):48–50.

15 Ginevičienė V, Pranculis A, Jakaitienė A, Milašius K, Kučinskas V. Genetic variation of the human ACE and ACTN3 genes and their association with functional muscle properties in Lithuanian elite athletes. *Med Investig Med.* 2011; **4747**(55):284–90.

16 Eynon N, Hanson ED, Lucia A, Houweling PJ, Garton F, North KN, et al. Genes for elite power and sprint performance: ACTN3 leads the way. *Sport Med.* 2013; **43**(9):803–17.

17 Swaroop A, Branham KEH, Chen W, Abecasis G. Genetic susceptibility to age-related macular degeneration: a paradigm for dissecting complex disease traits. *Hum Mol Genet.* 2007; **16**(Spec No. 2):R174–82.

18 Stranger BE, Stahl EA, Raj T. Progress and promise of genome-wide association studies for human complex trait genetics. *Genetics.* 2011;**187**: 367–83.

19 Bouchard C, Sarzynski MA, Rice TK, Kraus WE, Church TS, Sung YJ, et al. Genomic predictors of the maximal O_2 uptake response to standardized exercise training programs. *J Appl Physiol.* 2011; **110**(5):1160–70.

20 Rankinen T, Fuku N, Wolfarth B, Wang G, Sarzynski MA, Alexeev DG, et al. No evidence of a common DNA variant profile specific to world class endurance athletes. *PLoS One.* 2016; **11**(1):1–24.

21 Willems SM, Wright DJ, Day FR, Trajanoska K, Joshi PK, Morris JA, et al. Large-scale GWAS identifies multiple loci for hand grip strength providing biological insights into muscular fitness. *Nat Commun.* 2017; **8**:16015.

22 Bird A. Perceptions of epigenetics. *Nature.* 2007; **447**:396–8.

23 Weinhold B. Epigenetics: the science of change. *Environ Heal Perspect.* 2006; **114**(3):160–7.

24 Rooney J. Further thoughts on mercury, epigenetics, genetics and amyotrophic lateral sclerosis. *Neurodegener Dis.* 2011; **8**:523–4.

25 van Dijk SJ, Molloy PL, Varinli H, Morrison JL, Muhlhausler BS. Epigenetics and human obesity. *Int J Obes (Lond).* 2015; **39**(1):85–97.

26 Waddington CH. Genetic assimilation of the bithorax phenotype. *Evolution (N Y).* 1956; **10**(1):1–13.

27 Alberts B, Johnson A, Lewis J, Morgan D, Raff M, Roberts K, et al. *Molecular biology of the cell.* 6th ed. New York: Taylor & Francis Group; 2014. pp. 412–3.

28 Ptashne M. Epigenetics: core misconcept. *Proc Natl Acad Sci U S A.* 2013; **110**(18):7101–3.

29 Katan-Khaykovich Y, Struhl K. Dynamics of global histone acetylation and deacetylation in vivo: rapid restoration of normal histone acetylation status upon removal of activators and repressors. *Genes Dev.* 2002; **16**(6):743–52.

30 Radman-Livaja M, Liu CL, Friedman N, Schreiber SL, Rando OJ. Replication and active demethylation represent partially overlapping mechanisms for erasure of H3K4me3 in budding yeast. *PLoS Genet.* 2010; **6**(2):e1000837.

31 Ringrose L, Paro R. Polycomb/Trithorax response elements and epigenetic memory of cell identity. *Development.* 2007; **134**(2):223–32.

32 Felsenfeld G. A brief history of epigenetics. *Cold Spring Harb Perspect Biol.* 2007; **6**(1).

33 Denham J, Marques FZ, O'Brien BJ, Charchar FJ. Exercise: putting action into our epigenome. *Sports Med.* 2014; **44**:189–209.

34 Denham J, O'Brien BJ, Harvey JT, Charchar FJ. Genome-wide sperm DNA methylation changes after 3 months of exercise training in humans. *Epigenomics.* 2015; **7**(5):717–31.

35 Rönn T, Volkov P, Davegardh C, Dayeh T, Hall E, Olsson AH, et al. A six months exercise intervention influences the genome-wide DNA methylation pattern in human adipose tissue. *PLoS Genet.* 2013; **9**(6):e1003572.

36 Nitert MD, Dayeh T, Volkov P, Elgzyri T, Hall E, Nilsson E, et al. Impact of an exercise intervention on DNA methylation in skeletal muscle from first-degree relatives of patients with type 2 diabetes. *Diabetes.* 2012; 61:1–11.

37 Lindholm ME, Marabita F, Gomez-Cabrero D, Rundqvist H, Ekstrom TJ, Tegner J, et al. An integrative analysis reveals coordinated reprogramming of the epigenome and the transcriptome in human skeletal muscle after training. *Epigenetics.* 2014; **9**(12):1557–69.

38 Robinson MM, Dasari S, Konopka AR, Johnson ML, Manjunatha S, Esponda RR, et al. Enhanced protein translation underlies improved metabolic and physical adaptations to different exercise training modes in young and old humans. *Cell Metab.* 2017; **25**(3):581–92.

39 Rowlands DS, Page RA, Sukala WR, Giri M, Ghimbovschi SD, Hayat I, et al. Multi-omic integrated networks connect DNA methylation and miRNA with skeletal muscle plasticity to chronic exercise in Type 2 diabetic obesity. *Physiol Genomics.* 2014; **46**(20):747–65.

40 Sanchis-Gomar F, Luis Garcia-Gimenez J, Perez-Quillis C, Gomez Cabrera MC, Pallardo FV, Giuseppe L. Physical exercise as an epigenetic modulator. Eustress, the "positive stress" as an effector of gene expression. *Strength Cond J.* 2003; **25**(1):66–7.

41 Denham J, Marques FZ, Brien BJO, Charchar FJ. Exercise: putting action into our epigenome. *Sports Med.* 2014; **44**(2):189–209.

42 Ehlert T, Simon P, Moser DA. Epigenetics in sports. *Sport Med.* 2013; **43**(2):93–110.

43 Voisin S, Eynon N, Yan X, Bishop DJ. Exercise training and DNA methylation in humans. *Acta Physiol.* 2015; **213**(1):39–59.

44 Barrès R, Yan J, Egan B, Treebak JT, Rasmussen M, Fritz T, et al. Acute exercise remodels promoter methylation in human skeletal muscle. *Cell Metab.* 2012; **15**(3):405–11.

45 Bajpeyi S, Covington JD, Taylor EM, Stewart LK, Galgani JE, Henagan TM. Skeletal muscle PGC1alpha -1 nucleosome position and -260nt DNA methylation determine exercise response and prevent ectopic lipid accumulation in men. *Endocrinology.* 2017; **158**(July):2190–9.

46 Lamon S, Russell AP. The role and regulation of PGC-1(alpha) and PGC-1(beta) in skeletal muscle adaptation. *Plast Skeletal Muscle.* 2017; 1–292.

47 Sharples AP, Stewart CE, Seaborne RA. Does skeletal muscle have an "epi"-memory? The role of epigenetics in nutritional programming, metabolic disease, aging and exercise. *Aging Cell.* 2016; **15**:603–16.

48 McKinsey TA, Zhang CL, Lu J, Olson EN. Signal-dependent nuclear export of a histone deacetylase regulates muscle differentiation. *Nature.* 2000; **408**(6808):106–11.

49 Smith JA, Kohn TA, Chetty AK, Ojuka EO. CaMK activation during exercise is required for histone hyperacetylation and MEF2A binding at the MEF2 site on the Glut4 gene. *Am J Physiol Endocrinol Metab.* 2008; **295**(3):E698–704.

50 McGee SL, Fairlie E, Garnham AP, Hargreaves M. Exercise-induced histone modifications in human skeletal muscle. *J Physiol.* 2009; **587**(24):5951–8.

51 McGee SL, Hargreaves M. Exercise and skeletal muscle glucose transporter 4 expression: molecular mechanisms. *Clin Exp Pharmacol Physiol.* 2006; **33**(4):395–9.

52 McGee SL, Hargreaves M. Histone modifications and exercise adaptations.pdf. *J Appl Physiol.* 2011; **110**(258–63).

53 Liu Y, Randall WR, Schneider MF. Activity-dependent and -independent nuclear fluxes of HDAC4 mediated by different kinases in adult skeletal muscle. *J Cell Biol.* 2005; **168**(6):887–97.

54 Li B, Carey M, Workman JL. The role of chromatin during transcription. *Cell.* 2007; **128**:707–19.

55 Howlett KF, McGee SL. Epigenetic regulation of skeletal muscle metabolism. *Clin Sci.* 2016; **130**(13):1051–63.

56 Hargreaves M. Exercise and gene expression. *Prog Mol Biol Transl Sci.* 2015; **135**:457–69.

5   Systematically searching and reviewing the literature

Nirav Maniar, Kathryn Duncan and David Opar

Aims of this chapter

The aims of this chapter are to provide a brief reference guide for those who are attempting a systematic literature review for the first time and to provide an awareness of the issues involved with effective literature searching.

Introduction

Reviewing the literature is a critical step in the research process. A well-conducted literature review can help to generate new knowledge, can serve as a resource for yourself (and others) to quickly accrue knowledge in a specific area and can help identify areas for further research. Indeed, a review of the literature should set the foundation for any original research by helping to determine gaps in the current evidence base. In turn those gaps identified should be answered by defining a research question that guides original research.

Whilst the focus of this chapter will be on systematic reviews of the literature, a quick overview on the different types of review articles is a nice place for us to get started.

What's in a name?

A *systematic literature review* involves a defined (one might even say a systematic!) methodology around the strategy for searching articles, the process by which articles were either included or excluded and how the quality and risk of bias of included articles was determined. The methodology used to complete a systematic literature review, often referred to as the protocol, requires sufficient detail so that if someone was to replicate the steps reported they would find the same information you did. From the information discovered during the search, data is extracted and synthesized to draw conclusions.

Along with a systematic literature review the other most common type of review is a *narrative literature review*. The narrative literature review shares some common elements with the systematic review, in that it involves an organized and reproducible approach to searching the literature. However, narrative reviews entail less rigour around reporting of the protocol, do not require clearly defined reasons for why articles were included and excluded from the review and how the quality and risk of bias of included articles was assessed (if this was assessed at all). To a large extent narrative reviews can be influenced by something known as selection bias, whereby the authors of the narrative review are able to select articles for inclusion with some degree of subjectivity. This subjectivity can mean that articles, which are relevant to the review topic, could be overlooked and as a result this could influence the conclusions of the review. In spite of the issues around article selection, narrative reviews, particularly when written by those with expertise in the field, can provide "intuitive, experiential and explicit perspectives" on a specific topic.[1]

The final type of literature review is the emerging *scoping literature review*.[2] Given its recent eminence, a consensus definition for a scoping literature review (and even consensus around its appropriate naming) is yet to be described. In brief, scoping reviews tend to focus on broad topic areas of interest not necessarily with the purpose of addressing a specific research question, but instead to chart and summarize relevant literature and to determine gaps and limitations of the evidence base. As such scoping reviews attempt to capture a larger breadth of information, although not necessarily with the same depth as the other review types mentioned.

So now you know a little more about the types of literature reviews out there, let's set our sights on the systematic literature review.

If I have to complete a systematic review . . . where do I start?

For those performing a systematic literature review for the first time the task can, at the outset, seem somewhat daunting. As a starting point we recommend the Preferred Reporting Items for Systematic Reviews and Meta-Analyses Checklist, otherwise known as the PRISMA Checklist and the accompanying PRISMA flow diagram (Figure 5.1).[3,4] The PRISMA Checklist provides authors with 27 items that should

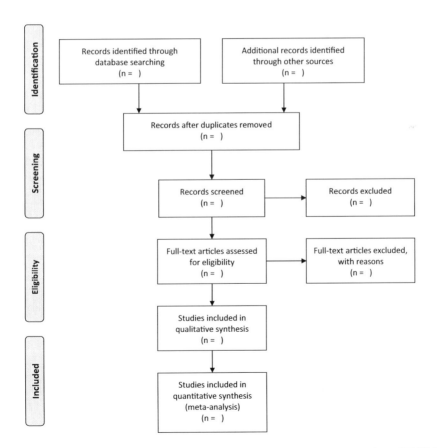

Figure 5.1 The Preferred Reporting Items for Systematic Reviews and Meta-Analyses (PRISMA)[5,6] flow diagram.

appear in any systematic literature review, whilst the PRISMA flow diagram is a visual summary of the outcomes of your systematic search strategy.

The PRISMA Checklist is not designed to spoon-feed you the process of conducting the review but is an essential document to read (and re-read) prior to developing the protocol for a systematic review. Being cognizant of all the information that is required to be reported at the end of your systematic review before you even start will help guide you throughout the entire process and means that you are less likely to get to the end of your review (and the hours and hours of work required to complete it) only to realize that you have left out critical pieces of information (that will take even more hours of work to rectify!).

Once you have read the PRISMA Checklist the next step is to start developing your systematic review protocol. The development and use of a protocol is a hallmark of a high-quality systematic review as it provides the transparency of reporting methods *a priori*, an important standard to set as it ensures accountability and research integrity for the authors. The PRISMA for Protocols (also known as PRISMA-P) provides a road map to assist researchers in developing and reporting their systematic review protocol.[7,8]

Using the PRISMA-P as a template, the remainder of this chapter will walk you through some of the basics of developing and executing your systematic review protocol. We will refer to relevant additional resources where required, but we also recommend you liaise with someone experienced in conducting systematic reviews, particularly your institutional library staff, as well as peers, colleagues and research supervisors. For the purposes of providing a working exemplar, at various stages throughout the chapter we will refer to content adapted from the systematic review and meta-analysis conducted by Maniar et al.[9] on hamstring strength and flexibility following injury.

Rationale and objectives

Besides some simple administrative information, the first step of developing your systematic review protocol is to determine and describe the rationale for your systematic review. Think of this a little bit like the introduction section of a scientific paper. You must rationalize the need for your review in line with what is currently known and what is unknown based on the literature. This may require some background reading (perhaps even a scoping review) or guidance by an expert in the field to help focus and define your research question. You might find that a systematic review answering your research question (or a very similar question) already exists. Scoping might also inform you if there is any literature available to answer your question and this might require you to adapt or reshape the emphasis of your review.

Your research questions must be clearly articulated. It should inform as to what your review will aim to address, which at a minimum should include reference to the PICO framework (Patient/problem/population; Intervention/Issue; Comparison/control/comparator; Outcome).[10]

Eligibility criteria

Eligibility criteria will ultimately determine which articles will be included in your systematic review. Eligibility is determined through the application of inclusion and/or exclusion criteria that will be guided by your research question. Your eligibility criteria should leave you with relevant studies based on study design, population of interest (possibly including age ranges and gender), geographical location of interest and your outcomes of interest. For example, you may have eligibility criteria to include studies that report data on (1) adolescent females who are overweight (population); (2) that were exposed to an exercise-based weight loss programme (intervention); (3) compared to a control group, which could be defined by only including randomized control trials (control); (4) to determine the impact on body composition measured through dual-energy x-ray absorptiometry (outcome).

Information sources

Determining the information sources from which you will search for literature will depend on your research question and the likely research disciplines that will have conducted the relevant work. For the areas of physical activity and health, we have provided some electronic databases to consider, along with a brief description of each in Box 5.1. To help frame your possible information sources it is also useful to look at previously published systematic literature reviews in your area of research and to examine the information sources that were used. Depending on your field of research you will need to think about whether searching the grey literature (research that is unpublished or published in a non-commercial form) will be relevant. Such grey literature could include reports or policy statements from government and industry or bodies such as the World Health Organisation.

Box 5.1 Description of common electronic databases that contain literature in physical activity and health

Medline is the premier bibliographic database from the US National Library of Medicine for biomedical and health literature. It covers 1946 to the present with citations from 5,600 journals. www.nlm.nih.gov/pubs/factsheets/medline.html

SPORTDiscus is a sport and sports medicine database including subject areas such as exercise science and fitness, coaching and education, kinesiology, nutrition and sports science. It covers 1930 to the present with citations from nearly 970 journals. www.ebscohost.com/academic/sportdiscus-with-full-text

CINAHL is a nursing and allied health database including physical therapy, nutrition, general health and rehabilitation. It covers 1937 to the present and includes citations from over 5,400 journals. www.ebscohost.com/nursing/products/cinahl-databases/cinahl-complete

PsycINFO from the American Psychological Association is the largest database covering literature in behavioural science and mental health. It has extensive coverage from the 1800s to the present and indexes more than 2,500 journals as well as dissertations and books. www.apa.org/pubs/databases/psycinfo/index.aspx

Embase is a biomedical and pharmacological literature database including drug, disease and device information. It covers 1974 to the present and indexes over 8,500 journals. www.elsevier.com/promo/rd-solutions/embase?p2=embase&term=embase&pscid=cm_ps_100000188

Education Resources Information Center (ERIC) is a database of journal articles, conference papers, grey literature and books covering education literature. It is sponsored by the Institute of Education Sciences of the US Department of Education and covers 1964 to the present with over 1.6 million records. https://ies.ed.gov/ncee/projects/eric.asp

Scopus is an interdisciplinary database of journals, books and conference papers across medicine, science, technology, social sciences, arts and humanities. It covers 1996 to the present and has over 67 million records including citations from over 22,700 journals. www.scopus.com/home.uri

Web of Science Core Collection is an interdisciplinary citation database across science, social sciences and arts and humanities. It covers 1900 to the present and includes citations from over 12,000 journals as well as conference proceedings and book citations. https://images.webofknowledge.com/images/help/WOS/hp_database.html

Search strategy

First steps

The best way to organize your search strategy is to start with your research question. Think about breaking your research question into a number of concepts, but exactly how many concepts depends on your research question (we will use three in our worked example). You could use the PICO framework (Population, Intervention/Issue, Comparison, Outcome) or alternatively a simple concept table (see Table 5.1).

Using our worked example from Maniar et al.[9] the research question/aim is "to systematically review the evidence base related to hamstring strength and flexibility in previously injured hamstrings". This leads to the division of three concepts: (1) a focus on a particular muscle group, in this case the hamstrings; (2) a focus on injury to that muscle group and (3) a focus on injuries that is dependent on time, that is, they are injuries that are retrospective or in the past. Using those three divisions we can create our concept table, which can be further developed by adding synonyms for each concept (Table 5.1).

Your concept table (or similar type strategy) will form the basics of your search strategy so it is a good idea to spend some time determining your concepts and expanding

Table 5.1 A concept table, with each column representing a concept based on the aim/research question of the systematic review. Each concept is expanded to include synonyms.

Muscle Group	Injury	Time
Hamstring	Injury	Past
Semitendinosus	Strain	Prior
Semimembranosus	Tear	Retrospective
Biceps Femoris	Rupture	Previous
Thigh	Pull	Recent
	Trauma	History
	Torn	

your synonyms and then having it reviewed by a colleague or research supervisor. Once you are happy with your concept table the next step is to design your search strategy. To do this you will need an understanding of the key search tools available to you and how best to use them.

Truncation and wildcard

Truncation is a search tool which allows a search term to be used once but to capture the many forms of the word including, most commonly, the plural form. It is almost universally represented with a * at the end of the word stem. For example, *injur** will search *injury* OR *injured* OR *injuring* OR *injuries*. It is also very useful to search words with variant spellings such as behavi* (behavior OR behaviour). When truncating a word it is important to think of other words which may inadvertently be captured. For example, a search term such as rat* to find rat studies where rat* is designed to capture rat OR rats. However, the letters 'rat' are the beginning of words such as 'rationale' which would be included, incorrectly, in your search results. In cases such as this using both forms of the word (rat OR rats) in the search string provides the necessary sensitivity and precision (for more information on sensitivity and precision in the context of literature search strategy see Box 5.2).

Box 5.2 Sensitivity and precision in search structure[11]

Sensitivity vs. precision

When designing a search for a systematic review you need to consider the balance between sensitivity and precision.

Sensitivity (comprehensiveness). This is the percentage of relevant articles located in comparison to the percentage of relevant articles in existence. A systematic review aims to retrieve all relevant articles in existence.

Precision (relevance) is the number of relevant articles retrieved in relation to the total number of articles retrieved.

A search strategy which is more sensitive (or comprehensive) will be less precise, meaning the number of non-relevant articles retrieved will be higher. However, the result will also include a greater percentage of all relevant articles in existence which is critical for a rigorous review. A systematic review search strategy should aim for high sensitivity despite the resulting low precision.

An example of achieving a balance for our muscle group concept would be to use the term *hamstring* for precision, as well as the term *thigh* for increasing sensitivity. However, including the term *leg* in the muscle group would produce too many additional results, outweighing the benefit of any possible additional relevant articles retrieved.

Spelling variations in the middle of words are searched with a wildcard symbol which replaces one or more letters, for example, p#diatric. However, the wildcard symbol varies from database to database (e.g. ? or # or $) so it can be easier to just type all forms of a word into the search string (such as paediatric OR pediatric).

Phrase and proximity searching

When searching a concept with more than one term it is necessary to enclose the phrase in quotations marks (''). Enclosing a search phrase, for example, 'physical activity', in inverted commas instructs the database to search for the terms together, in that order. This helps to increase the relevance (precision) of results for this search term. If the word *physical* as well as the word *activity* are present in the article title or abstract, but not next to each other, in that order, they will not be expressing the concept of 'physical activity' and hence will not be returned in your search. It is important to also consider that sometimes it is preferable to AND the terms. For example, the phrase 'hamstring injury' will exclude instances where the terms are used in a different order, such as *injury to the hamstring*. Another way to combine terms is proximity or adjacency operators such as near (regardless of word order) or within (in the word order written). For example, hamstring N3 injur* will find results where the word 'hamstring' is within three words of injur* regardless of the order of the words. The symbols for proximity operators vary from database to database and can be located on the database help pages.

Boolean operators (AND, OR, NOT)

Boolean operators are used to connect search terms together to broaden, narrow or exclude elements in a search and produce the most relevant set of results possible.

OR is used to expand a concept (sensitivity) and ensure all articulations of it which may be included in the article title, abstract or subject headings are used in the search. OR is used to combine ideas that are the same. For example, to fully articulate the concept of the injury it would be searched with a range of terms such as injury OR strain OR tear OR rupture OR pull OR trauma OR torn (Table 5.2).

AND is used to narrow search results (precision) to those which include all relevant concepts. It is used to combine ideas that are different or the separate columns in a concept table (Table 5.2).

NOT is used to exclude specific concepts or terms from a search but in systematic review searches is generally best avoided.[11] It can be used after an initial search has been conducted and reviewed and there is seen to be a large, non-relevant subset of

Table 5.2 Concept table incorporating key search tools such as truncation, phrase searching and Boolean operators

Muscle Group		Injury		Time
Hamstring*		Injur*		Past
OR	AND	OR	AND	OR
Semitendinosus		Strain*		Prior
OR		OR		OR
Semimembranosus		Tear		Retrospective*
OR		OR		OR
'Biceps Femoris'		Rupture*		Previous*
OR		OR		OR
Thigh		Pull		Recent*
		OR		OR
		Trauma		Histor*
		OR		
		Torn		

results, such as animal studies. However, it is important to remember that using NOT may inadvertently remove relevant studies. For example, *male* NOT *female* will exclude studies which include both males and females.[11] In cases such as this it is best to exclude papers as part of the screening process (which will be discussed in more detail later).

Search fields

To balance sensitivity and precision a search should be conducted using both free text keywords and controlled vocabulary terms in the search.[11] The best-known form of controlled vocabulary is Medical Subject Headings (MeSH), which is a standardized set of terminology, used by Medline, that can be assigned to articles. Subject headings, of which MeSH headings are just one example, are assigned by databases from the list of standardized terms, to capture the many different ways a concept may be described, beyond the syntax used in the search.[11] For example, the MeSH heading 'Sprains and Strains' is described as "A collective term for muscle and ligament injuries without dislocation or fracture. A sprain is a joint injury in which some of the fibers of a supporting ligament are ruptured but the continuity of the ligament remains intact. A strain is an overstretching or overexertion of some part of the musculature".[12] Articles which use terms such as injury, strain, tear, rupture, pull or torn may have a subject heading such as 'Sprains and Strains' assigned to them by respective databases. It is worth noting that not all databases use a single universal controlled vocabulary so your search strategy will have to account for variations across databases. For an example of incorporating controlled vocabulary, including exemplars from two different databases, into a concept table and search strategy see Table 5.3. To

Table 5.3 Developing a concept table to search terms in the title and abstract as well as the use of Medical Subject Headings (MeSH) used in the Medline database

	Muscle Group		*Injury*		*Time*
Title and abstract search terms	Hamstring* OR Semitendinosus OR Semimembranosus OR 'Biceps Femoris' OR Thigh	AND	Injur* OR Strain* OR Tear OR Rupture* OR Pull OR Trauma OR Torn	AND	Past OR Prior OR Retrospective* OR Previous* OR Recent* OR Histor*
MeSH terms for Medline	'Hamstring Muscles' OR 'Hamstring Tendons' OR 'Thigh'	AND	'Wounds and injuries' OR 'Sprains and Strains' OR 'Rupture'	AND	*(no relevant MeSH term)*

(Continued)

Table 5.3 (Continued)

	Muscle Group		Injury		Time
SPORTDiscus subject headings	'HAMSTRING muscle – Wounds & injuries' OR 'HAMSTRING muscle – Physiology' OR 'HAMSTRING muscle' 'THIGH' OR 'THIGH – Muscles' OR 'BICEPS femoris'	AND	'WOUNDS & injuries' OR 'OVERUSE injuries' OR 'SOFT tissue injuries' OR 'STRAIN (Physiology)' OR 'RUPTURE of organs, tissues, etc.'	AND	*(no relevant SPORTDiscus subject heading)*

assist in determining what controlled vocabulary to include in your search strategy you might consider using text mining tools (see Box 5.3).

Box 5.3 Text mining tools to assist with developing controlled vocabulary for your search strategy

There are tools such as PubReMiner (http://hgserver2.amc.nl/cgi-bin/miner/miner2.cgi) or the Yale MeSH Analyzer (http://mesh.med.yale.edu/help) which use PubMed to help find relevant MeSH terms using text mining. A key term is entered or a list of articles selected and subject headings associated with the resulting articles are listed. This guides you to MeSH terms which may be relevant for inclusion in your search.

To execute your concept search you will search the title as well as the abstract, using the alternative words and synonyms that describe your concept combined with OR. This is further combined, using OR again as this is still part of the same concept search, with a search of MeSH terms (or other examples of controlled vocabulary) to provide a comprehensive (sensitive) search. The combined articles returned from this search represent the results for a concept column from Table 5.3. Once each concept column has been searched separately (following the above steps) the concepts are combined using AND to produce a manageable (precise) number of results for screening. An example of an executed search strategy in Medline can be found in Table 5.4.

In Table 5.4, searches 1–3 represent the Muscle group concept column, searches 4–6 represent the Injury concept column and search 7 represents the Time concept column. The results for Search 8 consist of both the Muscle group and Injury concepts using the Boolean operator AND. Search 9 combines all three concepts and is your total number of results for this search strategy.

Table 5.4 Example execution of a Medline database search strategy

Search	Search Terms	Results
S1	(MH 'Hamstring Muscles') OR (MH 'Hamstring Tendons') OR (MH 'Thigh')	(10,949)
S2	AB (hamstring* OR semitendinosus OR semimembranosus OR 'biceps femoris' OR thigh) OR TI (hamstring* OR semitendinosus OR semimembranosus OR 'biceps femoris' OR thigh)	(32,852)
S3	S1 OR S2	(38,259)
S4	(MH 'Wounds and Injuries') OR (MH 'Sprains and Strains') OR (MH 'Soft Tissue Injuries') OR (MH 'Rupture')	(101,359)
S5	AB (injur* OR strain* OR tear OR rupture* OR pull* OR trauma OR torn) OR TI (injur* OR strain* OR tear OR rupture* OR pull* OR trauma OR torn)	(1,521,749)
S6	S4 OR S5	(1,228,273)
S7	AB (past OR prior OR retrospective* OR previous* OR recent* OR histor*) OR TI (past OR prior OR retrospective* OR previous* OR recent* OR histor*)	(4,312,115)
S8	S3 AND S6	(6,982)
S9	S7 AND S8	(1,928)

MH = MeSH heading, AB = abstract, TI = title

Preparing an appropriately sensitive and precise systematic search is essential to ensure relevant articles are located. It can be time consuming but, relative to the time committed to your review, it represents time well spent and ensures a rigorous basis for the review. A health sciences librarian can provide expert advice on developing a search strategy as well as guidance on how to use individual databases so seeking assistance at the beginning of the review's search process is recommended.

Search filters

The methodology of studies to be included can be an inclusion/exclusion criteria but can also be part of the search. The type of study can be controlled language in fields such as the subject heading or publication type.

Search filters are optimal search strategies which have been developed for particular study types (e.g. RCT) or review focuses (prognosis, aetiology) on specific databases. They can help to reduce the number of results when it is large and are particularly helpful when the review is based on a single study type. For example, several search filters have been developed by the Cochrane Community.[13]

Searching is an iterative process and a search is developed, expanded and changed based on the relevance and number of articles being retrieved. One method to explore how well a search has been constructed is to confirm that any known relevant articles are being retrieved. Limiters such as language and date range can be added to a search using the tools available in the database.

All database searches should be structured, modified for the requirements of each database such as relevant subject headings, specific fields to be searched for publication type or age range, and prepared and saved before your final searches are run. Title/Abstract search language is used consistently across each database but subject headings vary. For example, the subject headings for hamstring vary across databases and there are no relevant subject headings for the Time concept (see Table 5.3). The search date is recorded for the reporting in review methodology. A detailed search history and numbers of results must be saved for each database and included in the PRISMA flow diagram.

Data management, selection process and data collection process

Once completed, search results can be exported to bibliographic software such as EndNote (www.endnote.com) keeping a record of how many were located on each database. Records can be de-duplicated, as the same article will have been located on different databases, and a final number of results are confirmed for screening.

All retrieved articles need to be screened and the process for selecting articles for inclusion needs to be explicitly stated in the methods section of the review. You will also need to determine how the screening and selection process will be executed. For example, will all phases involve two independent reviewers and if there is conflict between reviewers, outline the strategy to resolve these (i.e. decision from third independent reviewer).

The initial screen of the title and abstract involves the removal of clearly irrelevant articles, leaving you with a curated list of articles for which you will need to source the full text articles. Eligibility is determined by a review of the full text article using the pre-defined inclusion/exclusion criteria. Articles excluded at this stage are assigned a reason for exclusion, which is required to be reported as part of the PRISMA flow chart. At the end of this process what is remaining are your included articles (a fist pump moment!). It is often common to review the reference list of your included studies, as well as any citations they have received, as this may reveal articles that could be considered for inclusion.

Screening can be done by hand, for example, by importing data into an Excel spreadsheet, but there are also products such as the web-based Covidence (www.covidence.org),[14] which can help make the process much smoother and faster. Covidence allows imported citations to be asynchronously screened by multiple reviewers, moves through the full text review and provides assistance for data extraction. The software keeps a record of the decision(s) on each article and pre-populates a PRISMA flow diagram for you.

Data items, outcomes and prioritization

Prior to executing your search you should also determine and define what data you plan to extract from your included articles. A minimum standard, particularly for systematic reviews which focus on randomized control trials, is to extract data on PICO (Population, Intervention/Issue, Comparison, Outcome); however, the information that you are required to extract will be guided primarily by your research question. It is important to "list and define all outcomes for which data will be sought" and to identify your primary and secondary outcomes, where necessary.[7]

Quality and risk of bias assessment of included studies

The purpose of assessing the quality and risk of bias of included studies is to determine if the findings from included studies are valid and specifically whether the study has internal validity. Think of the assessment of internal validity as trying to determine whether a study has answered the research question correctly in a way that is free from bias. Put another way, based on the way the study was conducted, what degree of trust can you have that the findings are reflective of the truth? For further information see the Cochrane Handbook Chapter 8.1.[15]

Whilst there is an abundance of information available on assessing article quality and risk of bias, this brings with it both positives and negatives. The breadth of information, most of which is freely available, enables anyone with access to a computer to read, learn and become informed in the area. There is, however, no universally utilized tool or checklist that is used across all disciplines of science to assess article quality and risk of bias, meaning that you will need to make your own (informed) decision about what is appropriate for your review. Your decision will be based on a number of factors, the most notable being what type of study design/s will be included in your review.

To delve into the necessary detail and depth on the assessment of quality and risk of bias would require a chapter (or maybe even an entire book!) all to itself. For the sake of brevity we have provided guidance on further reading and some freely available resources that will help you in determining how you should assess article quality and risk of bias for your systematic review (see Box 5.4).

Box 5.4 Resources to assist with developing your approach to assessing article quality and risk of bias for your systematic review

- Cochrane Handbook for Systematic Reviews of Interventions – Chapter 8[14]

  Compulsory reading to help understand what bias is and the different types of bias, why risk of bias needs to be assessed and how to assess risk of bias in randomized trials (Chapter 13 also examines assessing quality and risk of bias in non-randomised studies).[15]

- National Institute of Health: National Heart, Lung, and Blood Institute – Study Quality Assessment Tools (www.nhlbi.nih.gov/health-pro/guidelines/in-develop/cardiovascular-risk-reduction/tools)

  Provides quality assessment tools for six different study designs (including assessing the quality of systematic reviews and meta-analyses, which is worth a look). Each tool provides detailed guidance on how to complete the assessment.

- University of South Australia: International Centre for Allied Health Evidence – Critical Appraisal Tools (www.unisa.edu.au/Research/Sansom-Institute-for-Health-Research/Research/Allied-Health-Evidence/Resources/CAT/)

  A continually updated repository of available critical appraisal tools for seven different study designs, as well as a variety of other relevant tools for systematic reviews.

- Healthcare Improvement Scotland – Critical Appraisal of Medical Literature online tutorial (www.healthcareimprovementscotland.org/about_us/what_we_do/knowledge_management/critical_appraisal_tutorial.aspx)

  Free online tutorial on the critical appraisal of the literature, which involves a combination of pre-recorded presentations and self-directed learning.

Data synthesis

Distilling the information from the included literature and presenting the main findings from your systematic review occurs through a process called data synthesis. The three major types of data synthesis are: *meta-analysis, narrative or descriptive synthesis and meta-synthesis*. Depending on the structure of your review, the type of study designs included in your review and how similar (or homogenous) your final included articles are will depend on what type of data synthesis you might complete.

Meta-analysis

The most objective, robust and reproducible approach for data synthesis is a meta-analysis. In brief, a meta-analysis is a statistical approach used to combine the data from the included studies to provide an overall effect. Put another way, a meta-analysis brings together the results of lots of smaller studies and by combining them creates one big study. By doing this we assume that the results from our 'one big study' provide a better reflection of the true impact that an intervention has on an outcome measure.

Despite the benefits of performing a meta-analysis it is also important to appreciate when it is or isn't appropriate to perform a meta-analysis. As a general rule of thumb, when included studies differ a lot (i.e. they are different study designs, they are answering different research questions, they return a high I^2 statistic) then it is not appropriate to combine the results from these studies. In such situations it may be possible to perform a meta-analysis on a subset of the included studies which are of similar study designs and are answering the same (or similar) research questions. You will also need to consider the risk of bias of included studies, as a meta-analysis with many studies with a high risk of bias may lead to these bias (or errors) compounding, ultimately producing misleading data. Despite the objectivity of meta-analysis the decision making around whether to perform a meta-analysis involves a degree of subjectivity. As such a justification for the performance of a meta-analysis or otherwise should be provided where possible.

A detailed guide for the performance of a meta-analysis is not possible in the space provided for this chapter. For a step-by-step guide to performing a meta-analysis the authors recommend Chapter 9.4 and 9.5 from the Cochrane Handbook.[16]

Narrative or descriptive synthesis

In situations where meta-analysis is not possible, your approach to data synthesis might need to be narrative or descriptive in nature.[17,18] Invariably this approach is more subjective than a meta-analysis and is more oriented towards textual descriptions of the data. If you are of the view that your systematic review would be best suited to narrative or descriptive synthesis of the data, Box 5.5 provides suggestions of possible approaches to explore.

Box 5.5 Possible approaches for a narrative or descriptive synthesis for your systematic review

Weight of evidence[19]
Best evidence synthesis[20]
Grouping and clustering[17]

Meta-synthesis

More recently there has been growth in the application of synthesizing qualitative research, often referred to as a meta-synthesis (but also called 'qualitative meta-synthesis', 'qualitative meta-analysis', 'meta-ethnography'). Much like the narrative or descriptive synthesis approach the possible ways to perform a meta-synthesis are wide ranging and varied depending on the scope, aims and purpose of the study. If meta-synthesis is of interest we recommend reading "Methods for the synthesis of qualitative research: a critical review"[21] and "Conducting a critical interpretive synthesis of the literature on access to healthcare by vulnerable groups".[22]

Meta-bias(es)

Meta-bias refers to factors that could influence the finding of your systematic literature review that are not directly related to the conduct of included articles. The main sources of meta-bias are *publication bias* and *outcome reporting bias*. Publication bias refers to the phenomena whereby studies that report statistically significant results or positive findings are more likely to be published than studies with non-significant results or negative findings. Publication bias can skew the findings of your systematic review and/or meta-analysis and as a result you should report how you will look for the presence of publication bias. The most common approach to assess publication bias is to construct a funnel plot, which graphically represents the effect estimates from your included studies on the *x*-axis against a measure of study quality (most often sample size) on the *y*-axis. Generally speaking, you will need 10 or more studies to include in your funnel plot; however, if your included studies have a high degree of heterogeneity you may require even more studies to make your funnel plot.

Outcome reporting bias refers to "the selective reporting of outcomes based on their significance, magnitude or direction" in published literature.[23] It is more likely that statistically significant results will be published in full compared to non-significant results. One approach to examine the presence of outcome reporting bias is to compare the data reported in the published paper with study protocols that were published or submitted *a priori*, although this is most effective when examining randomized control trials. In the absence of an *a priori* protocol it is also possible to compare the outcomes reported in the methods to what is reported in the results.

Confidence in cumulative evidence

The final stage of your systematic review protocol is to describe how you will assess the confidence that you have in the data presented as part of your review (and in some cases meta-analysis). The most common method for determining the confidence in the evidence is the Grading of Recommendations, Assessment, Development and Evaluation (GRADE) approach, developed by the GRADE Working Group.[24–26] The Cochrane Training webpage has a series of slide casts to assist with completing the GRADE approach.[27]

My systematic review is finished . . . what do I do now?

Firstly, don't underestimate the enormity of your achievement. The process of completing a systematic review is long, involved and labour intensive. On the positive side of the ledger you have helped in the creation of new knowledge, by combining and synthesizing evidence in a particular field in an organized, reproducible and transparent way. The obvious question now is 'What's next?'. The reality is that the answer to that question is open ended. In most cases the completion of a systematic review is the first step in developing a programme of research. Not only will your review have provided (hopefully) answers to your research question, in all likelihood it would have also generated even more questions. These questions likely exist because the current evidence is of poor quality, or the evidence required to answer these questions does not exist in the current literature. So on reflection of your systematic review think about what have you learnt, what new knowledge has been generated and what questions still require further investigation. The findings from your systematic review should help define a research question which should be the platform to launch into original research. Moreover, your systematic review may also guide methodological considerations for original research, potentially highlighting where there is a need for the development of new innovative techniques.

You have now set the course for your programme of original research. If you are motivated to do so, it's time to take the next step and commence work on your research proposal, guidance for which is provided in Chapter 6.

References

1 Pae CU. Why systematic review rather than narrative review? *Psychiat Investig* [Internet]. 2015 [cited 2017]; **12**(3):417–9. Available from: www.ncbi.nlm.nih.gov/pmc/articles/PMC4504929/ DOI: https://doi.org/10.4306/pi.2015.12.3.417

2 Arksey H, O'Malley L. Scoping studies: towards a methodological framework. *Int J Soc Res Methodol* [Internet]. 2007 [cited 2017]; **8**(1):19–32. Available from: www.tandfonline.com/doi/abs/10.1080/1364557032000119616 DOI: https://doi.org/10.1080/1364557032000119616

3 Moher D, Liberati A, Tetzlaff J, Altman DG. Preferred reporting items for systematic reviews and meta-analyses: the PRISMA statement. *BMJ* [Internet]. 2009 Jul 21[cited 2017]; **339**:b2535. Available from: www.bmj.com/content/bmj/339/bmj.b2535.full.pdf DOI: https://doi.org/10.1136/bmj.b2535

4 Liberati A, Altman DG, Tetzlaff J, Mulrow C, Gøtzsche PC, Ioannidis JP, et al. The PRISMA statement for reporting systematic reviews and meta-analyses of studies that evaluate healthcare interventions: explanation and elaboration. *BMJ* [Internet]. 2009 Jul 21 [cited 2017]; **339**:b2700. Available from: www.bmj.com/content/bmj/339/bmj.b2700.full.pdf DOI: https://doi.org/10.1136/bmj.b2700

5 PRISMA [Internet]. [place unknown]: PRISMA; c2015. PRISMA checklist; 2015 [cited 2017]. Available from: http://prisma-statement.org/PRISMAStatement/Checklist.aspx

6 PRISMA [Internet]. [place unknown]: PRISMA; 2015. PRISMA flow diagram; 2015 [cited 2017]. Available from: http://prisma-statement.org/PRISMAStatement/FlowDiagram.aspx

7 Moher D, Shamseer L, Clarke M, Ghersi D, Liberati A, Petticrew M, Shekelle P, Stewart LA. Preferred reporting items for systematic review and meta-analysis protocols (PRISMA-P) 2015 statement. *Syst Rev* [Internet]. 2015 [cited 2017]; **4**(1):1. Available from: https://systematicreviewsjournal.biomedcentral.com/articles/10.1186/2046-4053-4-1 DOI: https://doi.org/10.1186/2046-4053-4-1

8 PRISMA [Internet]. [place unknown]: PRISMA; c2015. PRISMA for systematic review protocols (PRISMA-P); 2015 [cited 2017]. Available from: http://prisma-statement.org/Extensions/Protocols.aspx

9 Maniar N, Shield AJ, Williams MD, Timmins RG, Opar DA. Hamstring strength and flexibility after hamstring strain injury: a systematic review and meta-analysis. *Br J Sports Med*

[Internet]. 2016 [cited 2017]; **50**(15):909–20. Available from: http://bjsm.bmj.com/con
tent/50/15/909 DOI: http://dx.doi.org/10.1136/bjsports-2015-095311

10 Miller SA, Forrest, JL. Enhancing your practice through evidence-based decision making: PICO, learning how to ask good questions. *J Evid Base Dent Pract* [Internet]. 2001
[cited 2017]; **1**:136–41. Available from: www.sciencedirect.com/science/article/pii/
S1532338201700243 DOI: https://doi.org/10.1016/S1532-3382(01)70024-3

11 Lefebvre C, Manheimer E, Glanville J. Searching for studies. In: Higgins JP, Green SS,
editors. *Cochrane handbook for systematic reviews of interventions* [Internet]. Chichester West
Sussex: Wiley; 2008. [cited 2017]. pp. 95–150. Available from: http://onlinelibrary.
wiley.com/doi/10.1002/9780470712184.ch6/summary DOI: https://doi.org/10.1002/
9780470712184.ch6

12 US National Library of Medicine [Internet]. Bethesda, MD: US National Library of Medicine; c1993–2017. Medical subject headings 2017; 2017 [cited 2017]. Available from:
https://meshb.nlm.nih.gov/search

13 Cochrane Community [Internet]. London: Cochrane Collaboration; c2017. Search filters;
2017 [cited 2017]; Available from: http://community.cochrane.org/organizational-info/
resources/resources-groups/information-specialists-portal/key-resources/search

14 Higgins JP, Altman DG. Assessing risk of bias in included studies. In: Higgins JP, Green SS,
editors. *Cochrane handbook for systematic reviews of interventions* [Internet]. Chichester West Sussex: Wiley; 2008 [cited 2017]. pp. 187–241. Available from: https://onlinelibrary.wiley.com/
doi/10.1002/9780470712184.ch8 DOI: https://doi.org/10.1002/9780470712184.ch8

15 Reeves BC, Deeks JJ, Higgins JP, Wells GA. Including non-randomized studies. In: Higgins
JP, Green SS, editors. *Cochrane handbook for systematic reviews of interventions* [Internet]. Chichester West Sussex: Wiley; 2008 [cited 2017]. pp. 389–432. Available from: https://onlineli
brary.wiley.com/doi/10.1002/9780470712184.ch13 DOI: 10.1002/9780470712184.ch13

16 Deeks JJ, Higgins JP, Altman DG. Analysing data and undertaking meta-analyses. In: Higgins
JP, Green SS, editors. *Cochrane handbook for systematic reviews of interventions* [Internet]. Chichester West Sussex: Wiley; 2008 [cited 2017]. pp. 243–96. Available from: https://onlineli
brary.wiley.com/doi/10.1002/9780470712184.ch9 DOI: 10.1002/9780470712184.ch9

17 Snilstveit B, Oliver S, Vojtkova M. Narrative approaches to systematic review and synthesis
of evidence for international development policy and practice. *J Dev Effect* [Internet]. 2012.
[cited 2017]; **4**(3):409–29. Available from: www.tandfonline.com/doi/pdf/10.1080/19439
342.2012.710641 DOI: https://doi.org/10.1080/19439342.2012.710641

18 Narrative Synthesis in Systematic Reviews [Internet]. Lancaster: Lancaster University;
2009. Publications: Guidance; 2006. [cited 2017]. Available from: www.lancaster.ac.uk/
shm/research/nssr/research/dissemination/publications.php

19 Gough D. Weight of evidence: a framework for the appraisal of the quality and relevance
of evidence. *Res Pap Educ* [Internet]. 2007 [cited 2017]; **22**:213–28. Available from: www.
tandfonline.com/doi/abs/10.1080/02671520701296189 DOI: https://doi.org/10.1080/
02671520701296189

20 Slavin RE. Best evidence synthesis: an intelligent alternative to meta-analysis. *J Clin Epidemiol*
[Internet]. 1995 [cited 2017]; **48**(1):9–18. Available from: www.sciencedirect.com/science/
article/pii/089543569400097A DOI: https://doi.org/10.1016/0895-4356(94)00097-A

21 Barnett-Page E, Thomas J. Methods for the synthesis of qualitative research: a critical review.
BMC Med Res Methodol [Internet]. 2009 [cited 2017]; **9**(1):59. Available from: https://bmc
medresmethodol.biomedcentral.com/articles/10.1186/1471-2288-9-59 DOI: https://doi.
org/10.1186/1471-2288-9-59

22 Dixon-Woods M, Cavers D, Agarwal S, Annandale E, Arthur A, Harvey J, et al. Conducting a
critical interpretive synthesis of the literature on access to healthcare by vulnerable groups.
BMC Med Res Methodol [Internet]. 2006 [cited 2017]; **6**(1):35. Available from: https://bmc
medresmethodol.biomedcentral.com/articles/10.1186/1471-2288-6-35 DOI: https://doi.
org/10.1186/1471-2288-6-35

23 Shamseer L, Moher D, Clarke M, Ghersi D, Liberati A, Petticrew M, et al. Preferred reporting items for systematic review and meta-analysis protocols (PRISMA-P) 2015: elaboration and explanation. *BMJ* [Internet]. 2015 [cited 2017]; **349**:g7647. Available from: www.bmj.com/content/349/bmj.g7647 DOI: https://doi.org/10.1136/bmj.g7647

24 Guyatt GH, Oxman AD, Kunz R, Falck-Ytter Y, Vist GE, Liberati A, et al. Going from evidence to recommendations. *BMJ* [Internet]. 2008 [cited 2017]; **349**:1049–51. Available from: www.bmj.com/content/336/7652/1049 DOI: https://doi.org/10.1136/bmj.39493.646875.AE

25 Guyatt GH, Oxman AD, Vist GE, Kunz R, Falck-Ytter Y, Alonso-Coello P, et al. GRADE: an emerging consensus on rating quality of evidence and strength of recommendations. *BMJ* [Internet]. 2008. [cited 2017]; **336**(7650):924–6. Available from: www.bmj.com/content/336/7650/924 DOI: https://doi.org/10.1136/bmj.39489.470347.AD

26 Guyatt GH, Oxman AD, Kunz R, Vist GE, Falck-Ytter Y, Schünemann HJ. What is "quality of evidence" and why is it important to clinicians? *BMJ* [Internet]. 2008 [cited 2017]; **336**(7651):995–8. Available from: www.bmj.com/content/336/7651/995 DOI: https://doi.org/10.1136/bmj.39490.551019.BE

27 Cochrane Training [Internet]. London: Cochrane Collaboration; c2018. GRADE approach to evaluating the quality of evidence: a pathway; 2010 [cited 2017]. Available from: http://training.cochrane.org/path/grade-approach-evaluating-quality-evidence-pathway

6   Producing the research proposal

Marie Murphy and Catherine Woods

Chapter aims

The aim of this chapter is to help you write a research proposal for a range of different audiences.

Introduction

A research proposal is a concise summary of your proposed research. It represents the formal starting point for a research project and is frequently the culmination of reading the literature and discussions with colleagues. Research proposals are commonly required: to assign undergraduate dissertation titles; as part of applications for post-graduate study; and as part of an application for research funding. Writing a research proposal is a valuable process to go through. It will familiarize you with your topic area and it will help you to clarify the aims and objectives of your study. Importantly, completing a research proposal will highlight problematic areas that need attention. Your proposal will also become a significant part of any ethics application and after data collection is complete it may also form the basis for the introduction and methods sections in any reports, publications or dissertations. Hence, the more comprehensive your proposal, the easier it will be in the long run. Additionally, you will find it useful as a reference when you confront difficult times, and just a glance will keep you focused.

Purpose of a research proposal

A research proposal outlines the research question(s) you seek to address and the methods you intend to use to answer this research question(s). This needs to be written in language that can be easily understood by a reader who may have general knowledge of the broad subject area, but may not be an expert in your chosen topic (see Know your audience below).

The length, format and level of detail required in a research proposal will depend on the purpose of the proposal. Research proposals can vary from short 1- or 2-page summaries to seek approval for an undergraduate or post-graduate dissertation, to a longer and more detailed explanation as part of an application for ethical approval right through to a lengthy document including details of the resources required to complete the project, and the planned timeline for completion of the research within an application for research funding. Before you begin to draft a research proposal it is important that you know the purpose of the proposal, and have carefully reviewed any forms or guidance provided to ensure that you include the information that is required.

Know your audience

In addition to knowing the format for the proposal, you should put yourself in the shoes of the person who is likely to be reading and perhaps assessing your research proposal. Are they lay people who have little knowledge of the broad subject area in which you work (e.g. a lay member of an ethics committee or a public or patient representative on a grant review panel); do they know your broad area of work but not the specific methods to be used (e.g. dissertation supervisor) or are they subject and topic specialists who are researchers in your topic and likely to have a detailed knowledge of the literature, theories or methods used? In some funding applications you may be asked to summarize your proposals for different audiences – so it is important that you know who the likely readership is for your proposal and write accordingly.

If you are unsure who will be reading your proposal – or it may be read by a number of different people – then it is best to err on the side of lay language. This means explaining your plans in clear non-technical language, using as little subject-specific jargon as possible. This style of writing is perhaps the most challenging for someone who has read extensively on a topic and is immersed in the subject area. Salita[1] provides excellent guidelines and practical examples of how to write for a lay audience. The best way to check you have written in sufficiently lay language is to ask a friend or relative with no knowledge of the area to read the proposal and check their understanding of why you want to undertake the study and what you plan to do.

Components of a research proposal

As discussed above, the specific contents of a research proposal will depend on the audience and so reading the guidelines for a proposal will ensure that you meet the requirements in terms of content, structure, format and length. However, most proposals will require the following information:

   Title: This should be succinct (10 words or less), but provide information on the project topic. Avoid redundant words such as: "An investigation into . . ." or "A description of . . .". The title should avoid jargon and abbreviations; these can be introduced in the background or introduction if required. The title can be formed at the beginning or the end of the project, for some a 'working title' serves initially and this is then finalized before submission.

   Background: Using a small number of the key references (4–6) you should introduce the reader (who knows little about your chosen topic) to the area of interest, describing why it is important and highlighting what is known already, what is not known, and gaps in the literature. Your proposal should aim to build on previous research, and for this an outline of the theoretical framework you will be adopting to help you build new knowledge should be identified. The background should conclude with the purpose of your project. In a well-written background the reader should know the purpose or aim of the proposed work before they even read it, because you have guided them through your rationale for proposing the study.

   Aims/objectives of the study: In addition to the overall aim or purpose, you should define clearly the objectives of the proposed study. For example, if the aim is to consider the effects of high-intensity exercise on the cardiovascular system, then the objectives might include determining the time course of changes in blood pressure during and after a high-intensity exercise bout. Another example might have an aim of increasing physical activity in inactive adults aged 65+ years. The specific objectives might include developing an intervention to increase walking behaviour in the target age group, and then assessing change in minutes of physical activity from baseline to follow-up in order to determine if any change occurred.

Research question(s): Whether you include these in the proposal or not may depend on the specific guidelines you are given but articulating the specific research question(s) that your proposed research will answer is a very useful way of clarifying the aims and objectives of the study. Stating your research questions will help to justify the study.

Research design: You will need to select an appropriate research design to allow you to collect the evidence to answer your research question. Several different types of research design exist, your challenge is matching the best design to your research question given the time, resources and expertise available to you. Designs differ depending on whether you will collect qualitative data e.g. Action Research Design, Case Study Design, or quantitative data e.g. Cross-Sectional Design, Experimental Design. For more information on research design and the specific pros and cons for each one, see Thomas et al.[2] and other chapters within this text.

Hypothesis/null hypothesis: For student project proposals, in some disciplines, you may be asked to state a hypothesis or a null hypothesis. An hypothesis is a tentative answer to your research question based on what you think might occur. This is usually based upon your reading of the literature. A null hypothesis is a hypothesis that you are trying to disprove. An hypothesis from the study of high-intensity exercise example above might be "Blood pressure will remain elevated above baseline levels for 2 hours following a bout of high-intensity exercise". A null hypothesis might be "There will no elevation of blood pressure 2 hours after a bout of high-intensity exercise". For further details see Chapter 17.

Proposed methods: This section should articulate the approaches and methods used in your research. It will allow others to evaluate your chosen methodology and how this might influence the validity or reliability of your results. Sufficient information to allow replication of your study should be given. You should describe where you will get your data/participants (recruitment), how you will collect and analyse your data and how you will present your results. Detailed information on the study procedures includes each step in the execution of the research, how instructions were given to participants, how ethical approval was obtained etc. You may not have to specify equipment makes and models, but should include details of all measurements (protocols), inventories or questionnaires to be used. For questionnaires, identify the specific instrument used and its psychometric properties. If you are examining the effect of an intervention, include all relevant details on the design of the intervention within this section. The description of the analysis should explain what you will do with the raw data, what statistical analysis techniques you will use and how you might present the findings to make the best use of the data.

Limitations: For student project proposals you may be asked to outline any potential limitations to the proposed study or problems that you might encounter (participant drop out or lack of recruitment) and any contingency plans you have for coping with these problems. This is an opportunity to show that you have thought through the practical challenges that you might encounter when you begin to carry out your proposed project. If you are new to research or to the methods to be used, then speaking to other researchers (PhD students, post-docs, academic staff) may alert you to the types of problems you might encounter and potential solutions. Being knowledgeable on the strengths and weaknesses of your chosen methodology and the potential implications this may have on your results shows your depth of understanding of the research process.

References: Like all pieces of academic writing, a research proposal should include details of the key references used to develop your project proposal. Specifically, if you have cited another study in the body of the proposal you must ensure that full details of the study are contained in the reference list. Remember to format references consistently and according to the referencing convention used by your discipline/department or stated in the guidance notes.

Writing a research proposal for a funding application

Although the structure and components of a research proposal are likely to be similar for a research proposal submitted as part of a funding application, there are several additional considerations that you will need to take into account.

Firstly consider where the funding is coming from and write with the funder in mind. Make sure you are familiar with aims or objectives of the funder and understand what type of projects they are willing to fund. This is often called the 'scope' and will be found on the funder's website or in the guidance material issued with a funding application call. You must ensure that your proposed research fits the scope of the funder/call. However excellent the research proposal, it is likely to be rejected without consideration if it sits outside the scope of the funder.

Secondly consider who will be reviewing your proposal. Funders usually have decision-making panels comprising experts and lay people, but will usually send proposals to at least two 'expert reviewers' who will be asked to comment on the scientific merit of the proposed study. These individuals are likely to have detailed understanding of the theories and methods proposed, up-to-date knowledge of the literature and are probably active researchers in the area. When preparing your proposal for such expert reviewers be sure that you have read the latest studies in the area and are familiar with the most up-to-date methods. If you are proposing a challenge to existing thinking or a novel method for examining a research question make sure you explain and justify this clearly.

In addition to the subsections described above, it is likely that a research proposal for funding will need to include information/sections on some or all of the following:

Public and patient involvement

In recent years there has been a shift in thinking from doing research 'on' or 'about' people or patients, to doing research 'with' them. This important distinction means that where possible, research should be developed in conjunction with them or representatives of the group you intend to include as participants in your study. This involvement should start early and include seeking input on all aspects of the research including the purpose of the study, the research design and the methods to be used. Involving lay members in your research team will help you gain an insight to how easy/difficult it might be to recruit individuals to your study, how acceptable they will find the methods you propose and how clear your guidance to participants and consent procedures are. Most funders will expect you to have involved the public in the development of your proposal and will ask you to provide information on how you did this. Boote et al.[3] conducted a review of seven studies, which have used public involvement in designing a research proposal. In most cases this involvement consisted of focus groups or consultation meetings with lay individuals who are similar in characteristics (age/gender/ethnicity) to the population to be studied.

In addition to involving members of the public in the development of your proposal, many funders will expect you to demonstrate how they will continue to be involved at all stages of the project. This can include being part of the project steering group, commenting on or helping to develop recruitment material for the study and contributing to the dissemination of the findings. The UK organization INVOLVE (www.invo.org.uk/) provides guidance on best practice in involving the public in developing your research proposal, including information on writing plain English summaries and avoiding jargon.[4]

Justification for the research team

When preparing a proposal for a research funder, you will need to ensure that you have the appropriate expertise to deliver the project. A funder will want to be confident that the project team will be able to deliver the proposed project as planned. In this section you should refer to who will lead each element of the project and what expertise and experience they have in this area. Your team will need to include researchers with experience in all stages of the project including project management, recruitment, specific methods to be used, statistical analysis, public and patient involvement and dissemination. When deciding upon your team it is useful to consider who will bring which element of expertise to the proposal. Researchers often develop their proposals through discussion with other researchers who have similar interests and skills. When writing a proposal for funding, particularly when seeking funding for staff costs, you will need to explain the unique contribution of each member of the team avoiding overlap between team members.

Budgets and costs

In any research proposal it is wise to consider the costs of completing the research. When the proposal forms part of a funding application you will need to justify each cost. The budget needs to be sufficiently detailed and realistic to convince a funder that you have thought carefully through the project from start to finish and anticipated all of the costs likely to be incurred. Pain provides a useful summary of the advice on preparing a budget for a research proposal from a number of successful international researchers.[5] Depending on the funder and what they deem eligible you may need to consider the costs of facilities and equipment, salaries and benefits, travel (researcher, participant and lay public), administrative and dissemination (events and open access publications) costs. When developing the budget it is also essential to consult with the financial personnel of your institution, as they will know the rates and charges used by the institution and any 'on-costs' that you may previously have been unaware of.

Timelines

When writing your proposal for a funder you will need to outline how long each stage of the research will take and when each task will be completed. This is likely to include recruiting any project staff, gaining ethical approval, recruiting participants, collecting data, analysing data and disseminating results and findings. You will also need to specify the milestones or deliverables for the project including interim and final reports and publications and indicate when each of these will be completed. One way of representing all of this information in a single diagram is by using a Gantt chart which is a bar chart designed to illustrate the full schedule for a project. A Gantt chart can be prepared as a table with rows indicating the tasks to be undertaken and columns showing all of the months of the project. By shading in the appropriate cells, you can indicate when each task will occur and allow a reviewer to see how the project will be delivered. An example of a basic Gantt chart for an 18-month project is included in the case study presented later in this chapter.

Dissemination

This section of your proposal, more applicable to those seeking research funding, will involve you articulating how you intend to communicate the findings of the research. Different methods of dissemination will need to be highlighted depending on the target audience and the tools or resources you have at your disposal. So your first task is to identify who you will share your findings with. Once known, the most appropriate methods for each audience will need to be defined. Audiences typically include: the research funders, academic peers, local stakeholders or lay audiences. Funders will require a research report documenting an introduction, brief description of method, results, discussion and implications of your findings; you will also need to explain how the research budget was spent. Academics will consult peer-reviewed journal articles and conference presentations to find out more about your work. Local stakeholders or lay audiences are probably the most challenging to reach, yet essential in achieving impact. Strategies for dissemination to lay audiences include brief 1-page lay summaries, study website, blogs, articles in local community bulletins, newspapers or via other local media.

Other inclusions in your proposal

Your proposal will also form the basis of any ethics application. Ethics submissions will require all of the above information on the objectives of the research, recruitment and methods of data collection. They will also require details of how the data will be stored, privacy, confidentiality, perhaps any procedures should the participants become physically injured or distressed. Furthermore they will require copies of any recruitment material, screening questionnaires, and information and consent forms. More details of these are provided in Chapter 7 on the ethics process.

Box 6.1 Case study: a research proposal for a public sector funder

The case study below provides an example of how a research proposal for a funding body might be developed.

Study Title

Participation in sport and physical activity among 12- to 18-year-old youth

Study Background and Rationale

The increasing prevalence of overweight and obesity, coupled with reports of type 2 diabetes in children and adolescents highlights the importance of promoting a physically active lifestyle among youth (1, 2, 3). Current physical activity guidelines (PAGL) recommend that adolescents participate daily in ≥60 min of moderate to vigorous intensity physical activity that is developmentally appropriate, involves a variety of activities and is enjoyable (4, 5). However, in adolescents (13–15 years) from 105 countries worldwide, 80.3% do not meet the PAGL (7), the proportion meeting the PAGL appears to be decreasing (8, 9), and those who walk or cycle to school, a source of daily physical activity, has also declined dramatically (12). The purpose of this study is to assess participation in physical activity, physical education and youth sport in the target age range.

Objectives of the Research

The study objectives are to:

- Collect and analyse information on the levels of participation in physical activity, physical education and youth sport using both self-report and device-based measures.
- Collect and analyse information on the complex interactions of multiple correlates: sociodemographic, physical and psychological of sport participation, physical education and physical activity.
- This information will then be used to inform Physical Activity strategies for young people.

Study Hypothesis

We hypothesize that:

- Girls will be less physically active, receive less minutes of physical education per week and engage in less sport than boys.
- Older children will be less active than younger children.
- Participation in team sports will be more prevalent in boys than girls.
- Participation in individual sports will be more prevalent in girls than boys.
- Children with high levels of identified specific study correlates of interest will be more active than children with low levels of identified correlates of interest.

Research Design Overview

A cross-sectional research design.

Methodology

A mixed methods approach will be employed where self-report measures and accelerometer data will be used to meet the study objectives.

Recruitment: To estimate the sample size needed a power calculation is required (this is covered in Chapter 17). You will need to consult published literature on the outcome of interest, for example, research shows that approximately 20% of 12- to 18-year-olds meet the PAGL (6–11). Using this data as a guideline, a sample size is estimated, in this case of approximately 4,700 participants. This allows for over-sampling and adjusting for design effect.

Participants will be students in full-time post-primary education. The sampling frame would be all eligible post-primary schools, and a proportion of these would be randomly selected e.g. 10–15%. In Ireland there are 700 eligible post-primary schools, this would yield a sample of between 70 and 105 schools. Screening and recruitment will occur at the school and individual participant level. It is unfeasible to extract children from class groups so a systematic, one-stage cluster (school) sampling method will be used to obtain a representative sample of the target population. Clusters will be based on: (i) school type (National, Secondary School, Community College, Comprehensive College, Vocational School etc.), (ii) geographic location (Urban, Rural), (iii) gender (Male, Female, Mixed) and (iv) school classification (Free Education, Fee Paying).

Inclusion criteria: All pupils in the relevant years will be invited to participate in the study.

Exclusion criteria: Children without parental consent or informed assent.

Outcome measures:

The specific primary and secondary outcome measures and method of assessment are identified in Table 6.1:

Table 6.1 Outcome measures for the project

	Description (All measures have established reliability and validity.)	Source
Primary Outcome Measures		
Physical Activity, physical education and sport	% meeting the national physical activity guidelines.	Self-report questionnaire (10) ActivPAL accelerometer.
	Daily minutes of moderate to vigorous physical activity, undertaken in bouts of 10 minutes or more.	Self-report questionnaire, cross-validated with school timetable.
	Minutes of physical education per week	Self-report questionnaire on frequency, duration and type of participation.
	Level of participation in extra-curricular and community-based sport.	
Secondary Outcome Measures		
Correlates of physical activity	Your measures need to be specific to your research question. Instruments could focus on children's perceptions of competence, enjoyment, efficacy, social support etc.	Identify a valid and reliable measure to address your research question.
	For example, to determine if perceived level of enjoyment is related to participation level in physical activity or physical education.	

Demographic details	Age, sex, year in school and school type. Area of residence (urban/ rural). Parent/guardian employment status etc.	Questionnaire.

Procedures

Ethical and legal considerations: As the participants are under 18 years approval for the study will be sought from the Research Ethics Committee of the University, as well as approval from the schools involved and local education board.

A recruitment visit to each school will provide information on the study and informed consent forms. Data collection will involve three stages:

- School principals will receive an invitation to take part in the study. Following their agreement, study information and ethical requirements will be put in place.
- An accelerometer will be given to each child who provides both informed consent and participant assent and they will be asked to wear it for a total of 7 days, including a minimum of 1 weekend day.
- One week later all students will complete a self-report questionnaire about their week's physical activity, via a low-cost android tablet. To ensure quality and to minimize error in data collection, all questionnaire administration will be supervised by trained researchers. In each school, the study will be briefly explained and instructions will be provided on how to complete the questionnaire. In order to protect confidentiality, each participant will be given an ID number. Physical activity will be clearly defined to avoid confusion between sport, structured exercise and/or general physical activities. Moderate and vigorous intensity levels will be clearly explained to the students and they will be given an opportunity to ask questions. Participants will be informed that their responses will be treated in strictest confidence, and that their names will not be associated with the data. They will be encouraged to take time, reflect on their answers and to be as honest as possible.

Data analysis

All data will be collected and stored on a password protected SPSS 23 statistical package. Once the data has been cleaned, descriptive statistics will be presented through the use of frequencies, proportions, means, medians, standard deviations and (IQR) or ranges. Depending on the specific research question, appropriate statistical tests will be used to make comparisons between subgroups (e.g. girls and boys) or to investigate association between two or more parameters (e.g. levels of physical activity and socioeconomic class).

The project team

This research programme will be led by academic staff [name location, and individuals involved, plus a brief outline of their relevant expertise and experience in carrying out similar research or working as part of a research team on similar projects].

Project budget

Detailed budget sheet		
Staff costs Post-doctoral researcher Research assistants X 2 Final Year project students X 6		
Consultancy costs		
Equipment		
Travel costs		
Collaboration costs		
Dissemination costs		
Subtotal		
Institutional overheads		
TOTAL		

Timeframe

Research Plan and Timeline

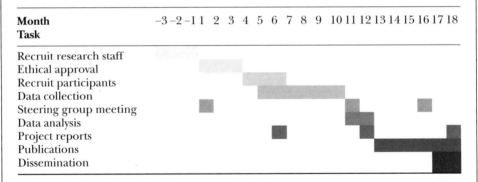

Month Task	–3 –2 –1 1 2 3 4 5 6 7 8 9 10 11 12 13 14 15 16 17 18
Recruit research staff	
Ethical approval	
Recruit participants	
Data collection	
Steering group meeting	
Data analysis	
Project reports	
Publications	
Dissemination	

Figure 6.1 Example of a Gantt chart for an 18-month project.

Implications of this research

This study will provide an anonymized database on the participation levels of 12- to 18-year-olds in physical education, extra-curricular sport, community-based sport and general physical activity. This database will include subjective self-report data that provide important information on type, location and suggest determinants of activities that children participate in. It will also be augmented by accelerometer data, important for validity and for fine-grained analysis of the sporadic physical activity that this age group participates in, beyond the structured school or club-based participation. This highly detailed, valid and reliable database will provide information to inform policy decisions, practice and planning and to evaluate progress on key outcome variables.

Dissemination

Dissemination will be via published report, advocacy documents and peer-reviewed publications.

A published report: we will provide funders with a detailed analysis on participation, suggest determinants of participation and recommendations for change. This report has the potential to inform targets as part of the National Physical Activity Plan, it may also inform sport policy and service provision.

Advocacy documents: we will produce 2-page summaries of the main findings, and these will be sent to teachers, administrators, communities to facilitate opportunities for children and youth to partake in sport, physical education and physical activity.

Peer-reviewed publications: we will publish 3 papers in peer-reviewed academic journals. These will describe the protocol, survey and fitness and health findings.

Presentations: we will make presentations at domestic and international conferences to advance research knowledge. We will also give presentations to stakeholders and policy makers to improve physical activity opportunities for children and youth.

Other: social media (Facebook, Twitter etc.) and a project webpage will be used to increase awareness about the study and its findings. Some educational material or video could be generated for the participating schools.

Case study references

(1) Kohl HW, Craig CL, Lambert EV, Inoue S, Alkandari JR, Leetongin G et al. The pandemic of physical inactivity: global action for public health. *The Lancet.* 2012; **380**:294–305.

(2) Lee I-M, Shiroma EJ, Lobelo F, Puska P, Blair SN, Katzmarzyk PT. Effect of physical inactivity on major non-communicable diseases worldwide: an analysis of burden of disease and life expectancy. *The Lancet.* 2012; **380**:219–29.

(3) Hallal PC, Victora CG, Azevedo MR, Wells JC. Adolescent physical activity and health. *Sports Med.* 2006; **36**(12):1019–30.

(4) Strong W, Malina R, Blimkie CJR, Daniels SR, Dishman RK, Gutin B et al. Evidence based physical activity for school-aged youth. *Journal of Pediatrics.* 2005; **146**:732–37.

(5) Department of Health and Children. The national guidelines on physical activity for Ireland. Health Services Executive and the Department of Health and Children. Dublin. 2009. Available from: http://health.gov.ie/wp-content/uploads/2014/03/active_guidelines.pdf

(6) Hallal PC, Andersen LB, Bull FC, Guthold R, Haskell W & Ekelund, U. Global physical activity levels: surveillance progress, pitfalls, and prospects. *The Lancet.* 2012; **380**:247–57. DOI:10.1016/S0140–6736(12) 60646–1

(7) Sleap M, Tolfrey K. Do 9- to 12-yr-old children meet existing physical activity recommendations for health? *Med Sci Sports Exerc.* 2001; **33**(4):591–96.

(8) Metcalf BS, Hosking J, Jeffery AN, Henley WE, Wilkin TJ. Exploring the adolescent fall in physical activity: a 10-yr cohort study (EarlyBird 41). *Med Sci Sports Exerc.* 2015; **47**(10):2084–92.

(9) Riddoch CJ, Bo AL, Wedderkopp N, Harro M, Klasson-Heggeb L, Sardinha L et al. Physical activity levels and patterns of 9- and 15-yr-old European children. *Med Sci Sports Exerc.* 2004; **36**:86–92.

(10) Hardie Murphy M, Rowe DA, Belton S and Woods CB. Validity of a two-item physical activity screening measure for assessing attainment of physical activity guidelines in Irish youth. *BMC Public Health.* 2015; **15**:1080.

(11) Woods CB, Tannehill D and Walsh J. An examination of the relationship between enjoyment, physical education, physical activity and health in Irish adolescents. *Irish Educational Studies.* 2012; **31**(3):263–80.

(12) Motl RW, Dishman RK, Saunders R, Dowda M, Felton G and Pate RR. 2001. Measuring enjoyment of physical activity in adolescent girls. *American Journal of Preventive Medicine.* 2001; **21**(2):1107.

References

1 Salita JT. Writing for lay audiences: a challenge for scientists. *Eur Med Wri Assoc.* 2015; **24**(4):183–9.

2 Thomas J, Nelson J, Silverman S. Research methods in physical activity. 7th ed. Leeds, UK: Human Kinetics; 2015.

3 Boote J, Baird W, Beecroft C. Public involvement at the design stage of primary health research: a narrative review of case examples. *Health Policy.* 2010; **95**(1):10–23.

4 Involve NIHR. *Briefing notes for researchers: involving the public in NHS, public health and social care research.* Eastleigh, UK: INVOLVE Eastleigh; 2012.

5 Pain E. How to budget your grant proposal. 2017. Available from: www.sciencemag.org/careers/2017/09/how-budget-your-grant-proposal

7 Ethical issues in health and physical activity research

Valerie Cox

Chapter aims

Many researchers find the ethics approval process daunting and confusing. In this chapter we hope to explain the different factors you need to consider when planning your research and clarify the information that you need to provide for your ethics application. We also cover the information you need to give to participants and considerations around consent.

History of research ethics

The idea of medical/research ethics is not new, with Hippocrates proposing the idea of 'do no harm' as long ago as 500 BCE. The drive to establish principles for modern research ethics grew from various atrocities, including forced human experimentation in the Second World War. In 1964, the World Medical Association established recommendations for medical research in the Declaration of Helsinki. This has been updated several times since and most countries are signatories.[1]

Nowadays, most scientific journals require evidence of ethical approval before they will accept your work for consideration. For example, the *Journal of Sports Sciences* states that authors "must include a statement that the study received institutional ethics approval". They also require specific confirmation that appropriate consent was obtained from the participants.

Most Universities have had some form of ethics and safety approval system for sport and exercise-based research in place for many years, as the risk from physical activity, blood tests etc. has always been obvious. However, other risks, such as potential psychological traumas and thinking about the safety of the researcher when off-site, were often not so well considered. More recently much more comprehensive coverage of ethics and risk has been put in place by most Higher Education institutions.

As illustrated in Figure 7.1, the modern ethical approval processes seek to ensure that research:

- Respects the autonomy of the participants
- Is of scientific value
- Minimizes risk of harm

Every year I receive complaints from some researchers that corrections needed on their ethics applications relate to 'research design not ethics'. However, research cannot be ethical unless the design is appropriate and safety issues have been considered.

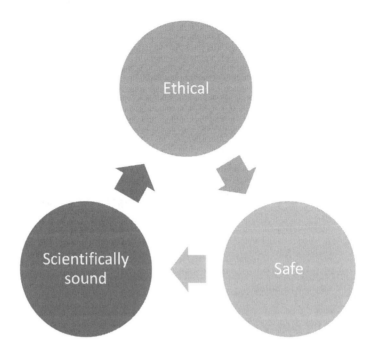

Figure 7.1 Studies must be ethical, scientifically sound and safe.

Poorly designed studies produce information that is scientifically unsound and wastes participants' time and effort.

Types of ethical issues

Possible ethical issues in physical activity and health

In the area of physical activity and health, examples of likely ethical conflicts/problems include (but are not limited to):

- Risk of physical injury or discomfort
- Risk of psychological distress
- People taking banned/illegal or potentially dangerous supplements
- Giving potentially health-benefiting interventions to some but not all participants
- Risk of giving scientific credibility to practices with little scientific evidence
- Inappropriate coercion/misuse of power to persuade people to participate
- Excluding groups from research such as homeless people or females – especially if those are the groups in most need of health improvements
- Cultural insensitivity causing upset, offence or embarrassment etc. to some groups

Although most countries have legislation/regulation in place around research ethics, it is not always possible to give prescriptive advice. "No code can replace the need for [scientists] to use their professional and ethical judgement".[2]

Deliberate scientific malpractice

Sometimes ethical issues are related to deliberate malpractice by scientists including:

- Plagiarism
- Fraudulent results
- Withholding information from publication

It should be obvious that all of these are unethical and most institutions have procedures in place for appropriate investigation and disciplinary action if such practises are suspected.

Reporting misconduct and ethical concerns

If you believe misconduct has taken place, or there is an ethical concern about a study, it is important that you act to report this, or you may be complicit. You should check what procedures are in place for reporting your concerns. This will depend on your organization and the relative positions of the suspect and yourself. For example, you may be suspicious about one of your students and report this to the course director or equivalent, but the procedures would be different if you suspected another staff member. Most Universities and healthcare organizations have clear whistle-blowing policies that you will be able to follow. In some cases you may also be able to get advice from an appropriate professional body or union representative.

In most cases there will be time for you to take appropriate advice on how to handle the matter, but if you believe researchers or participants are in immediate, significant danger you must act immediately to stop the work.

Ethics review and approval processes

All research should go through an appropriate ethics and safety review process. The key principles of this are that the people reviewing the applications:

- Are independent of the specific research being considered
- Have appropriate competence

It is also common policy for ethics review committees to be formally constituted to include members of different 'categories', such as: Researchers, Legal experts, Lay people and those with pastoral and/or caring roles.

Research Councils UK (2009) recommend that all organizations undertaking research should have:

- Clear and full policies on ethical standards
- Clear procedures for obtaining ethical approval for research, which are communicated effectively to all relevant staff
- Appropriate procedures for considering and advising on the wider ethical concerns connected to the research or its potential outcomes
- Appropriate procedures to obtain and record clearly informed consent from research participants

Most organizations such as Universities will have ethics approval procedures in place, but in some cases additional approval may be needed. For example, in the UK the Integrated Research Application System (IRAS) is used to apply for the permissions and approvals for health and social care/community care research. A specific online tool is available to help people decide if they do need this approval.[3] Likewise, if the project is with Prisons or Probation Trusts approval from Her Majesty's Prison and Probation Service (HMPPS) is needed. Note that these approvals are to work with participants but also to access data/samples already collected. Other countries will often have similar systems in place. Some studies in physical activity, for example with clinical or incarcerated populations may also need to apply via these systems. It is important to always check exactly what permissions are needed for your studies.

Individuals, who are not associated with an organization with an ethics committee structure in place, should try to find an appropriate body who can review their work for them.

Recruitment, informed consent and permissions

Recruitment

As part of your ethics application you need to include details of how you will recruit participants. This may be via a specific organization (with appropriate gatekeeper permission; see below) or by approaching individuals. The use of social media in particular needs to be given careful consideration. A message via the account of an organization, for example, a walking group, might be appropriate but using personal accounts should always be discouraged due to the risk of inappropriate messages and online abuse. Extra care needs to be taken to ensure that any vulnerable groups are being recruited appropriately.

Informed consent

Consent is fundamental to ethics and this must be INFORMED consent. This means that participants:

- Understand exactly what they are being asked to do
- Understand any predictable risks
- Consent to take part and to accept these risks

Over the last few years there has been a push to replace the term 'subjects' with 'participants'. The latter is felt to better convey the idea that these people are autonomous and play an active role in research, rather than the more passive idea of subjects. Indeed, in many aspects of physical activity and health it is appropriate for the participants to be involved in research design as co-creators.

Clearly there are potential problems if there is deliberate DECEPTION of participants and/or VULNERABLE groups who cannot give consent. These are dealt with separately below.

Participant information sheet

In order to obtain consent, participants need to be given clear information about the activities and the risks. This will usually be in the form of a written document, which should contain all the information listed in Figure 7.2. This information sheet must be written in language that will be understood by the participants (lay language) and avoid technical jargon or terminology – see later example. Participants must have a paper copy of the information that they can keep, or be provided with access to the information electronically. The contact for queries should be a member of the research team but the contact for complaints must be someone not directly involved in the research study. Usually this is a module leader or course director for student projects, the Head of Department or similar for staff research projects, or an official of the institution's constituted ethics committee.

Consent form

The consent form will be signed by the participant to confirm they have received the participant information, they agree to take part and consent to any risks or disclosures etc. In some cases you need the researcher and/or an independent witness to sign the forms too. The consent form must be kept by the RESEARCHER not the

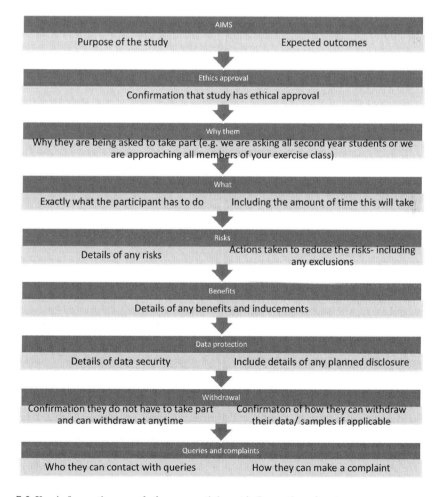

Figure 7.2 Key information needed on a participant information sheet.

participant, although they may be provided with a copy. Since consent forms contain people's names they must always be kept securely.

There will usually be specific requirements for how long the consent forms need to be kept, so make sure you are aware of how long this is. If your data collection includes any photographing or recording of participants you need to obtain explicit consent for this. It is often better to have a number of specific statements for participants to initial as well as signing the overall form.

For example

- Confirmation they have been given full information including risks and any benefits
- Confirmation they know what will happen to any data – including any disclosures
- Confirmation they consent to images, recordings etc.
- Confirmation they consent to the use of specific quotes from interviews etc.

Sometimes getting a signed, paper consent form from each participant is not possible, for example, if you have an online questionnaire. Where there is a low risk of your questionnaire resulting in any harm it may be appropriate for you to have an initial page that explains the participant information and a simple 'click yes' box if they agree to continue. However, this will be at the discretion of your ethics approval team.

Language in consent and participant information sheets

Consent forms and participant information forms must be written so that they can be understood by the participants. In most cases this means language that an adult with no specific scientific expertise can understand. For example, writing that "You will be working at 90% of $\dot{V}O_2$ max" will be fairly meaningless to most people. Instead wording should be something like "You will be cycling at a high intensity, so that you will feel out of breath". Clearly for other groups, such as children, different language would need to be used. You may also need translated documents if you are working with people with different language fluencies. Always pilot these sheets to check they work well with the population you will be working with.

Withdrawing

A key principle of research ethics is that the participant is free to withdraw consent at any time and stop taking part. If a participant does decide to withdraw you should not ask them to provide any reasons for this, as this might be considered a form of coercion/unreasonable persuasion.

If participants decide to withdraw after they have completed any actual activities they participate in, they should also be able to withdraw any samples/data they have already provided from analysis in your study.

- You need to consider this requirement when planning any anonymization, as you may need to code samples/data so that you can identify who it belongs to if necessary. For example, you can put a code number on the participant information sheet and on the data. If a participant gives you their number you can then identify

their data, but it is otherwise anonymous. Make sure participants know they need to keep their number safe for this purpose. In online data collection you can usually set up systems to issue a code number to participants in a similar way.
- It is reasonable for you to set a time limit after which samples/data can no longer be removed, since it would not be reasonable to recall research publications for data re-analysis. However, this deadline must be clear in the information given to participants.

For some studies where data is anonymized as it is collected, particularly for questionnaires asking for information that is not very personal, your ethics approval system may be happy for you to tell participants that data cannot be removed after it is submitted. However, this needs to be clear in the information given to participants before they consent.

Gatekeeper permission

If you are obtaining data or samples that are already collected, or if you are accessing participants via an organization like a school or a sports club, you may need evidence of approval for this. This is usually called 'Gatekeeper' permission and should be in the form of a written document signed by an appropriate person. Similar principles apply as with participant consent and you need to ensure you can demonstrate that the gatekeeper was fully aware of what they were being asked to provide and any risk and/or benefits.

You do need to check that the gatekeeper does have the authority to give the permission you are seeking. For example, if they are giving you access to data you may need to check what consent was given when the data was collected. This is particularly important where data you are receiving is not anonymous.

Compulsion

Sometimes participants are being compelled to take part in activities that form part of the research data set. For example, pupils may have to participate in a physical education class at school or professional sportspeople or army recruits may have to complete a set of fitness tests. It is important in these situations to be clear what is happening ONLY for the research project and what would be happening even if the research was not taking place.

You also need to consider if you have consent to use any data for research. For example, the army recruits may have signed a contract that says they have to take part in fitness tests, however, unless the contract specifically states that results will be used in research you may still need to get consent to use the data in this way.

The risk of 'compulsion' or perceived compulsion on the part of the participant may also occur in scenarios such as students being recruited by their lecturers into a project or an athlete being recruited by their coach.

Consent to publish

Generally it should be a principle of research that the findings can be made public. Sometimes work relates to a commercial product and may impose limitations on publication of the results. If this is due to protection of commercial intellectual property rights this may be appropriate. However, there may be ethical problems if a company simply wants to ensure that any negative findings can't be made public. Researchers should consider any such limitation on publication very carefully and this must be fully declared in any ethics application.

Confidentiality and data protection

Most researchers do consider ethics in the data collection stage of their project. However, it also covers analysis, storage and disposal of data.

Legislative requirements

In many countries there is specific legislation in place relating to data protection. This specifically covers certain types of information that can be identified to individual living people. In 2018 tightened data protection regulations, the General Data Protection Regulation (GDPR),[4] came into place across the European Union, including the UK.

Since data protection generally only applies where individuals can be recognized, regulations do not usually apply to anonymous data. Note that data protection requires that information collected should be necessary for your research. You should not ask for demographic data unless it is directly related to your specific research questions. Having multiple demographic data also risks individuals being inadvertently identifiable in anonymous data.

Note that in the UK, data that is in the 'public domain' is also not covered by data protection legislation. This includes any information that is available to anyone, even if there is a charge to access it. For example, certificates of births, marriages and deaths can be searched for a fee, so are not covered by the data protection legislation. Information on websites, social media etc. is also in the public domain. However, you still have a responsibility to ensure material is correct, and has been legally disseminated, before you include it in your research.

Data protection means ensuring that data is kept secure. A quick internet search will show you multiple examples where organizations such as government departments and private companies have been fined for breaches of this. You need to put appropriate measures in place to make sure data is stored, and if necessary archived, appropriately. Always check how long you are required to keep documents like consent forms for after the end of the research project. You may also need to keep a formal record of when and how the documents were disposed of.

As well as considering data identifiable to individual people, it is important to consider information that might identify companies and other organizations. You may need to take legal advice if your work will do this.

Disclosure

Any disclosure of information that is identifiable to an individual person must have consent. This needs to be part of your participant information sheet and consent form. For example, if results from your testing will be given to a teacher or coach, your participants must be explicitly told this and give consent.

You must consider whether inadvertent disclosure is likely. For example, if you are carrying out fitness testing on a group of people they may well see each other's results. You need to either put procedures in place to ensure this cannot happen or include a statement in the participant information that makes it clear that this may happen and ask the participants to consent to this.

Protection issues

In some projects there is a risk that participants may disclose they are at risk of harm. For example, they may disclose eating disorders or inappropriate actions by coaches. As part of your research design and your ethics application you must identify there is a risk of such disclosures and explain how they will be handled appropriately.

The researcher must also be aware of the risk of inadvertently becoming aware of illegal activity and know how they should proceed should this occur. The ethics committee granting approval for the research is likely to have guidelines on this, particularly where there are legal issues, such as the compulsory reporting of serious illegal activity, such as child abuse.

Risks

Minimizing risks

In terms of making ethical decisions about a study we are deciding if any benefits outweigh the potential risks. Good design should always seek to increase benefits and minimize risks (Figure 7.3). It is unlikely that projects with a high degree of risk will get approval.

The British Psychological Society recommends that risks should be "no greater than encountered in everyday life",[5] which depends on what participants normally do. With physical activity in particular the risks depend on factors such as habitual activity and physical fitness. For example, carrying out a maximum exertion test on

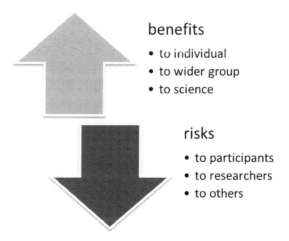

benefits
• to individual
• to wider group
• to science

risks
• to participants
• to researchers
• to others

Figure 7.3 Good research design seeks to maximize benefits and minimize risks.

an athlete who completes similar activity every week might be fine, but would not be allowed with a frail elderly participant.

Types of risks

Figure 7.4 shows some of the types of risks that may be encountered. In some cases your participant information can provide links/sources of support/information if psychological or other issues do arise.

Screening and exclusions to reduce risks

Appropriate screening and/or exclusion criteria can reduce the risks in many cases. Some examples are given below.

*   Ask about previous physical injury/medical conditions, or test that blood pressure is normal before physical exercise
*   Ask about known psychological/mental health problems before administering some psychological tests
*   Ask about use of illegal/dangerous substances before taking part in physical activity if they may lead to problems
*   Ask about habitual exercise levels/fitness status before administering physical activity

These should always be included in detail in your ethics application and risk assessment documents. Additionally the information sheet should include directions to the relevant support services, so that the participants can contact them if they need to during or following their involvement in the research.

Reputational risk

As well as risk of harm to individuals, researchers need to consider reputational harm. This does not mean that you cannot carry out research that challenges claims made by a company, for example, investigating if a particular supplement does give all the

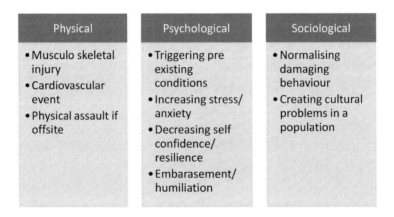

Physical	Psychological	Sociological
• Musculo skeletal injury • Cardiovascular event • Physical assault if offsite	• Triggering pre existing conditions • Increasing stress/ anxiety • Decreasing self confidence/ resilience • Embarasement/ humiliation	• Normalising damaging behaviour • Creating cultural problems in a population

Figure 7.4 Some examples of types of risks in physical activity research.

benefits the advertising claims. However, when naming particular organizations in any publications it is important to seek appropriate legal advice.

The reputational risk we are considering for ethics is the impact on an organization of an inappropriate study being carried out or of research misconduct. Reputational risk may also apply where sources of funding would lead to embarrassment.

Liability insurance

In any situation of risk it is important to ensure appropriate liability insurance is in place. While many individual practitioners have professional indemnity coverage this may not specifically cover research, so it is important to check.

Large organizations such as Universities will usually have insurance that does cover research, but this may have important limitations on it. Every few years I am involved when our University insurers carry out an audit of the type of research activities that we undertake to check they are happy to cover these. You may need to specifically check this, especially if you are planning research in a new subject area or with a vulnerable group. You also need to check the insurance situation carefully for any research that is not taking place in your home country.

Where liability lies for each particular activity usually depends on the primary purpose for which it is happening. If an activity such as an exercise class or walking group would be happening anyway and not just for your research the risk assessment and liability may lie with the people organizing the event. However, you should always make sure that it is fully clear who is responsible.

Deception and covert observations

Ethical research must be based upon mutual respect and trust between the researchers and the participants. Transparency and honesty are obviously key research principles. However, sometimes in research, especially in psychology-based studies, deception is essential. There will need to be consideration of what deception is reasonable.

Placebos

Some studies, especially those involving the administration of supplements etc. will need to use a placebo. Usually the subject is told that they will receive treatment or placebo, so this is not really deception. It is important to ensure there is no risk to the subject in them not knowing which treatment they have received.

Misleading participants about study aims and hypotheses

The most common form of deception is probably misleading the subjects about the study aims. For example, you may tell them it is a study on motivation when actually you are looking at self-confidence or self-efficacy. The ethics approval process will consider if there are any risks in the deception.

Not telling participants the actual procedure

Studies where participants are not accurately told what will happen to them are less common and more problematic. For example, you may want to 'startle' people with a loud noise during physical activity to see how they cope with unexpected interruptions. Risk and safety are important here and this will not usually be allowed if there are any risks associated with the procedure. In the example above we might allow a loud noise if someone is putting a golf ball indoors, but would not allow it if they were riding a horse and might fall as a result.

Debrief following use of deception

In any case where deception has been used, a full debrief, explaining to the participants the nature of the deception, is necessary. This should be done as soon as is practicably possible. Usually a written debrief sheet is provided for this purpose.

Covert observation

If you are going to make covert observations of individuals you need to ensure you are aware of any relevant legislation. Observing people, even in public places, has some restrictions in most countries. This is especially true in potentially sensitive situations, such as observing people attending a medical facility or observing children.

From a physical activity context, relatively non-invasive activities, such as observing if people use the lift (elevator) or stairs might be appropriate. However, remember to consider the need for gatekeeper approval from the owner of the premises.

Illegal and banned activities

Studying illegal and banned activities

Great care needs to be taken in research into any illegal or banned activities. The researchers may find themselves in a situation where they would need to disclose this information to law enforcement or other bodies. For example, studying the use of banned steroids or underage drinking in children.

From an ethical point of view, studies should not normalize or endorse illegal, banned or dangerous activities. For example, the ACSM code of ethics specifically states that members should not "advise, aid or abet any athlete to use prohibited substances".[6]

This does not mean we can never research such activities, and indeed it is important that we do understand the potential harm many of these activities lead to. However, it does mean that such research requires careful planning and sometimes appropriate legal advice.

Inadvertent revelation of illegal activity and/or banned substances

Researchers should take care that they do not inadvertently collect information about illegal activities. For example, you may need to exclude people who take prohibited supplements from your study. Rather than ask a specific question about this put all your exclusions in one question and tell them to tick if ANY apply. That way you do not specifically know they do anything illicit. Additionally if a study reveals possible issues of sexual abuse with children there may be a legal requirement to report this. Guidelines should be obtained from the ethics committee through which the research was approved.

Identifying breaches by organizations

Care needs to be taken if studying activities that have statutory requirements, such as if staff have appropriate qualifications to run physical activity events or health and safety compliance. Within the ethics application there needs to be a clear plan for how any breaches of regulations that are discovered will be dealt with and this must also be clear to the individuals or organizations taking part in the research.

Incentives, coercion, interests and influence

Clarity of the source of funding and other relevant information that demonstrates an interest is of paramount importance in research. For example, the *Journal of Sport Science* requires that authors provide "a declaration of interest statement".[7]

Incentives

Any sort of incentive for participants could potentially unduly influence someone to take part. This is especially problematic where the study is high risk. For most physical activity research, physical and psychological risks to participants are relatively modest and low-value incentives will sometimes be offered. Some incentives are in the form of information/services, such as the participants receiving a fitness report and exercise plan, or there may be payment. The issues around this are discussed by Grant and Sugarman,[8] who suggest that "An amount of money that is not excessive and is calculated on the basis of time or contribution may, rather than constitute an undue inducement, be an indication of respect for the time and contribution that research subjects make". Whilst Grady discusses the implications of incentives upon consent.[9]

Coercion

As mentioned above, participants must act autonomously to freely give informed consent. Researchers need to take care that they are not inadvertently coercing participants by virtue of a power or dependency relationship. This applies in situations such as lecturer and students or with coaches and their team.

Commercial interests

Clarity of the source of funding and other relevant information that demonstrates a commercial interest in the work must always be clear when applying for ethical approval and in subsequent publication. Typically this would be included in the written information provided to the participant during recruitment and when attaining consent. As mentioned above it is also important to declare any limitations on publication imposed due to commercial or other interests when applying for ethical approval.

Political influence

As I write this in 2018 we have seen a lot of comment about the influence of politics on scientific matters, notably the political challenges to the idea of man-made climate change and claims that some scientific organizations are being prevented from using terminology that is considered politically difficult. The areas of physical activity and obesity can also become embroiled in political arguments, such as selling school playing fields for house building and banning advertising of potentially unhealthy food to children.

Funding for physical activity research may be under political control and this may lead to some degree of bias in the type of studies that can be performed. Researchers need to be careful that they are not acting to further a specific political agenda rather than to further scientific knowledge in a more dispassionate way. A key principle of research ethics is that the benefits of research should be distributed fairly and not just to benefit the elite or one gender or ethnic group. Consider if your research helps to increase social justice and social equality.

Vulnerable groups

Research with vulnerable groups is dealt with in more detail in Chapters 21–29 of this book. In physical activity and health it is common for research to involve potentially vulnerable groups such as children and older adults.

You need to note that vulnerable groups, including children, may not be able to give consent themselves. This usually needs to come from next of kin or someone with a legal power of attorney. In some cases your ethics review team may approve consent being given by someone in a position of care such as a teacher, but you will need to check carefully that this will be sufficient and that you do not need next of kin approval as well. The British Association of Sport and Exercise Sciences has a specific expert statement on research with young people that you may find useful.[10]

Although some vulnerable groups cannot consent themselves, you should still seek confirmation they do want to participate in the form of ASSENT. Consent is defined as "the positive agreement of an individual" while providing assent is "to go along with".[11] When working with vulnerable groups you should be aware of any signs of distress or discomfort that may mean they no longer want to participate.

In most countries specific procedures are in place to ensure that any research involving people who are incarcerated does not involve coercion and working with such populations will usually require extensive approval processes.

Providing participants with study results

It is generally considered good practice to have procedures in place to allow participants to know what the overall findings of your research are. These should be provided in lay language without the use of complex jargon or terminology.

Giving participants their own results

In some studies participants are given some of their own data. For example, they may be given their physical activity levels or fitness scores. It is important to make sure that information given is accurate and that any advice accompanying this is correct and checked by someone with appropriate qualifications. It is also important to consider any risks this might pose, for example, when working with people with psychological issues relating to body composition.

Diagnostic tests, medical screening and professional advice

Some of the tests used in research are also used diagnostically in medical practice. For example, blood pressure measurements or some types of psychological psychometric tests. In most cases the researchers are not using these to provide medical screening or care and are often not medically qualified to act on the results. However, it is not really appropriate for us to conceal a potentially damaging medical issue from a participant.

Often the best course of action is to clearly indicate in the participant information form that such tests are being used and MIGHT mean they have a problem, but that the test may be incorrect, the researchers are not qualified to give clinical advice and that if their result is potentially abnormal they will be advised to seek advice from their doctor or other suitably qualified person. As part of the ethics application the researchers must indicate what values they will use to say a test is abnormal, usually related to guidelines used clinically in their own country. They also need to consider the potential stress this might cause to participants and if this is reasonable.

Using existing data/samples

Secondary data and consent

Some research uses data that already exists (secondary data) and/or samples that have already been collected. In all these cases it is important to consider any issues of consent. Where the individual person who gave the data/samples will be identifiable, you will usually have to obtain consent from those individuals for the further work you plan unless this was explicitly covered in the original consent given. Where the data/samples will be provided to you in a genuinely anonymous format your ethics approval process may allow the person who holds the data/samples to give you gate-keeper approval to use them. However, this may still depend on what analysis you plan and whether this was covered in the original consent given. There are also problems where the data includes considerable amounts of demographic or other information that mean individual people can be inadvertently identified.

Audit of services

Not all analysis of data needs ethical approval and using data to report on services and inform local practice is usually not classed as research. For example, if you are using information on how many male and female children attended a community exercise programme to help the people running the programme to target low participation groups, this may be viewed as service development/audit not research. They might also use the information to help them in a specific funding application. In most cases this sort of analysis will not need ethical approval, although you should always confirm this with your local ethics team. However, if you plan to disseminate the findings more widely, for example, at a conference or in a publication, then that is research and should have ethical approval.

Ethics and animal work

The use of animals in research is governed by legislation in most countries. In the UK this is highly regulated for many species by the Home Office under the Animals

(Scientific Procedures) Act 1986. Detailed consideration of animal-based research is outside the scope of this book, but in addition to ensuring all legal requirements are met researchers should consider the following ethical principles in all animal work:

- Replacement – can the work be done in a different way without using animals?
- Reduction – how can you reduce the number of animals you need to use?
- Refinement – can you use methods that reduce suffering and improve welfare?

Some sources of further information

Professional body guidelines

- The BASES Expert Statement on Ethics and Participation in Research of Young People Produced on behalf of the British Association of Sport and Exercise Sciences by Prof Craig A. Williams FBASES, Rev Mark Cobb, Prof Thomas Rowland and Prof Edward Winter FBASES www.bases.org.uk/Ethics-and-Participation-in-Research-of-Young-People
- American College of Sports Medicine (ACSM) code of ethics www.acsm.org/membership/membership-resources/code-of-ethics
- British Psychological Society (BPS) code of research ethics www.bps.org.uk/sites/default/files/documents/code_of_human_research_ethics.pdf
- Royal College of Paediatrics and Child Health: Ethics Advisory Committee. Guidelines for the ethical conduct of medical research involving children. *Archives of Disease in Childhood*. 2000; **82**:177–82.

Other useful links

- UK Medical Research council (MRC) tool to determine if you need NHS ethical approval http://hra-decisiontools.org.uk/ethics/
- UK Research Integrity Office (August 2008) "Procedure for the Investigation of Misconduct in Research" http://ukrio.org/wp-content/uploads/UKRIO-Procedure-for-the-Investigation-of-Misconduct-in-Research.pdf
- Research Councils UK (RCUK, March 2009) "Policy and Code of Conduct on the Governance of Good Research Conduct". www.rcuk.ac.uk/publications/researchers/grc/
- *Journal of Sports Science* information about disclosure of interests for authors www.elsevier.com/journals/journal-of-sport-and-health-science/2095-2546/guide-for-authors
- General Data Protection Regulations (GDPR) for EU www.eugdpr.org/
- Australian Government, National Health and Medical Research Council, Human Research Ethics Committees (HREC). www.nhmrc.gov.au/health-ethics/human-research-ethics-committees-hrecs

References

1 Available from: www.wma.net/policies-post/wma-declaration-of-helsinki-ethical-principles-for-medical-research-involving-human-subjects/
2 BPS code of research ethics. Available from: www.bps.org.uk/sites/default/files/documents/code_of_human_research_ethics.pdf

3   UK Medical Research council (MRC) tool to determine if you need NHS ethical approval. Available from: http://hra-decisiontools.org.uk/ethics/

4   Available from: www.eugdpr.org/

5   BPS code of research ethics. Available from: www.bps.org.uk/sites/default/files/documents/code_of_human_research_ethics.pdf

6   ACSM code of ethics. Available from: www.acsm.org/membership/membership-resources/code-of-ethics

7   Available from: www.elsevier.com/journals/journal-of-sport-and-health-science/2095-2546/guide-for-authors

8   Grant R, Sugarman J. Ethics in human subjects research: do incentives matter? *J Med Philos.* 2004; **29**: 717–38.

9   Grady C. Money for research participation: does it jeopardize informed consent? *Am J Bioeth.* 2001; **1**:40–44.

10 Available from: www.bases.org.uk/Ethics-and-Participation-in-Research-of-Young-People

11 Royal College of Paediatrics and Child Health: Ethics Advisory Committee. Guidelines for the ethical conduct of medical research involving children. *Arch Dis Child.* 2000; **82**:177–82.

8 Observational (cross-sectional and longitudinal) studies

Christopher S. Owens, Diane Crone, Christopher Gidlow and David V.B. James

Aims of the chapter

This chapter explores observational studies and their application in physical activity research with a particular focus on cross-sectional and longitudinal approaches. Considerations in the design and use of both types of studies are considered and the chapter concludes with a case study which utilized both a cross-sectional and longitudinal observational study design.

The aims of the chapter are to:

- Provide an understanding of observational studies with a specific focus on cross-sectional and longitudinal designs.
- Demonstrate how cross-sectional and longitudinal observational studies are used in physical activity research.
- Provide guidance and considerations on how to design and undertake cross-sectional and longitudinal observational studies to ensure the collection of high-quality data.
- Provide illustrative examples using a case study of a longitudinal and cross-sectional observational study.

What are observational studies?

Observational studies involve the researcher observing without intervention, thus making them distinct from intervention or experimental studies. In this chapter, we focus on two specific forms of observational study: cross-sectional studies and longitudinal studies, where physical activity is the outcome variable (also known as the dependent variable).

Longitudinal observational studies involve studying participants over time with repeated or continuous measurements.[1] In particular, prospective longitudinal studies involve the same participants being followed up as time elapses. Prospective longitudinal studies have the particular benefit of measuring changes in health behaviours, such as physical activity and possible predictor variables (also known as the independent or explaining variables) that might be associated with a change in behaviour. In contrast, cross-sectional observational studies involve measurements at a single time point, providing a 'snapshot' of a health behaviour like physical activity at that particular point in time. In cross-sectional observational studies, the associations between the outcome and predictor variables is through a 'between' participant analysis.

How are cross-sectional and longitudinal studies used in physical activity?

Longitudinal observational studies in physical activity research involve measuring physical activity with the same participants at more than one time point, which could be over a period of weeks, months or years. These types of studies focus on the change in physical activity levels as the outcome variable over a period of time.[2–4] For example, Taylor et al.[5] objectively measured physical activity using accelerometers (over five days) in a cohort of children in New Zealand, at the ages of 3, 4, 5, 5.5, 6.5 and 7 years to monitor changes over time. Some studies also focus on the factors (i.e. predictor variables or independent variables) associated with physical activity as the outcome variable from a longitudinal perspective.[6,7] For instance, Owens et al.[8] investigated factors associated with the change in adolescents' physical activity over time (the case study provides an example of this approach).

Cross-sectional studies in physical activity are the more common study design, comparing across (between) participants at a single point in time. They focus on physical activity levels as the outcome variable and factors associated with physical activity levels.[9–13] The inclusion of potential factors associated with physical activity levels within observational studies can be informed by an extensive theoretical evidence base. This 'theoretical framework' is important in attempting to mitigate limitations due to potential confounding and moderating factors.

One example of this is Salvo et al.[14] who measured physical activity levels and the relationship with a number of sociodemographic variables (e.g. socioeconomic status) among adults in Mexico. They used accelerometers for physical activity measurement and a survey for sociodemographic data at a single point in time (i.e. participants wore an accelerometer for a seven-day period only). Mytton et al.[15] adopted a similar approach, using a cross-sectional observational study design with physical activity levels in adults as the outcome variable (in relation to recommended guidelines) and using a self-report questionnaire, investigated the association with independent variables such as green space.

Considerations for the design and use of cross-sectional studies

There are a number of key considerations when designing and using cross-sectional studies in physical activity research. For example:

- Cross-sectional studies are less time consuming and cheaper to conduct than longitudinal studies. As they are only undertaken at one point in time, the issue of losing participants at follow-up (as is the case with longitudinal studies) is avoided.
- As data is only collected at one time point (i.e. a 'snapshot'), it is important to be aware of the difference between an association and causality. More specifically, it is not possible to draw any causal inferences from associations between independent variables and the outcome variable in a cross-sectional study.[16]
- As cross-sectional studies can identify associations between the independent variables and the outcome variable, they can be the starting point for further investigation through, for example, a longitudinal study.

Considerations for the design and use of longitudinal studies

There are a number of key considerations when designing and using longitudinal studies in physical activity research. For example:

- Longitudinal studies are expensive and they are resource-intensive because they require follow-up at multiple times, of the same individuals, over a sustained period of time (e.g. months, years, decades).
- Loss of participants to follow-up, also referred to as attrition, is a main limitation of this study design because it can create selection bias in results and reduce the power of the findings.[17] This is because loss to follow-up is unlikely to be random and those more likely to remain engaged with a study are likely to be different to those who drop out in terms of a behaviour such as physical activity.[4] To reduce loss to follow-up it is important to devise a strategy for retaining participants within the study.[18] For instance, this could include updating contact address details regularly and being aware of potential changes over the study period such as job changes of participants. Failure to develop and implement a strategy will result in fewer participants at follow-up point(s).
- Measurements must be made at each data collection point, especially where they are likely to change and are not fixed (e.g. body mass).
- In longitudinal studies, despite finding an association, the issue of a causal relationship (i.e. establishing a cause and effect) between predictor variables and the outcome variable is complex. Although it is possible for causal inferences to be made, which is not possible in cross-sectional studies, issues such as bias and confounding factor(s) are elements that must be considered fully in relation to the associations found. This should be followed by considering elements such as strength of association, temporality, dose-response relationship and plausibility (e.g. biological) in relation to the association being potentially causal.[19] Overall, the strongest study designs in terms of determining a direct cause and effect relationship are in experimental studies, in particular a randomized controlled trial.[20] Longitudinal studies do however provide the opportunity to explore mediating and moderating factors, once potential confounding factors have been accounted for.

Case study example

Owens et al.[8] provides an example of an observational longitudinal prospective study. In adolescents, the change in physical activity levels was investigated over time, along with factors potentially associated with any change, in the period of transition from compulsory education to post-compulsory education. Data were collected at two time points (baseline and at 6–9 months later), which allowed cross-sectional analysis of baseline data, as well as longitudinal analysis of changes over the transition period.

Variables included physical activity (as the outcome variable) and a range of potential predictor variables which included gender, ethnicity, socioeconomic status, area of residence, educational attainment and school type. Screen time was also measured as a proxy for sedentary behaviour, as a further outcome variable, but this is not discussed in this chapter (please see Owens et al.[8]). Data were initially collected through a self-administered questionnaire at baseline (Year 11 at school, aged 15/16 years). The questionnaire collected data in relation to participants' levels of physical activity (outcome variable) and potential predictor variables. At baseline, participants ($n = 2{,}204$ pupils) from 24 schools agreed to complete the questionnaire. Significant time and effort ensured an efficient recruitment process. The same participants were followed up approximately 6–9 months later, using the same questionnaire when participants were either in sixth form (at school), in further education college, in employment, training or were unemployed. At follow-up, $n = 886$ of the original cohort completed the questionnaire representing a 40.2% response rate, and of those $n = 663$ participants (30.1% of the original cohort) resulted in complete data as 223 were omitted from the main analysis due to missing data. Although 30.1% of the original cohort was sufficient for meaningful analysis in the main analysis, the high level of 'attrition' (59.8%) was a limitation of the study despite designing and implementing a loss to follow-up strategy. This attrition rate is similar to that of other longitudinal studies in physical activity research (e.g. Hagstromer et al.[21]).

From a longitudinal perspective, Owens et al.[8] were interested in whether or not there was a change in physical activity levels between baseline (in full-time compulsory education) and follow-up (post-compulsory full-time education). Change was measured using a dichotomous outcome of either 'meeting physical activity guidelines' or 'not meeting these guidelines' (in line with recommended guidelines for physical activity from the Department of Health[22]) at each time point. 'Significant' change between baseline and follow-up was determined using a McNemar test for significance of changes. A significant reduction in physical activity was found from baseline to follow-up. Binary logistic regression was then used to investigate factors associated with the 'significant change'. A dichotomous outcome (outcome variable) was created for the binary logistic regression; "did not change from meeting to not meeting guidelines through the transition" or "did change from meeting to not meeting guidelines through the transition" (i.e. did decline). Predictor variables (i.e. gender, ethnicity, socioeconomic status, area of residence [urban/rural], education attainment and type of school [private/state]) were included in the regression to explore their association with the reduction in physical activity level. Findings revealed that gender was associated with the reduction in the physical activity level, with females being approximately 42% less likely to reduce their physical activity, compared with males. It is, however, important to recognize the potential influence of confounding and moderating variables on this finding. For instance, although gender (the predictor variable) was found to be significantly associated with change in physical activity level (the outcome variable), there could be other factors that were contributing to this association that were not controlled for (e.g. body image as it is potentially related to physical activity [the dependent variable] and gender [the predictor variable]).

From a cross-sectional perspective and using the data collected at baseline, an analysis (Owens et al., not published) was undertaken into whether or not participants were meeting or not meeting guidelines for physical activity (as explained above) at baseline (i.e. in line with recommended guidelines as above at one time point) and what factors were associated with meeting these guidelines. From the original 2,204 participants who completed the questionnaire at baseline, only 1,427 participants had complete data that could be included in analysis. Findings revealed that compliance with physical activity guidelines (i.e. meeting guidelines) was low (13.2%). In relation to factors associated with compliance with guidelines, binary logistic regression was undertaken. Results showed that participants were more likely to meet recommended physical activity guidelines if they: took active modes of transport (compared to passive modes of transport); met guidelines for screen time (compared to not meeting guidelines); were in the less deprived compared to the most deprived quartile for socioeconomic status; or were male (compared to female).

Overall, although this study has limitations relating to loss to follow-up and possible effects of confounding or moderating factors, these are common limitations in longitudinal studies. Despite this, the study had the benefit of being able to examine the data from both a cross-sectional and longitudinal perspective, with the choice of included predictor variables informed by a significant body of literature. The challenge for researchers planning longitudinal studies is to be fully aware of potential limitations and where possible develop strategies to ensure their limited impact on outcomes.

Conclusions and summing up

This chapter provides an overview of observational studies, with a specific focus on cross-sectional and longitudinal design. Through the inclusion of the case study which utilized both approaches, the reader can now appreciate some of the important considerations for these study designs. Furthermore, the chapter has included key information to enable the reader with insight and knowledge to design and undertake this type of research, ensuring both the most appropriate design and collection of high-quality data. Readers may also wish to refer to Chapters 9–12 in this text, for related information on research designs and tools that may be used in observational studies.

References

1   Caruana EJ. Roman M, Hernandez-Sanchez J, Solli P. Longitudinal studies. *J Thorac Dis.* 2015; **7**(11):E537–40.
2   Sigmund E, Sigmundova D, El Ansari W. Changes in physical activity in pre-schoolers and first grade children: longitudinal study in the Czech Republic. *Child Care Health Dev.* 2009; **35**(3):376–82.
3   Aires L, Andersen LB, Mendonca D, Martins C, Silva G, Mota J. A 3-year longitudinal analysis of changes in fitness, physical activity, fatness and screen time. *Acta Paediatr.* 2010; **99**:140–4.
4   Eime RM, Harvey JT, Sawyer NA, Craike MJ, Symons CM, Payne WR. Changes in sport and physical activity participation for adolescent females: a longitudinal study. *BMC Public Health.* 2016; **16**:533.
5   Taylor RW, Williams SM, Farmer VL, Taylor BJ. Changes in physical activity over time in young children: a longitudinal study using accelerometers. *PLoS One.* 2013; **8**(11):e81567.
6   Uijtdewilligen L, Twisk JW, Chinapaw MJ, Koppes LL, Van Mechelen W, Singh AS. Longitudinal person-related determinants of physical activity in young adults. *Med Sci Sports Exerc.* 2014; **46**(3):529–36.
7   Eime RM, Casey MM, Harvey JT, Sawyer NA, Symons CM, Payne WR. Socioecological factors potentially associated with participation in physical activity and sport: a longitudinal study of adolescent girls. *J Sci Med Sport.* 2015; **18**(6):684–90.
8   Owens CS, Crone D, De Ste Croix MBA, Gidlow CJ, James DVB. Physical activity and screen time in adolescents transitioning out of compulsory education: a prospective longitudinal study. *J Public Health.* 2014; **36**(4):599–607.

9 Pan SY, Cameron C, DesMeules M, Morrison H, Craig CL, Jiang X. Individual, social, environmental, and physical environmental correlates with physical activity among Canadians: a cross-sectional study. *BMC Public Health.* 2009; **9**:21.

10 Ding D, Sallis JF, Hovell MF, Du J, Zheng M, He H, Owen N. Physical activity and sedentary behaviours among rural adults in siuxi, china: a cross-sectional study. *Int J Behav Nutr Phys Act.* 2011; **8**:37.

11 Ortlieb S, Schneider G, Koletzko S, Berdel D, von Berg A, Bauer CP, et al. Physical activity and its correlates in children: a cross-sectional study (the GINIplus & LISAplus studies). *BMC Public Health.* 2013; **13**:349.

12 Godino JG, Watkinson C, Corder K, Sutton S, Griffin SJ, van Sluijs EMF. Awareness of physical activity in healthy middle-aged adults: a cross-sectional study of associations with sociodemographic, biological, behavioural, and psychological factors. *BMC Public Health.* 2014; **14**:421.

13 Cai Lian T, Bonn G, Si Han Y, Chin Choo Y, Chee Piau W. Physical activity and its correlates among adults in Malaysia: a cross-sectional descriptive study. *PLoS One.* 2016; **11**(6):e0157730.

14 Salvo D, Torres C, Villa U, Rivera JA, Sarmiento OL, Reis RS, Pratt M. Accelerometer-based physical activity levels among Mexican adults and their relation with sociodemographic characteristics and BMI: a cross-sectional study. *Int J Behav Nutr Phys Act.* 2015; **12**:79.

15 Mytton OT, Townsend N, Rutter H, Foster C. Green space and physical activity: an observational study using Health Survey for England data. *Health Place.* 2012; **18** (5):1034–41.

16 Sedgwick P. Cross-sectional studies: advantages and disadvantages. *Br Med J.* 2014; **348**:g2276.

17 Wolk D, Waylen A, Samara M, Steer C, Goodman R, Ford T, Lamberts K. Selective drop-out in longitudinal studies and non-biased prediction of behavior disorders. *Br J Psych.* 2009; **195**(3):249–256.

18 Faden VB, Day NL, Windle M, Windle R, Grube JW, Molina BSG, et al. Collecting longitudinal data through childhood, adolescence, and young adulthood: methodological challenges. *Alcohol Clin Exp Res.* 2004; **28**(2):330–40.

19 Bradford Hill A. The environment and disease: association or causation? *Proc Roy Soc Med.* 1965; **58**(5):295–300.

20 Bauman AE, Sallis JF, Dzewaltowski DA, Owen N. Toward a better understanding of the influences on physical activity: the role of determinants, correlates, causal variables, mediators, moderators, and confounders. *Am J Prev Med.* 2002; **23**(Suppl 2). 1:5–14.

21 Hagstromer M, Kwak L, Oja P, Sjostrom M. A 6 year longitudinal study of accelerometer-measured physical activity and sedentary time in Swedish adults. *J Sci Med Sports.* 2015; **18**(5):553–7.

22 Department of Health. *At least five a week: evidence on the impact of physical activity and its relationship to health. A report from the chief medical officer.* London: Department of Health; 2004.

9 Interviews and focus groups

Diane Crone and Lorena Lozano-Sufrategui

Aims of the chapter

This chapter explores and explains how to design and undertake qualitative studies using interviews and focus groups. It covers key aspects regarding the issues associated with using these methods and ensuring high-quality data are collected, along with a case study example provided to illustrate how these techniques can be used. The aims of the chapter include:

- To explore and explain the designing and undertaking of interviews and focus groups in qualitative research.
- To explain how to prepare the interview and focus group data for analysis.
- To provide details on the analysis of data and the series of steps used to ensure rigour in qualitative data analysis.
- To provide an illustrative example of using interviews and focus groups in physical activity research.

What are interviews and focus groups?

An interview is a guided conversation between an interviewer and one or more participants which aims to explore the ways in which the participants view their world, described in their own words, guided by the interviewer.[1] The term 'interview' is a collective term and includes a range of types of interviews including one-to-one interviews and focus groups. Focus groups are a type of group interview in which the researcher facilitates discussion between participants, and her role generally involves moderating conversations between participants. In this facilitating role, they draw out discussion of both similar and differing perspectives between group participants, and furthermore enable understanding on why, how and what is of importance regarding the issue under discussion.[2] It is therefore not merely the recording of a collection of viewpoints from participants, but also the study of the social interactions and group dynamics that occur in the setting.

Semi-structured interviews and focus groups are methods of data collection that include open-ended, neutral, sensitive and understandable questions that aim to yield as much information about the phenomenon of interest as possible.[3] Their semi-structured, i.e. flexible, nature allows for the discovery of information that is important to participants in terms of their experiences, and this may not have been considered by the researcher or identified in previous literature.[4]

In this chapter, the term 'interview' is used to denote a one-to-one interview between a participant and a researcher, and a focus group is a form of group interview between a researcher and a group of 3 or more participants. Generally speaking one-to-one interviews aim to explore people's personal experiences, views and beliefs on specific matters and focus groups are useful to explore questions about group norms and meanings.[5]

Interviews

Interviews involve one or sometimes two people, for example a couple, and can be undertaken face to face, or via electronic mediums such as the telephone, Skype® or FaceTime. Interviews undertaken via electronic mediums often require more experience due to the difficulty of establishing rapport with a participant, but can be effective in respect to time resource, or accessibility of participant and/or researcher, i.e. interviewing people who are located a distance from the researcher, or have limited time availability to travel to meet for a face-to-face interview.

Focus groups

Focus groups are a type of interview but include more participants and usually range in size from between 4 and 12 people.[6] The uniqueness of focus groups is that they allow interaction between participants and this often enables a range of perspectives and opinions to emerge through those discussions with other participants and not solely the researcher, as in one-to-one interviews. The researcher aims to focus the participants on a particular topic to explore their opinions, experiences, perspectives etc. on that topic.[1] Differing perspectives are welcomed, as they facilitate discussion between participants, and not solely between a participant and the researcher. However, focus groups are more challenging to manage due to the nature of group discussions, and ensuring that everyone has their say and does not feel intimidated by, for example an over-dominant participant. Often, between three to five focus groups are needed to facilitate the collection of adequate data and reach data saturation.[7,8]

How are interviews and focus groups used in sport and physical activity research?

Interviews and focus groups can be used in a variety of ways in physical activity and sport research. They can be used independently or together. For example some researchers may use follow-up interviews with the same participants, for example when evaluating the long-term impact of physical activity interventions over time, for example a year, or when the participant and/or researcher consider that a further interview is needed to elaborate, explain or clarify further aspects of a previous discussion.[9] Sometimes researchers may use focus groups to find out initial understandings of a phenomena and then follow-up with individual interviews with participants who have presented what is deemed an information-rich case.[10] This is when the participant has a perspective or experience related to the phenomena that is of interest to the researcher, who wants to understand more about what is happening for the participant, through a more focused individual interview.[11] An example of this can be found in Crone et al.,[12] who investigated the mental health and physical activity relationship phenomena using both focus groups and individual interviews.

Table 9.1 presents some examples of how interviews and focus groups have been used in published research in this area.

Table 9.1 Examples of the uses of interviews and focus groups in physical activity and sport research

Type of use for an interview and/or a focus group	Area of research	Types of participants	Frequency of method
One-to-one interviews	Physical activity (walking programme) and mental health as an adjunct to care in a mental health service (Crone, 2007)[13]	People with severe mental illness who participated in an off-site walking programme (context: secondary mental healthcare)	A one-to-one interview with participants, following the duration of the walking programme
One-to-one interviews	Understanding the social and physical environmental factors influencing adolescents' physical activity in urban public open spaces (Van Hecke et al., 2016)[14]	Participants were young people who were interviewed whilst walking in a public open space (context: community)	A one-to-one interview with the researcher, undertaken whilst walking in the open space
Focus group	The use of sports therapy as an adjunct to treatment in mental health services (Crone & Guy, 2008)[15]	Participants were users of mental health services who had taken part in sports therapy as part of their treatment plan (context: secondary mental healthcare)	Two focus groups were undertaken with two groups of participants
Focus group	The use of technology for health information in adolescents (Skinner, Biscope, Poland, & Goldberg, 2003)[16]	Canadian male and female adolescents	27 focus groups with 210 youths from across Ontario, Canada
Interviews and focus groups	Physical activity and mental health (Crone et al., 2005)[12]	Patients referred from primary care onto a programme of exercise via their General Practitioner (context: primary healthcare)	Three sites were identified and a focus group conducted at each one, a selection of individuals were followed up from each site for one-to-one interviews
Interviews and focus groups	Pediatric diabetes training for healthcare professionals in Europe (Kime et al., 2017)[17]	Healthcare professionals who care for children and young people with type 1 diabetes and their families	One survey questionnaire, one focus group, one individual semi-structured interview with those who did not attend the focus group discussion

Typically, these methods are used to investigate the participant's perspectives, opinions, experiences and perceived outcomes, or to understand processes involved in physical activity and sport experiences that have not been fully understood previously. Both interviews and focus groups can be used in a number of ways. Some examples are summarized below:

- Undertaken with the same participants, pre- and post-intervention (interviews or focus groups), to investigate both processes (i.e. how a participant travelled through the intervention) and outcomes (i.e. perceived benefits of participation, experiences) of an intervention and its related processes.
- Undertaken as a series of interviews with the same participants, over a period of time, for example a year. This could be used to track and understand longitudinal engagement or perceived change, over a period of time. Usually this would be undertaken using individual interviews, but this could also be undertaken as a recurring focus group. However, there may be problems ensuring the same people attend, if over an extended period of time.
- With a group of people where there is little known about, or where they have a unique characteristic or need. For example a recently established migrant community, or a specific population where a new intervention has been developed, such as older men and walking football. This could be undertaken using interviews or focus groups.

There are many approaches to using both interviews and focus groups and which method(s) to use must be determined by the research questions and aims of each research project.

Designing interviews and focus groups

Researchers use interview guides to structure the interview and/or focus group, and to help guide the interviewer about what to ask and in what order.[3,6] They are particularly useful to help the researcher stay on track and also to guide a novice researcher through the process of the interview to ensure that no areas of interest are forgotten, should a schedule not be used.

The interview guide initiates the discussion with questions that can be answered easily and comfortably, and then proceeds to more complex topics.[11] Using questions that are comfortable and easy to answer will give time for the participant and researcher to build trust and rapport at the beginning of the interview, and this building up of confidence can lead to the generation of rich i.e. quality data, especially when discussing sensitive topics.[18] The interview schedule includes open-ended questions allowing the participant to elaborate and explain their feelings, experiences, thoughts, opinions etc. It is developed and directly linked to the research questions and aims. Specific questions/topics and prompts are developed with a view to elicit the information the researcher needs to address in their research questions or phenomena under investigation. The schedule (or guide) should be flexible enough to allow a range of experiences and/or opinions to be presented, and can also include prompts to assist the researcher to find out more about specific topics. The following excerpt is taken from the interview schedule used in Crone,[13] where she investigated the experiences of people with mental health problems when attending a walking programme.

Table 9.2 Example interview schedule adapted from Crone[13]

You are currently taking part in the walking programme, can you start off by telling me about how you came to be on the scheme, when and where you are now?

Can you tell me about your past experiences of doing anything like this before?

Why did you decide to participate in the walking project?

What were your thoughts or feelings of the project before you started, when it was first mentioned to you?

What are your thoughts or feelings of the project now you have participated in the walking groups for several weeks/months?

Note: if there has been a change in opinion, ask 'why have your opinions changed?'

What did you expect to experience on this project?

Prompts: physically? mentally? socially? Anything else?

Have you experienced what you expected?

Prompts: physically? mentally? socially? Anything else?

What, in your opinion, has helped you to experience these?

Has there been anything that you have experienced that you didn't expect? What was this?

Can you describe your experiences on the walking project?

- What has been most memorable? Why do you remember that?
- What has been most enjoyable? Why do you remember that?
- What has been most scary or nerve-racking? Why do you remember that?

What do you think about the walk leader? The project itself? The other people you have met? The environment that you go walking in?

Have any of these aspects had an influence on your experiences? If so how have they/it influenced you?

Can you tell me what you feel whilst you are participating in the walking group? Why do you think you feel that way?

Looking back into the role that exercise or activity has played in your life, how does this experience of activity relate to that?

Do you think you are likely to continue participating in this walking project?

Prompt: if yes, why? If no, why not?

And finally, is there anything that you would like to tell us that would help us to improve the project in the future for other people?

The length of interview and focus group can depend on many factors but, on average, interviews often last between 20 and 60 min and focus groups between 40 and 90 minutes.[19]

Preparing interviews and focus groups

In the preparation phase, the interview guide should be piloted to help researchers prepare for the demands related to interviewing,[3] to check the order in which questions will be asked and to ensure there is not repetition. Rehearsing interviews with an experienced colleague can be a valuable opportunity for feedback on the type of questions being asked and interviewing style.[19] These rehearsals should be voice recorded (with permission), so that interviewers can reflect on their interviewing style and adjust it if needed. Besides piloting, researchers also need to think about a suitable location to conduct the interviews (for both themselves and the interviewee) and inform participants about the study using a participant information sheet and consent form. These documents include information about the aims of the study and methods; as well as other ethical issues related to voluntary participation, confidentiality, anonymity and right to withdraw.[20] It is also important to ensure that participants know the interview or focus group will be recorded prior to the event, so that they consent. If for example a participant in a focus group declines for the discussion to be recorded, then none of the discussions can be recorded and the quality and richness of the data is therefore compromised as the researcher can only rely on hand-written notes during the session.

If researching physical activity interventions, it is advisable for researchers to do on-site observations before conducting interviews or focus groups.[3] This can help them build trust and rapport with participants, which can positively impact subsequent interviews, as participants may feel more comfortable talking to someone they 'know'. Spending time in the field can also help researchers identify 'information-rich' cases and decide about the type of group mix for focus groups and the number of participants.[6,10] The group must be small enough for everyone to have an opportunity to contribute, and large enough to allow for a variety of views to be discussed.

Undertaking interviews and focus groups

Skilled interviewers support participants to share their perspective on the phenomenon of interest as seen by participants.[21] Being respectful, non-judgmental and non-threatening can facilitate this process.[3] Besides, adopting an 'active listening' attitude by using non-verbal cues, short responses and/or back channels utterances such as 'right' or 'hmm' can help assist the complex interactions between researcher and participants.[22] Follow-up probes can also be used to gain additional information from participants and go deeper into their accounts, responses and stories.[23] Keeping silent, i.e. not jumping in at the point the conversation seems to dry up, can also help to facilitate people to continue to share their experiences.

Generally, interviews and focus groups are digitally recorded to ensure that everything said is preserved for analysis[3]. Digitally recording interviews enables researchers to give full attention to the participants' accounts, and it can also help capture the production of meaning, as the researcher's voice is also recorded.[24] However, some participants may feel uneasy with being recorded. In this instance, researchers should offer the option of turning the voice recorder off as and when requested by participants. In this case, researchers can ask participants for permission to take notes about what is being said.

When undertaking focus groups, it is a good idea to ask the group to introduce themselves in the order in which they are sitting, for the purposes of the recording and of course introductions (even though they may know the researcher and each other). This ensures that when the recording is transcribed, it is easier to identify the owner of a voice and the researcher knows whose voice belongs to whom. This is especially important if the group members are not known to the researcher. It is important for example to know who is speaking if they are a woman of 20 years, or for example a woman of 60 years. Without a reference point it may not be able to determine this.

Whilst undertaking the focus group, researchers should not only listen to participants' responses to the questions, but they should also carefully observe how participants interact with each other.[6] These lively collective interactions can bring forth "more spontaneous expressive and emotional views" than interviews.[19] Focus groups can create spaces where participants support or challenge others, and this can reveal unarticulated group norms that would not otherwise arise in a one-to-one interview. Focus groups can also be empowering and encourage change within the group, as L Lozano-Sufrategui, McKenna, Carless, Pringle and Sparkes et al. (2016), showed in their study of weight stigma.[25]

At the end of the focus group, it is important to ensure that participants are thanked for their time and contribution. Furthermore, this is an ideal time to explain next steps, i.e. if there is a process of member checking, or a planned sharing of summary findings, these are explained. Should participants wish to know more, or be informed of where the research will be going next, this must be made available to them in a format that they will be able to comprehend. Layperson summaries and/or infographics of findings are a good example of how this can be done.

Preparing, managing and analysing interviews and focus groups data

The digital recording of the interview or focus group is transcribed verbatim (word for word) into a word document. It is advisable at this stage to change all proper nouns to pseudonyms, for example participants' names, places and any other identifying information. Once transcribed, the analysis process is a series of steps. One of the most common methods that has been well documented and used in physical activity research is Thematic Analysis.[26,28] This involves a series of six steps which are summarized in Table 9.3. For an example from physical activity research which uses this method please refer to L Lozano-Sufrategui et al.[29]

Ensuring trustworthiness in interviews and focus groups

Lincoln and Guba (1985) believed that the quality criteria used to judge quantitative studies were not appropriate for judging qualitative research.[30] As a result, Lincoln and Guba provided alternative criteria to judge the quality of qualitative studies,[30] which included the notions of credibility, dependability, transferability and confirmability.

Table 9.3 Summary of Thematic Analysis adapted from Braun & Clarke (2006), p. 87[26]

Phase	Brief description
Phase 1: Familiarization	Transcribing, reading and re-reading the transcripts. Identify some initial ideas.
Phase 2: Generating initial codes	Codes of interest are generated by extracting and collating pertinent excerpts of the data that are connected/related.
Phase 3: Searching for themes	Emerging codes are organized into broad themes that reflect the content and meaning of the data, and reflect the research aims and objectives.
Phase 4: Reviewing themes	Themes are reviewed and refined in relation to the generated codes, and the entire data set.
Phase 5: Defining and naming themes	Themes are labelled and defined, attempting to capture the essence of the data it contained, within the context of the research questions and aims.
Phase 6: Producing the report	Themes are presented in a written report including an explanation of each theme supported by quotations from the transcript to enable the voices of participants to be represented in the findings.

However, these criteria are still underpinned by the positivistic notions of 'truth', 'internal validity', 'reliability', 'generalizability' or 'external validity' and 'objectivity'.[31] The parallelisms between Lincoln and Guba's criteria approach have been criticized because they have generated ontological and epistemological contradictions that are inappropriate for qualitative studies.[32,33] Further, the use of universal criteria has been deemed inappropriate for judging qualitative studies given the diversity and uniqueness of genres and forms of qualitative inquiry (e.g. ethnography, phenomenology, narrative research, autoethnography). Thus, an evaluative approach that acknowledges the diversity and uniqueness of each tradition in qualitative research has been suggested. This is what has been identified as a 'relativist approach', where specific criteria are applied in ways that are contextually situated,[33] hence aligned with an ontological relativism and epistemological constructionism. In practice, this would mean that qualitative researchers have to "make informed decisions and ongoing judgments about which criteria reflect the inherent properties" of their studies.[31] Sometimes, this may involve making decisions as the study progresses and applying alternative criteria in situ to assess their work.[33]

For these reasons, ensuring trustworthiness in interviews and focus groups will depend on many contextual and situational factors, and therefore we are unable to provide a definite list of universal criteria. This being said, researchers may want to consider or adapt the list of alternative criteria provided by Smith and Caddick to judge qualitative work.[34]

Case study of a project using interviews and focus groups

Introduction

L Lozano-Sufrategui et al. (2016) provide an example of an ethnographic study which aimed to understand hard-to-reach men's health behaviours during and 6 months after attending a men-only weight management programme. Ethnography is a methodology which requires the researcher to be immersed into the world of the participants. As such, the lead researcher attended a full cycle of the programme (12 weeks) and in addition to interviews and focus groups, also utilized participant observation throughout as a method of data collection.[35] Immersion in the field by observing, participating in the activities and learning the culture in addition to having informal conversations with potential participants was critical to understanding their perspectives. To collect the breadth and depth of data that was required a range of methods was used. However, for the purpose of this chapter, the focus will be on the use of interviews and focus groups. As with most ethnographic studies the case study is presented in the first person, from the perspective of the lead researcher, who is Spanish, the reason for this disclosure is relevant as the case study develops. For a fuller explanation of the method and findings see Lozano-Sufrategui.[9]

Case study

Identifying 'hard-to-reach' men was a challenge, by the very nature of them being 'hard-to-reach'. To assist with this a questionnaire was used as a sampling strategy at the weight management programme to get a general overview of 'who' the participants could be. 'Hard-to-reach' is not a visible characteristic, therefore questionnaire data enabled the researchers to identify the men who met the criteria for this characteristic which is: those who 'never' use traditional health services despite self-reporting 'poor' heath. Initial sampling to identify who would be invited to the subsequent focus groups and interviews took place early on during fieldwork i.e. first 2 weeks of fieldwork. During this time, participants identified me as a 'tourist': someone different but who was interested in learning their culture. Therefore, asking personal questions about their health behaviours in a one-to-one interview or focus group at this stage would have been inappropriate as some of these men never, or only very rarely, talk about these health or weight matters, let alone discuss these with a so-called tourist.

From the questionnaires, I identified some 'hard-to-reach' men, or 'information-rich cases' who I believed could provide insight into understanding and answering my research question. Part of the selection of these participants included that they seemed willing to talk to me. During this phase – from week 3 to week 8 approximately – my interactions with participants became more frequent, especially when they realized that I was able to talk about the things they were interested in, for example Spain, paella, the European economic crisis and football. Having been a football player previously, I know about the sport. Because of these interactions, I became more involved in the field, i.e. the world of the participants, and the men began to invite me to participate in their activities during the programme, mainly playing football, and thus I adopted the role of participant-as-observer. This reduced the social and physical distance that separated participants and myself, and they even granted me a nickname of 'Torres', the Spanish international footballer who had also played in the English Premiership. During this phase, I invited male participants to participate in 2 themed focus groups.

The aim of using focus groups was twofold. First, I used them as 'ice-breakers' so that I could get to know participants in a more formal research setting, i.e. in an interview room. Second, I invited men who I saw integrated with others on the programme as I thought this would enable me to explore participants' interactions, group meanings and norms. The following fieldnote elucidates how group norms were expressed within the dynamics of the group:

> [Fieldnote, 24th July 2014] During a focus group, Matthew referred to his belly as 'the beer belly'. He seemed to be proud when he talked about it. While he stroked his belly, he laughed and said: "it has cost me a few pints and burgers to get this!". It seems that eating unhealthy food and drinking excessive amounts of alcohol reflects what Matthew thinks is a socially accepted form of masculinity. Other men responded to Matthew's comment by laughing or stroking their bellies, which suggests that Matthew's view of masculinity is generally accepted as a norm by this group of men.

Once I felt I had developed a closer relationship with the men based on trust and rapport, I felt ready to undertake one-to-one interviews with participants who I believed could share relevant information with me. My observations, field conversations and focus groups data informed my decisions to invite participants to one-to-one interviews. However, before starting these "conversations with a purpose",[36] I refined the interview guide, as a result of the questions that arose during a preliminary analysis of focus group data. For example, the fieldnote above generated the following, new question:

> [Fieldnote, 3rd August 2014] If participants say they are proud of their 'beer bellies', why do they want to lose weight by attending this weight management programme? What does this contradiction mean?

These new questions generated insights that I had not anticipated before the focus groups, and are an example of how a focus group can help focus the individual interview schedule. For example, when I interviewed Matthew in a one-to-one interview, I asked:

LORENA: You seemed to be proud of your belly the other day, can you please explain what this means to you?

MATTHEW: I am not proud of it. I am embarrassed. I am fat, I know I am fat, and I know other people know. In the past they have taken the piss out of me, for being fat, so now I make the comment before anybody else so that nobody can say anything about it afterwards. It's just a defensive mechanism, I hate my belly, but I don't want anyone to say anything about it.

The use of the focus group and the subsequent interview enabled me to understand more about the personal lives of participants, and the individual meanings they attached to these.

Conducting interviews often requires the researcher to ask the participant to recollect events in the past. One strategy to assist people with that recollection of events and factors associated with them is through using a life history approach to understand, in this case, the participants' journey to the programme. However, some participants found it difficult to remember some events and their accounts seemed disorganized, incoherent and disjointed. To help participants elicit talk, by deviating their attention from themselves towards an object, I used strategies such as timelining and participant-generated photo-elicitation. For example, Figure 9.1 shows a combination of a participants' timelining graph combined with the photographs he brought to the interview. The horizontal axis shows the participant's age, and the vertical axis shows the participant's weight. The crosses show key events in the participant's life that resulted in a change in weight or health behaviours. By linking the crosses together, the line that was generated shows participants' weight fluctuation across time. This graph was the basis for a more coherent, organized and complete story to understand participants' journey to the weight management programme. This is one strategy that could be used when investigating life course phenomena.

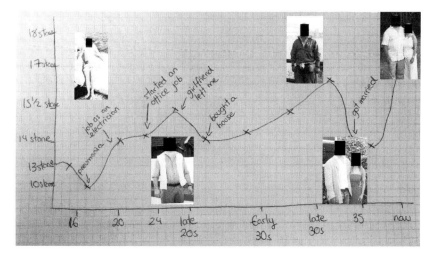

Figure 9.1 Timelining graph with photographs.

This case study provides an example of a number of strategies to understand a 'hard-to-reach' group. These included:

- Prolonged engagement in the field (environment of the research, i.e. the weight management programme) as participant observer.
- Informal conversations during the programme with participants, using topics that were meaningful to them.
- Gathering data using multiple methods and using these methods at the right time and place, depending on the types of relationships I had with the men.
- Using tools to help elicit talk with men who found it difficult to give an account of their lives (timelining).
- Providing opportunities such as focus groups for participants to feel empowered and supported by other men.
- Adjusting my interview schedule to further explore the specific needs, interests and concerns of the group of men who voluntarily decided to participate in my research.

Conclusions and summing up

This chapter has presented an explanation of interviews and focus groups and how they can be used in qualitative, physical activity research. It has presented detail regarding the preparation of the interview schedule, and subsequent data analysis to undertake to present trustworthy findings in a report, dissertation, thesis or article. The chapter concludes with an illustrative case study where both focus groups and interviews were used with a hard-to-reach group. Through the inclusion of the case study which utilized both approaches, it is hoped that the reader now appreciates and understands the considerations for this study design. Furthermore, it is hoped that the reader has the insight and knowledge to design and undertake this type of research to ensure the collection of high-quality data, in their own interest area of physical activity research.

References

1 Kvale S. *Doing interviews.* Thousand Oaks, CA: Sage; 2008.
2 Gibbs A. Focus groups and group interviews, Chapter 26. In: Arthur J, Waring M, Coe R, Hedges LV, editors. *Research methods and methodologies in education.* London: Sage; 2012. pp. 186–92.
3 Merriam SB, Tisdell EJ. *Qualitative research: a guide to design and implementation.* San Francisco: John Wiley & Sons, Inc.; 2015.
4 Gill P, Stewart K, Treasure E, Chadwick B. Methods of data collection in qualitative research: interviews and focus groups. *Br Dent J.* 2008; **204**(6):291–5.
5 Hennink MM. *Focus group discussions.* Oxford: Oxford University Press; 2013.
6 Krueger R, Casey M. *Focus groups: a practical guide to applied science.* Thousand Oaks, CA: Sage; 2009.
7 Bryman A. *Social research methods.* 4th ed. Oxford: Oxford University Press; 2012.
8 Cleary M, Horsfall J, Hayter M. Data collection and sampling in qualitative research: does size matter? *J Adv Nurs.* 2014; **70**(3):473–5.
9 Lozano-Sufrategui L, Rowlands S. Men, health, & wellbeing: critical insights, leeds beckett university, city of leeds, United Kingdom, 7–8 July 2014. *Int J Men's Health.* 2015; **14**(3):201–3.

10 Patton MQ. *Qualitative research encyclopedia of statistics in behavioral science.* John Wiley & Sons, Inc.; 2005.

11 Patton MQ. *Qualitative evaluation and research methods.* Thousand Oaks, CA: Sage; 2015.

12 Crone D, Smith A, Gough B. "I feel totally alive, totally happy and totally at one": a psycho-social explanation of the physical activity and mental health relationship from the experiences of participants on exercise referral schemes. *Health Educ Res.* 2005; **20**(5):11.

13 Crone D. 'Walking back to health' a qualitative investigation into service users' experiences of a walking project. *Issues Ment Health Nurs.* 2007; **28**(2):167–83. DOI: 10.1080/01612840601096453

14 Van Hecke L, Deforche B, Van Dyck D, De Bourdeaudhuij I, Veitch J, Van Cauwenberg J. Social and physical environmental factors influencing adolescents' physical activity in urban public open spaces: a qualitative study using walk-along interviews. *PLoS One.* 2016; **11**(5):e0155686. DOI: 10.1371/journal.pone.0155686

15 Crone D, Guy H. 'I know it is only exercise, but to me it is something that keeps me going': a qualitative approach to understanding mental health service users' experiences of sports therapy. *Int J Ment Health Nurs.* 2008; **17**(3):197–207. DOI: 10.1111/j.1447–0349.2008.00529.x

16 Skinner H, Biscope S, Poland B, Goldberg E. How adolescents use technology for health information: implications for health professionals from focus group studies. *J Med Int Res.* 2003; **5**(4):e32.

17 Kime NH, Waldron S, Webster E, Lange K, Zinken K, Danne T, et al. Pediatric diabetes training for healthcare professionals in Europe: time for change. *Pediatr Diabetes.* 2017; DOI: 10.1111/pedi.12573. [Epub ahead of print].

18 Smith B, Sparkes AC. Interviews: qualitative interviewing in the sport and exercise sciences. In: Smith B, Sparkes AC, editors. *Routledge handbook of qualitative research in sport and exercise.* Oxon: Routledge; 2016. p. 123.

19 Sparkes AC, Smith B. *Qualitative research methods in sport, exercise and health: from process to product.* Abingdon, UK: Routledge; 2014.

20 Taylor SJ, Bogdan R, Marjorie L. *Introduction to qualitative research methods: a guidebook and resource.* Hoboken, New Jersey: John Wiley & Sons, Inc.; 2016.

21 Marshall C, Rossman GB. *Designing qualitative research.* 6th ed. London, UK: SAGE; 2016.

22 Mishler EG. *Research interviewing: context and narrative.* Cambridge, MA: Harvard University Press; 1986.

23 Glesne C, Peshkin A. *Becoming qualitative researchers: an introduction.* White Plains, NY: Longman; 1992.

24 Elliott J. *Using narrative in social research: qualitative and quantitative approaches.* London: Sage; 2005.

25 Lozano-Sufrategui L, McKenna J, Carless D, Pringle A, Sparkes A. 'Sorry mate, you're probably a bit too fat to be able to do any of this': men's experiences of weight stigma and its implications. *Int J Men's Health.* 2016; **15**(1):4–23.

26 Braun V, Clarke V. Using thematic analysis in psychology. *Qual Res Psychol.* 2006; **3**(2):77–101. DOI: 10.1191/1478088706qp063oa

27 Braun V, Clarke V, Weate P. *Using thematic analysis in sport and exercise research.* London: Routledge; 2016.

28 Clarke V, Braun V, Hayfield N. Thematic analysis. In: Smith JA, editor. *Qualitative psychology: a practical guide to research methods.* 3rd ed. London: Sage; 2015. pp. 222–48.

29 Lozano-Sufrategui L, Pringle A, Carless D, McKenna J. 'It brings the lads together': a critical exploration of older men's experiences of a weight management programme delivered through a Healthy Stadia projec. *Sport Soc.* 2017; **20**(2):303–15.

30 Lincoln YS, Guba EG. *Naturalistic inquiry.* Vol. 75. London, UK: Sage; 1985.

31 Burke S. Rethinking 'validity' and 'trustworthiness' in qualiative inquiry: how might we judge the quality of qualitative research in sport and exercise sciences? In: Smith B, Sparkes AC, editors. *Routledge handbook of qualiative research in sport and exercise.* Oxon: Routledge; 2016. pp. 330–39.

32   Sparkes AC. Validity in qualitative inquiry and the problem of criteria: implications for sport psychology. *Sport Psychol.* 1998; **12**(4):363–86.

33   Sparkes AC, Smith B. Judging the quality of qualitative inquiry: criteriology and relativism in action. *Psychol Sport Exerc.* 2009; **10**(5):491–7.

34   Smith B, Caddick N. Qualitative methods in sport: a concise overview for guiding social scientific sport research. *Asia Pacific J Sport Soc Sci.* 2012; **1**(1):60–73.

35   Wolcott HF. *The art of fieldwork.* Altamira: Rowman; 2005.

36   Burgess RG. Autobiographical accounts and research experience. In: Burgess RG, editor. *The research process in educational settings: ten case studies.* Lewes: The Falmer Press; 1984. pp. 251–70.

10 Questionnaires

Philip Hurst and Stephen R. Bird

Chapter aims

The aims of this chapter are to present the potential uses of questionnaires and the principles involved in developing an effective and valid questionnaire. It will consider some of the issues involved with the effective development and use of questionnaires as a research tool, their administration and ethical considerations. The information provided in this chapter is not set out to be definitive, but rather, it is presented as an introduction in the development and use of questionnaires in health and physical activity research.

Depending on the intended research methods, the reader may wish to read this chapter alongside Chapters 8, 9 and 11, on Observational studies, Interviews and focus groups, and Surveys as much of the information presented in these chapters relates and informs the others to provide a more comprehensive coverage. These chapters have been presented in this way to provide an informative coverage of the topic without excessive duplication and repetition of material.

Introduction

A questionnaire is a series of pre-set questions that are designed to address the research aims. This allows the researcher to collect a set of data of the same information, in the same format, from every participant in the sample. Given this, questionnaires are a convenient way to collect data from a large, heterogeneous sample on a wide range of issues.

Since their use in health and physical activity is prevalent, researchers often mistakenly assume that questionnaires are easy to design and use. However, without strong rationale, and a careful design, which is clearly thought through and explicitly defined, the use of questionnaires does not always equate with obtaining useful data. For these reasons, key principles must be followed if researchers are to be effective in collecting valid and reliable data, and considerable effort and planning is needed to ensure the data obtained is of sufficient quality to answer the research question(s). This is regardless of whether the questionnaire is the primary means for data collection in the research or is being used to collect just one item of data, for example, participants' perceived exertion during an exercise task or adherence to an intervention.

The use of questionnaires in research

Questionnaires may be used in many research contexts, for example:

- They could form the entire means by which data is collected in a survey, such as providing descriptive information, data for the determination of associations between factors and data for comparing groups or scenarios.

- As a screening tool for assessing whether a prospective participant meets the inclusion/exclusion criteria within a larger study design, such as a physical activity intervention.
- To elicit information relating to participants' behaviours, attitudes and beliefs.
- The collection of descriptive data on the characteristics and demographics of participants within a study that also collects data via other means, such as physiological health data.
- The method by which pre- and post-intervention data are collected to determine the effectiveness of an intervention, with the questionnaire providing all the data or being used alongside other measures of health and fitness, such as blood lipids;
- Used in conjunction with interviews and focus groups.

As can be seen from the above, almost every health and physical activity researcher is likely to use a questionnaire of some form at some time. Indeed even the "Participant Information and Consent Form" is a questionnaire.

Designing effective questionnaires

Designing effective questionnaires is important when ensuring precision and accuracy of data. Before a questionnaire can be designed, it is important that the researcher has a clear idea of what they want to investigate (i.e. the domain in question). This may seem relatively straightforward at first, but it can quickly become difficult when scrutinized. For example, if a questionnaire is being developed to measure participants' dependence to exercise, all concepts related to exercise dependency need to be identified and categorized (e.g. withdrawal effects, tolerance and intention). DeVellis (2003) and Lynn (1986) recommend identifying a domain through literature reviews and qualitative methods,[1,2] such as focus groups and semi-structured interviews (see Chapter 9). When combined, both methods can help generate a list of questions that fully represent the domain in question. After generating a list of items (i.e. questions) for the questionnaire, it is important the researcher check the reliability and validity of it prior to its use.

Validity of questionnaires

A questionnaire must have validity (i.e. the questionnaire measures what it is supposed to measure). It is well known that when asked about their exercise or dietary habits most people will recall one of their good weeks, and commonly over-report their level of activity. Hence the questionnaire may not provide data for a 'typical week'. With the advent and widespread availability of activity monitors the validity of responses can be compared against more objective measures. Although even this has issues, firstly the monitor itself needs to have a proven high validity and there is always the risk that when asked to wear the monitor the person will be more conscientious in their exercise habits – the 'Hawthorn effect', and hence will record activity levels for that week that are better than their typical week's activity. In order for a researcher to have confidence in the interpretation of their data, they must be assured that the questionnaire is valid. There are many forms of validity, with the most common types briefly addressed below:

- *Content validity*: Once a questionnaire has been designed, the researcher must determine whether the questionnaire actually measures what it is intended to measure. For example, if a questionnaire aims to determine changes in self-esteem following a bout of exercise, the items on the questionnaire should measure self-esteem. The most effective way of examining content validity is through expert opinion. Once a questionnaire is designed, experts within the field should examine the content validity of the items and ensure that the questionnaire measures what it intends to measure.

- *Criterion validity:* This refers to the effectiveness of the questionnaire in measuring what it is intending to measure. A newly developed questionnaire should be assessed against a direct and independent measure of what the new questionnaire is designed to measure. For example, if a questionnaire aims to examine participants' physical activity levels, the criterion validity of the questionnaire can be assessed by the actual amount of physical activity performed, which may be measured by accelerometer data, for example.
- *Construct validity:* This type of validity refers to the extent to which the questionnaire relates to existing constructs being measured. This type of validity represents one of the greatest challenges in questionnaire development. Convergent validity and discriminant validity are two forms of construct validity that can be assessed to demonstrate construct validity.

  - *Convergent validity:* This type of validity concerns the degree to which two measures of similar theoretical constructs relate to each other. For example, a questionnaire that measures clinical depression should be correlated with other questionnaires that measure depression. Convergent validity can be assessed by estimating the correlation coefficient between two questionnaires.
  - *Discriminant validity:* This concerns whether the questionnaire can indicate differences between two or more types of populations. For example, it could be hypothesized that people who exercise have more favourable attitudes towards exercise than those who don't. If the questionnaire indicates differences in attitudes between exercisers and non-exercises, the questionnaire exhibits discriminant validity.

- *Face validity:* While this does not really refer to validity, face validity generally refers to the appearance and how easy the questionnaire is to read and interpret. A questionnaire must be clear and unambiguous. The questions may take many forms and elicit a variety of responses (e.g. free text-boxes, a list of options, yes/no responses) and it is important that the participant can easily answer each question. The questionnaire should avoid the use of technical language or terms that may not be understood by the 'lay-person' who has not undertaken extensive study in the field of health and physical activity. Therefore, the format of the questionnaire determines how easy it is for participants to read and understand the questions.

While there are numerous methods in providing validity for questionnaires, there is no 'gold standard' by which questionnaires can be validated. Instead, the validation of any questionnaire requires multiple procedures, which are employed sequentially at different stages of its development. Validity is thus built into the test at the outset rather than being limited to the last procedure/stage of questionnaire development. Each of these stages can be seen as fundamental to the validity of a questionnaire.

Reliability of questionnaires

Reliability, or reproducibility, indicates accuracy or precision of a questionnaire and whether it performs consistently. We describe three forms of reliability in this chapter:

- *Cronbach's alpha:* The first and arguably most common form of reliability in questionnaire development is the calculation of Cronbach's alpha. This calculation provides an estimate of internal consistency that describes the extent to which all questions on the questionnaire measure the same construct. Cronbach's alpha is expressed as a number between 0 and 1, and can be calculated on most statistical software. The closer the number is to 1, the higher the internal consistency. However, higher Cronbach's alpha scores do not necessarily mean high degree of internal consistency. Generally, coefficients above 0.95 may suggest that the questions are very similar and may need modifying. Coefficients above 0.70 and close to 0.90 are suggested to have good internal consistency. Further, it is important to consider that the alpha scores reported on a questionnaire on one set of participants may be different to that of another sample. Therefore, researchers should calculate Cronbach's alpha each time the test is administered.
- Test-retest: This type of reliability measures the stability of responses over time. A questionnaire with good test-retest reliability will have similar results when administered to the same person on two separate occasions, when there has been no intervention, activities or events that may affect the responses occurring between the two testing occasions. To assess the test-retest reliability, researchers can calculate the correlation coefficient between the two administrations of the questionnaire.
- Split-half: This type of reliability examines the consistency within the questionnaire when questions are measuring a similar construct. The questions of the questionnaire are split into two equivalent halves (usually by odd and even numbers or by first and second half) and correlation between the two halves is assessed. The higher the correlation, the greater reliability. Researchers must be aware that the split-half method cannot be used when the questionnaire assesses more than one construct (e.g. vigour and self-esteem).

Deciding the type of response

Researchers must decide on how the respondent will answer each question. There are a range of response types that researchers can use in their questionnaire. In health and physical activity research, Likert-type and frequency scales are most commonly used.

Generally, a Likert-type scale attempts to quantify a person's attitude towards various statements on a scale from 1 to 5, with 3 being a neutral midpoint. The scale is often anchored from strongly disagree to strongly agree. For example, an item could ask participants to rank their agreement on a scale from 1 (strongly disagree) to 5 (strongly agree) with the following statement: "It is important that the food I eat keeps me healthy". Further items of a similar construct would be asked and the responses are either summed or averaged to produce a single value. Using Likert-type scales allows the researcher to economically administer the questionnaire with ease to a large sample and allows comparison between participants' final scores. However, despite this, the use of Likert-type scale constrains the research to numerical data, which may be difficult to translate into actual real-world practices.

Frequency scales are similar to Likert-type scales and can be used to understand how often a type of behaviour occurs. A question may ask "how often do you take part in moderate physical activity in a week". Respondents may be asked to provide numerical data (e.g. 4 hours) or to select a choice of responses (e.g. less than 1 hour, 1–3 hours, 3–5 hours etc.). An important aspect to consider for frequency scales is the wording of the question. Ambiguous statements may affect the quality and nature of responses and depending on how the question is framed, may influence responses in unintended ways. For example, if the question asks "how often have you exercised recently", participants may interpret 'recently' differently.

Other less common types of response formats include the Guttman and Rasch scale, which presents a number of items to which the respondent is asked to rank in order of agreement; the Thurstone scale, which measures attitudes of agreement towards specific statements; and knowledge-based questions, which can evaluate how well a person understands a certain topic.

Piloting of the questionnaire

Having developed a draft questionnaire, it's important to pilot with a 'convenience' sample who ideally should be from the same demographic group as the intended sample in the population. This should bring to light any issues with language, the clarity of the questions and how long the questionnaire takes to complete. For examples of questionnaire development and validation in health and physical activity, see examples from Armstrong and Bull (2006),[3] Craig et al. (2003)[4] and Hurst et al. (2017).[5]

Recruiting and ethical considerations of questionnaires

As with all forms of research the characteristics of participants will be determined by the nature of the research and the research questions being addressed. Consequently the eligibility and inclusion/exclusion criteria will need to be determined, which could include age, sex, existing injuries and known medical conditions. If a particular group is being targeted for the research, then the researcher(s) may collaborate with organizations such as hospitals, medical clinics or organizations that focus on a particular condition, such as heart disease or diabetes. However undertaken, the recruitment process needs to attain a representative sample of the targeted population, otherwise there is a risk of bias due to some members with particular characteristics being over- or under-represented. Indeed there is always a risk of bias in any research that involves recruitment as it is common for participants to volunteer for interventions in topics for which they already have a high interest. Thus to determine the representativeness of recruited participants, researchers may compare the characteristics of participants with databases on the demographics and patient characteristics of other groups reported in the literature, such as national surveys.

When planning the recruitment strategy the researcher must be cognizant of any ethical considerations. For example, if intending to recruit via a GP's surgery there may be a risk of unintended coercion or a power relationship between doctor/ researcher and potential participants. The same would apply if a university lecturer sought to recruit students of their university. Such relationships would not preclude these people from being recruited, but the design of the study and the recruitment process would need to build in a means by which the risk of coercion or perceived risk due to the power relationship was minimized.

The recruitment process will need to be approved by the relevant ethics committee. Many questionnaires will be deemed to be of low or negligible risk, although others that may involve sensitive topics, vulnerable groups and issues of privacy and confidentiality may be classified as more than low risk. Furthermore, as indicated above, the potential risk of coercion or power relationships in the recruitment process will need to be considered as part of the ethics review.

If a questionnaire deals with a sensitive topic, it is possible that it may cause the participant some distress or discomfort when answering the questionnaire. Researchers should be aware of this potential risk and have in place reasonable strategies to deal with it. This may include providing contact details within the questionnaire of organizations that specialize in the topic and/or distress, and have services available. A question checking that the questionnaire has not caused distress to the respondent could be included at the end of the questionnaire. Other possible risks associated with undertaking any research, including questionnaires, is that of uncovering illicit or illegal activities. Here again, the researcher should be aware of the procedures that they need to follow in these circumstances. Typically these can be attained through the relevant ethics committee/organization through which the research would be approved, and such safeguards would need to be written into the ethics submission.

Other issues for consideration are how consent is attained, and this will need to be incorporated into the questionnaire process, as will the participants final agreement for their responses to be used in the analyses. Hence at the end of the questionnaire there needs to be an option for them to withdraw their consent. As part of the consenting process, participants should be informed about how their data will be stored, how its security will be assured and how privacy will be maintained. Each ethics committee will have its own specific requirements for these. Common examples may be that data is stored on password-protected computers and servers, which are owned by the researchers' employing organization. In the case of hard copies these may be in locked cabinets that only the research team will have access to. Data will be required to be kept for a specified duration by the ethics committee and by any journal publishing a manuscript derived from the study. Health and medical data is commonly required to be kept for longer than other data, with 10 years being typical. For all of the above, the researcher needs to specify in the information and consent forms who will have access to the data, and this would typically be restricted to the research team. This may also specify when any data would be destroyed and provide the participant with the option of having their data destroyed if they so wish, although this may be limited to the point before it has been included in any publications.

Social desirability: a confounder in the responses to questionnaires

While use of questionnaires in health and physical activity can generate interesting data, the value of this data depends on how accurate it actually is. Ensuring the accuracy of data retrieved from questionnaires can be difficult when they are based on self-report. It is typical for participants in health and physical activity research to over- and under-report how healthy and physically active they are. For example, participants tend to under-report sensitive or embarrassing behaviours, such as illicit drug use, and over-report positively viewed behaviours, such as physical activity.

Asking participants about socially desirable responses may generate errors that influence the accuracy and precision of the data. To overcome social desirability, researchers can use a variety of techniques and procedures such as the random response technique, the bogus pipeline procedure and the unmatched count technique. While it is beyond the scope of this chapter to explain each one in detail, readers can refer to Krumpal (2013)[6] for more information.

Administering questionnaires

Questionnaires may be administered face to face, via the internet or through other media. Each of these has associated issues of time, accessing participants, number of participants and higher or lower response rates.

Face-to-face administration of questionnaires

Administering a questionnaire face to face should be undertaken at a location that is suitable, convenient and safe for both the participant and researcher. For the researcher this method may be quite time consuming in terms of travel to a location and then working through the questionnaire with the participant; however, it may also be the most productive as any issues with completing the questionnaire such as the clarification of a question can be resolved immediately and hence the researcher is almost guaranteed to attain usable data.

Online administration of questionnaires

Administering an online questionnaire over the internet is perhaps at the opposite end of the spectrum, in that it can be sent to many prospective participants at the click of a button, and the respondents do not have to be within convenient travelling distance of the researcher, but can be located anywhere in the world that has access to the internet. In similar vein, social media platforms such as Facebook and Twitter offer a medium in which to advertise and recruit participants from all over the world of different populations who would be difficult, if not impossible, to reach. Websites such as SurveyMonkey and Qualtrics can be used to upload the questionnaire and participants can complete this at a time and place convenient to them.

Online administration can increase anonymity of responses and subsequently improve validity of data. For sensitive topics, participants can sign up to the study without having to provide direct information about who they are. Obtaining informed consent in these circumstances can be achieved using an information letter in lieu of signing informed consent. Thus, researchers can provide all information about the study, including benefits, risks, voluntary nature of participation and any compensation, at the onset of the questionnaire. This anonymity can provide a greater sense of confidence among participants when responding to sensitive topics and decrease social response biases.[7] If the participant wishes to withdraw their involvement in the research at a later date, this can be achieved by providing contact details of the research team at the start and end of the questionnaire, or if an identifying code is linked to the participant's responses. The same principles will apply to face-to-face questionnaires, in which participants' data is removed without reprisal.

While there are numerous benefits of online questionnaires, the response rate using an online method is likely to be much lower, and issues such as the clarification of a question are more problematic. Hence it's likely that a much greater number of prospective respondents will need to be contacted in order to attain the same volume of valid data than if it was collected face to face. Similarly, participants may complete the questionnaire on more than one occasion and may not match the inclusion criteria of the study. To help overcome these issues, researchers could request participants to contact them to obtain a code prior to completing the questionnaire. This can ensure that the participant is who they say they are and that they meet all inclusion criteria for the study. While it may decrease the response rate of the questionnaire, it can minimize the risk of multiple responses from the same participant.

Response rates

Improving response rates of questionnaires can be achieved by providing advance notice, by raising awareness and interest in the research, personalizing the initial contact of the participant (e.g. addressing the participant by their name and stressing the importance of their contribution) and offering incentives for their participation (e.g. financial gains or prize draws). While this does increase the resources needed to collect the required sample size, researchers should consider this when administering questionnaires. Non-responses can introduce bias and affect the accuracy and precision of data collected. For further information on how to improve response rates for questionnaires, readers should refer to the Cochrane collaboration for a more in-depth review.[8]

Summary

Questionnaires provide the researcher with an opportunity to collect a large amount of data worldwide at a relatively low cost. Questionnaires can provide meaningful and rich data, which has the potential to inform and shape policy of a variety of topics across the health and physical activity sciences. While a wealth of knowledge can be gained through the use of questionnaires, particular attention should be given to their accuracy and precision. Prior to administration, researchers should check that the questionnaire is appropriate in answering the research question(s) and that it meets acceptable standards of validity and reliability. Researchers should be aware of the potential ethical risks associated with questionnaire use and the influence social desirability can have on participants' responses. Such an approach can help ensure that the data collected are meaningful, which in turn can help inform knowledge and understanding of issues relevant across health and physical activity settings.

References

1   DeVellis RF. *Scale development: theory and applications.* 2 ed. Thousand Oaks, CA: Sage; 2003.
2   Lynn MR. Determination and quantification of content validity. *Nurs Res.* 1986; **35**:382–6.
3   Armstrong T, Bull F. Development of the World Health Organization Global Physical Activity Questionnaire (GPAQ). *J Public Health.* 2006; **14**:66–70.
4   Craig CL, Marshall AL, Sjöström M, Bauman AE, Booth ML, Ainsworth BE, Sallis JF. International physical activity questionnaire: 12-Country reliability and validity. *Med Sci Sports Exerc.* 2003; **35**:1381–95.
5   Hurst P, Foad AJ, Coleman DA, Beedie C. Development and validation of the sports supplements beliefs scale. *Perform Enhanc Health.* 2017; 5:89–97.

6 Krumpal I. Determinants of social desirability bias in sensitive surveys: a literature review. *Qual Quant.* 2013; **47**:2025–47.

7 Cantrell MA, Lupinacci P. Methodological issues in online data collection. *J Adv Nurs.* 2007; **60**:544–9.

8 Edwards PJ, Roberts I, Clarke MJ, DiGuiseppi C, Wentz R, Kwan I and Pratap, S. Methods to increase response to postal and electronic questionnaires. *Cochr Database Syst Rev.* 2009, Issue 3. Art. No.: MR000008. DOI: 10.1002/14651858.MR000008.pub4.

11 Notes and tips on surveys

Philip Hurst and Stephen R. Bird

Chapter aims

The aims of this chapter are to introduce the reader to survey research and its application within health and physical activity. Depending on the reader's intended research
methods, it may be beneficial to read this chapter alongside Chapters 8–10 on observational studies, interviews and focus groups, and questionnaires, given that much of the
information presented in these chapters relates and informs the others to provide a more
comprehensive coverage. These chapters have been presented in this way to provide an
informative coverage of the topic without excessive duplication and repetition of material.

Introduction

A survey is a research tool that gathers information from a relatively large sample of
people to help provide inferences about a wider population. Survey data are cross-
sectional and can be collected in many formats, such as questionnaires, interviews
and focus groups. They are designed to provide a snapshot about a particular subject
at that particular time. Data obtained from these methods are essential to many types
of research in health and physical activity and offer the opportunity for innovative,
efficient and cost-effective research, which can help inform decisions in clinical and
applied settings.

Data collected from a survey can enable the researcher to: (1) determine whether
there are any associations between factors (e.g. exercise and gender); and (2) compare characteristics of different groups or situations (e.g. do females exercise more
than males?).

Surveys play a fundamental role in generating both quantitative and qualitative
data for health and physical activity. While researchers often favour the randomized
controlled trial (RCT) for its ability to determine cause and effect, surveys offer the
opportunity to generalize findings to a larger population – which is practically impossible to obtain via RCTs. Surveys are therefore a valuable research tool that can shape
policy guidelines and identify issues, and potential causes of physical activity and
health issues that may be further investigated via additional surveys or other techniques such as RCTs.

Designing the survey

The ultimate aim of a survey should be to gather valid, reliable, unbiased data from a
representative sample of participants.[1] While there is no universal recommendation

on best practice in respect to survey design, it is accepted that careful attention is given to how easy it is for respondents to understand and complete it. In short, the task required to interpret the survey and provide responses should be as easy as possible. Given this, the words used can significantly influence how well the reader will understand and interpret the questions on a survey. The use of jargon (i.e. any word or phrase that is difficult for a layperson to understand), such as medical terms, or abbreviations/acronyms, can influence the nature and quality of responses. For instance, LeBlanc et al.[2] reported that lay people may not understand common terms used in medical practice (e.g. malignant and tumour), and that ambiguous words such as 'growth' or 'ability' can be confusing for the reader.

Another factor argued to influence the quality and nature of responses is how long the survey takes to complete (otherwise known as response burden). It has often been suggested that if a survey takes longer to complete, it will result in lower response rates and reduced data quality. However, in a meta-analysis examining response rates and questionnaire length, Rolstad, Adler, and Rydén (2011)[3] indicated that response rates were not influenced by survey length but how easy it was to complete. Shorter questionnaires requiring more complex answers are more likely to have lower response rates than longer questionnaires with easier answer options. Thus, if a survey requires greater cognitive effort to complete, response rates and the quality of the data are more likely to be lower.

A survey will be designed on the basis of how it best answers the research question(s) and like other forms of research, will come to light from a literature search, previous research, a particular scenario and/or a need for an issue to be addressed. Furthermore, some consideration of how the data will be analysed will guide the study design (e.g. whether the data needs to be quantitative or qualitative). Indeed it is the relationship between the research question(s) and how best to answer it that will guide both data collection and how to interrogate the data. For this reason, it is important that the survey is carefully planned and piloted before any data are collected. The design, structure and order of questions can thus affect the responses obtained, and researchers should be aware of any biases that may influence responses. Further information regarding the design of other types of survey research is provided in the relevant chapters on interviews, focus groups and questionnaires.

The survey sample

Since most surveys will collect data from a proportion of a population (i.e. it would be impractical and unethical to collect data from every person of that population), a sample of the population has to be selected. To illustrate how this could be achieved, take the following hypothetical example. Public Health England wants to survey the physical activity levels of patients diagnosed with hypertension in the country. As it would be impractical and costly to survey every patient, a sample is selected. In this example, Public Health England could obtain a list of patients diagnosed with hypertension from hospitals in England and subsequently administer the survey to a proportion of this population.

The survey could also seek to determine whether there are differences between groups within a population. For example, this survey, which is targeted at hypertensives, is likely to include individuals who are aged between 18 and 80. In such cases the responses to questions on physical activity habits are likely to differ between an 18 year old and an 80 year old. Asking for key demographic data in the survey, such as age and gender, as well as other characteristics that may be pertinent to the topic being researched, enables important comparisons and may identify differences in physical activity levels between age groups, whereas aggregating the responses of all age groups may produce less meaningful data.

When defining the survey sample, it is important that the sample is representative of the larger population that it will infer too. If this is not achieved, accurate conclusions cannot be drawn about that population. In short, a sample should include participants who reflect the characteristics of that population, such as age, sex, BMI, disease history, socioeconomic status and others that may be relevant to the topic being investigated.

Recruiting a sample

A common issue within survey research is that those who are most likely to respond to it are those with an existing interest in the topic. Hence, even if researchers were to contact every person in their defined population, they may still get some bias in those who respond, unless they were to get a 100% response rate. In a more common scenario of researchers only having the capacity, time and resources to contact a sample of their defined population, they may need to take steps to ensure that it is representative. For these reasons, researchers need to consider the type of sampling strategy they use when recruiting.

Researchers can use two forms when recruiting a sample: random and non-random. Broadly speaking, surveys using quantitative methods will commonly use random sampling, for example when distributing a questionnaire to a sample of a larger population. Whereas surveys using qualitative methods such as focus groups and interviews commonly use non-random sampling. However, these distinctions are not absolute, nor are the quantitative and qualitative approaches solely used in questionnaires, focus groups and interviews. Indeed, a mixed-methods approach is often most informative.

Random sampling

Simple random sampling

The most common and stringent technique is simple random sampling. This should help to reduce the risk of bias within the sample at this stage, although as previously mentioned, bias may still occur through differing response rates. Using this method, participants are chosen by chance and the probability of a person being selected to the sample is equal for everyone. Using the Public Health England example above, after choosing the sample, each person could be given an ID number and random numbers are then selected for inclusion into the study. To randomly assign participants to the sample, a quick and cost-effective method could be to use an online, computer-generated software programme (e.g. www.randomizer.org/).

Stratified sampling

If the researcher was to use stratified sampling, they would divide the population into homogenous groups by factors, which are called strata (stratum is singular). The researcher would then separate the sample according to these factors and randomly select people from strata to be recruited to the study. The sample could be divided by a variety, or a combination of strata, such as gender, socioeconomic status and geographical location. For the Public Health England example, the researcher may divide the population into physical activity level and take a random sample from the stratum. For stratified sampling, it is important to note that the strata are representative of the entire population and that one person should not be included into multiple strata. If strata are overlapping, selection bias is increased as the probability of a person being selected is higher.

Cluster sampling

When a population is widely scattered, it may be difficult to select a sample that is representative of the population. Cluster sampling can combat this issue by dividing the entire population into 'clusters' or groups. These clusters can be divided by geographical areas, such as cities, schools, sports clubs and fitness groups. The clusters are chosen randomly and people within the clusters are sampled. Using the hypothetical example above, instead of sampling the entire population of England diagnosed with hypertension, the sample could be divided into clusters based on cities. The researcher would then randomly select a sample from within that cluster.

Non-random sampling

Non-random sampling purposefully targets people within a population. In qualitative research, this is often the most common form of sampling where participants who meet pre-selected inclusion criteria (e.g. age, gender, physical activity level) are recruited to the study. In survey research this is less common given that results from the data cannot be generalized beyond the sample. There are three main types: (1) *Convenience sampling*: researchers recruit anyone from the population if they are willing to take part in the research. (2) *Purposive sampling:* a population is identified and participants within this sample are recruited. (3) *Snowball sampling:* after a participant has completed the survey, the researcher may ask them to invite others to take part in the study.

Regardless of the type of sampling method used, researchers need to be aware of the strengths, weaknesses and statistical implications of each. All methods are not free of limitations. The aim of the researcher should be to use the most appropriate sampling method and ensure that the sample recruited is representative of the population they are inferring to.

Sample size

There is no definitive answer to what sample size is needed for survey research. As already suggested, the most representative sample would be one that included almost all members of a particular population group. However, to do this would be unethical, as the use of a sample that is larger than necessary is a waste of resources and participants' time, if the information collected could be obtained using a smaller sample size. On the other hand, the use of a sample that is smaller than necessary would provide uninformative results that do not reflect the population and may thereby also be a waste of resources and participants' time.

Researchers need to think pragmatically and consider what a reasonable level of representativeness and validity could be attained balanced against the amount of time and resources available. They will need to consider the study objectives and design, the anticipated endpoint, type of sampling used and the type of statistical analysis. There are methods by which a 'reasonable' sample size can be calculated and are akin to the statistical power calculations used in intervention studies. These calculations factor in the sampling error (i.e. the sample not being representative of the population), which will get smaller as the size of the sample gets closer to the whole population group. Statistical software such as G* power can be used to calculate sample size; however, if the researcher is unfamiliar with statistics a statistician should be consulted.

It is rare that everyone asked to complete the survey will actually complete it. Researchers should therefore anticipate non-responses in sample size calculations to ensure a sufficient sample size. The number of people who complete the survey as a proportion of the number of participants contacted or recruited should be reported in the results. While there is no agreed-upon standard for acceptable response rates for surveys, it has been suggested that an acceptable response is between 60% and 75%.[4] If response rates are lower than 60% it could be argued that the final sample may not reflect the population and indicate a higher likelihood of response bias. Researchers should therefore be aware that while a larger sample is desirable, high non-response rates can be more damaging to the credibility of the results than a smaller sample size.

In addition to the problems caused by potential bias resulting from some of the contacted sample not responding, further problems can arise if participants completing the questionnaire give responses that are what they deem to be socially desirable (i.e. participants present a favourable image of themselves). For example, participants responding to questions about physical activity levels may over-report how much they actually do, whereas questions about anti-social behaviours (e.g. drug use) may encourage participants to under-report their actual use. These types of surveys may therefore be susceptible to social desirability and affect the validity of the survey. To overcome these issues, researchers can use social desirability scales to detect and assess the extent of social desirable biases. Several social desirability scales have been developed since the first scale was published in 1957 (see Perinelli & Gremigni, 2016 for review)[5] with the most popular scales being the Marlowe Crowne Social Desirability Scale (MCSDS)[6] and the Social Desirability Scale-17 (SDS-17).[7]

Ethical considerations

Like any other form of research, surveys will need to be scrutinized by the relevant ethics committee before any data is collected. Researchers have an ethical duty to ensure they are respecting each respondent's autonomy when completing the survey and should ensure confidentiality of the data. Before a person completes a survey, they should be fully informed of the purpose of the study, including any risks and benefits, and consent to participate. Similarly, upon participation, persons should be made aware that they have the right to withdraw from the research without reprisal. This would be available to them throughout the stages of data collection, but not be possible after the data has been published – a point that may need to be stated in the information and consent documentation (see Chapter 7).

Particular concern is needed when involving vulnerable populations (e.g. children, people with learning difficulties or patients in care) and covering sensitive topics (e.g. body image). In these circumstances, researchers should ensure that participants from these groups are given ample opportunity to understand the nature, aims and anticipated outcomes of participation. For vulnerable groups, such as children, informed consent should be sought from persons legally responsible on their behalf. Parents or guardians should have the opportunity to understand what the research requires of their child and the benefits and risks associated with it. In cases involving sensitive topics, researchers should ensure to respect the privacy of participants and ensure that any information about them cannot be identifiable by other parties. Further information about the consent procedures for vulnerable populations and sensitive topics can be found on the American Psychological Association or British Psychological Society websites.

Reporting the results

Once the researcher has collected the data, they will need to consider how the data will be reported. Reporting the results of survey research should allow the reader to easily appraise whether or not the research is to have any impact on health and physical activity. For example, the results and reporting of survey research could allow other researchers to guide future investigations, applied practitioners to judge which treatment is best for their patients and policy makers to establish the best preventative and treatment strategies. Survey research therefore needs to be reported transparently so that the reader can follow what was planned, what method was used, what results were discovered and what conclusions can be made. To ensure clarity and appropriateness in the reporting of results, researchers should consider the STROBE (Strengthening the Reporting of Observational Studies in Epidemiology) statement, which consists of a 22-item checklist.[8]

Conclusion

Surveys allow the researcher to gather information from a relatively large sample of people to help provide inferences about a wider population. To ensure that the results from survey research are reliable and of quality, researchers need to maintain the same level of rigour as any other form of research. This requires systematic and thoughtful planning in the design, delivery and reporting of the survey. As mentioned in this chapter, there is no universal standard for best practice in respect to survey research, but there are certain steps that should be followed when sampling, designing and reporting the results. How this is achieved will depend on the aims of the research and the anticipated outcomes. In general, the aim of survey research should be to collect unbiased, valid and reliable data from a representative sample that can help provide further information about a wider population.

References

1   McColl E, Jacoby A, Thomas L, Soutter J, Bamford C, Steen N, et al. *Design and use of questionnaires: a review of best practice applicable to surveys of health service staff and patients. Health Technol Assess.* 2002; **5**(31):1–256.
2   LeBlanc TW, Hesson A, Williams A, Feudtner C, Holmes-Rovner M, Williamson LD, Ubel PA. Patient understanding of medical jargon: a survey study of us medical students. *Patient Educ Couns.* 2014; **95**:238–42.

3 Rolstad S, Adler J, Rydén A. Response burden and questionnaire length: is shorter better? A review and meta-analysis. *Value Health.* 2011; **14**:1101–8.

4 Draugalis JR, Coons SJ, Plaza CM. Best practices for survey research reports: a synopsis for authors and reviewers. *Am J Pharm Educ.* 2008; **72**:11.

5 Perinelli E, Gremigni P. Use of social desirability scales in clinical psychology: a systematic review. *J Clin Psychol.* 2016; **72**:534–51.

6 Crowne DP, Marlowe D. A new scale of social desirability independent of psychopathology. *J Cons Psychol.* 1960; **24**:349.

7 Stöber J. The social desirability scale-17 (Sds-17): convergent validity, discriminant validity, and relationship with age. *Eur J Psychol Assess.* 2001; **17**:222.

8 Von Elm E, Altman DG, Egger M, Pocock SJ, Gøtzsche PC, Vandenbroucke JP. The strengthening the reporting of observational studies in epidemiology (Strobe) statement: guidelines for reporting observational studies. *Int J Surg.* 2014; **12**:1495–9.

12 Qualitative research in physical activity and health

Brett Smith and Cassandra Phoenix

Aims of the chapter

The purpose of this chapter is to introduce the reader to qualitative research. The first section highlights the basic aims of qualitative research and the epistemological and ontological assumptions that guide it. The second section highlights various qualitative approaches. Section three and four focuses on methods of data collection and analysis. The final section attends to how we might judge the quality of qualitative research. Illustrative examples of qualitative research from the field of physical activity and health are provided throughout.

What is qualitative research?

Aims of inquiry, ontology and epistemology

Qualitative research is an umbrella term for capturing a complex, expansive, and continuously evolving field of inquiry, approaches, methods, and judgement criteria. As a field of inquiry, it aims to understand people's experiences and language use. Qualitative research also seeks to understand the meanings people themselves ascribe to events, thoughts, emotions, feelings, situations, behaviours, social relationships, and the material world as well as how matter acts and how material-discursive forces are co-implicated in what people can do.[1,2] For example, when interested in a topic like postpartum women and physical activity, qualitative methods could be used to produce rich and in-depth understandings of females' experiences of becoming physically active, the ways they talk about activity during social interactions, the meanings they give to their body, health, and family relationships, and how the material acts to constrain and open up different ways of becoming physically active.

Qualitative research can be further described through the ontological and epistemological beliefs that guide and serve as the substructure of any piece of research.[3] Ontology is a belief system that is concerned with the question, "What is the form and nature of reality and, thus, what is there that can be known about it?" Rather than believing that there is a singular truth that can be found independent of us and, however subtle or approximate, can be known (known as realism), ontologically qualitative researchers most often believe that there are multiple truths and our social reality is dependent on us. Epistemology is a belief system about the relationship between the inquirer and the known. Qualitative researchers largely hold to epistemological constructionism. That means they believe that the researcher inescapably influences the research and, no matter how hard one tries, the methods used are not objective or neutral. Thus, for qualitative researchers theory-free knowledge is a chimera and knowledge is not discovered but socially constructed. The ontological and epistemological beliefs a researcher holds, either knowingly or unknowingly, cannot be ignored. That is because these beliefs underpin and inform the whole of the research, from start to finish. For example, and as alluded to in examples below, our ontological and epistemological beliefs guide what questions can be created and answered, how the research is designed, the ethical practices engaged with, how methods are used, and how validity, reliability and generalizability are understood.

Qualitative approaches

Qualitative research can also be understood as an umbrella term for a wide variety of traditions or approaches. For instance, researchers who have studied health and physical activity have used ethnography,[3] different types of grounded theory,[4,5] differing forms of phenomenology, such as Interpretative Phenomenological Analysis,[6] and narrative research.[7] Community based participatory action research (CBPAR) is another qualitative approach that researchers in health and physical activity might utilize. CBPAR refers to scholarly work undertaken in partnership with communities.[8] The aim is to deliver useful solutions to problems that communities themselves have identified and to facilitate positive changes around, for example, the health and physical activity participation of local people.

Though CBPAR has been less commonly used in physical activity, a growing number of scholars have highlighted why this approach is valuable and, whilst never guaranteed, can work to improve health. The reasons for this lie in the characteristics of what constitutes CBPAR, which include the researcher: working *with* people *in* the community, rather than *on* them inside a setting *divorced* from their everyday lives (e.g. a university laboratory); engaging in grassroots participation, wherein community members bring forward their experiential knowledge and inform a locally resonant research agenda; they commit extensive time to each project (often years); working iteratively and fluidly with methods that favour local behaviours and affect, rather than using a rigid, linear, and controlled research design; seeking long-lasting solutions that are delivered by the community in a self-sustaining way; and eventually stepping back and then away from the research so that the work is left in the hands of the community.[9] Together, the aforementioned characteristics of CBPAR provide a very strong platform and means to make a difference in the long-term to people's health and quantity and quality of physical activity. One example of CBPAR can be found in the work of Robertson et al.[10] on health, men, and physical activity. A thematic analysis (see below) of the qualitative interview data revealed that building and sustaining trust amongst people was vital for positive physical activity change. In their analysis Robertson et al. also highlighted the various mechanisms that facilitated change. These were the physically vibrant and socially enjoyable aspects of being active with other people, the emotional space for reflection created during the project, and the improved self-efficacy-generating enthusiasm for further change.

Collecting qualitative data

A further way to understand what is qualitative research is to focus on the methods used. Methods include the techniques used for data collection and analysis. With regard to data collection, semi-structured interviews are the most commonly used within qualitative research. A detailed overview of interviewing that incorporates the various types of interview now available (e.g. mobile and internet interviewing), tips on how to interview well (e.g. on active listening), responses to commonly asked questions (e.g. how do you know your participant is telling the truth), and the problems that can arise when using interviewing and how to deal with these (e.g. a failure to consider interviews as social interaction) can be found in Smith and Sparkes.[11] Regarding interviews, Smith and McGannon also highlighted a misunderstanding frequently made in physical activity, sport and health research.[12] They noted that in many 'limitations' section within a qualitative research paper the authors state that recall bias or memory distortion is a limitation of interviewing. However, as Smith and McGannon argued,[12] for most qualitative researchers this is not the case. For example, epistemologically it is recognized that memories are partly socially constructed, knowledge is always historically contingent and partial, people's perceptions change and contradict, and our discourses constitute and become experience rather than transparently reflecting experiences. Thus, recall bias or memory distortion is not a limitation of interviewing but simply part of what is means to be a finite human.

Of course, some researchers might disagree with all this and still believe that recall bias or member recall is a problem of interviewing. However, as Smith and McGannon add,[12] to write in a paper that bias or memory recall is a limitation reflects a poor decision from the researcher to choose interviewing. *If* they do believe that a problem or limitation of interviews is bias or memory recall then they should not have chosen interviewing when considering which method to use from the start. Instead, *if* a researcher believes that a problem or limitation of interviews is bias or memory recall, then they should have chosen to collect naturalistic data (i.e. data that is generated without the influence of the researcher) from the start. The 'problem' and 'limitations' then lies with the methodological decision making of the researcher. Such issues are important to note because not only would many researchers argue that bias or memory recall are not limitations when using interviews.[11,12] It is also important because when it comes to collecting quality qualitative data via interviewing a researcher needs to appreciate that interviews are more than just a method. It is a craft that takes time to learn well, much practice, and deep intellectual engagement. As part of all this, researchers need to understand that to collect high quality data it can be useful to interview people extensively and multiple times, rather than use the typical 'drive-by-interview' (i.e. interviewing a person just once and for a short time, (e.g. 40 minutes).[11]

Whilst interviews are most commonly used to collect qualitative data, there are numerous other data collection methods available to researchers interested in physical activity and health. These include participant observation, media material, artefacts, diaries, autobiographies, and vignettes.[2] Another way to collect data is through visual methods, such as autophotography.[13] Autophotography, or what is sometimes called photovoice, refers to a method in which the participants take photographs that represent their senses of self, emotions, behaviours, or, for example, who they are in relation to a given phenomenon or topic (e.g. "what physical activity as a disabled youth means to me"). The photographs produced can be used as data in their own right, by which it is meant that the researcher can analyse each photograph taken. Alternatively, photographs can be used as a photo-elicitation device. This involves using the photographs participants have taken to elicit additional information, deeper thoughts, and more immediate feelings about a certain topic. They may also be used to help translate knowledge and engage the public.

Digital qualitative methods are a further way to collect data. Mindful of ethical dilemmas plus the digital divide, researchers might leverage the possibilities of collecting data using web-based and mobile technologies like email groups, websites, blogs, Facebook, Twitter and a multitude of other digital platforms.[14] A recent example of the use of digital methods within the context of health, sport and physical activity, and one that also is grounded in CBPAR, can be found in Bundon and Smith,[15] and Smith et al.[16] Adopting new technologies does not mean that traditional ways of collecting data, such as by interviewing, need to be jettisoned. For instance, in their physical activity and health research Bell et al.[17] asked participants to carry a small Global Positioning System (GPS) unit to gain insights into the locations of activity and to later use as an elicitation device to gather high quality data from interviews. The integrated location/activity data were first mapped with a Geographical Information System (Quantum GIS v.1.8, www.qgis.org) to provide a visual representation of participants' routine place interactions, depicting location and relative levels of physical activity. The subsequent personalized map – a geo-narrative – created was then used in interviews (including mobile interviews) to elicit talk and engage participants in the interpretation of their own GPS activity maps. Bell et al. noted numerous benefits of using such a geo-narrative map, including how it encouraged detailed accounts of participant's physical activity experiences in their own terms, offering subjective insights into participants' shifting wellbeing needs and priorities, and the ways in which they sought to meet them through diverse local place interactions. The maps provided a visual aid to discuss the importance of participants' routine, often pre-reflective practices.

Analysing qualitative data

Just as there are multiple traditions and data collection strategies, there are also various ways in which a qualitative researcher might analyse qualitative data.[18] These include a phenomenological analysis, grounded theory analysis, narrative analysis, critical discourse analysis, conversation analysis, and a meta-synthesis of qualitative research.[2] Given the value to develop health policy and provide more complex understanding of health, researchers might also consider an analysis of 'exceptions', as shown in the work on physical activity, ageing and health by Phoenix and Orr.[18] Another analysis available is the version of a thematic analysis as described by Braun et al.[19] As articulated by them, a thematic analysis is a "method for identifying patterns ('themes') in a data set, and for describing and interpreting the meaning and importance of those" (p. 191). In terms of how to do a thematic analysis, Braun et al. describe the process as involving several phases. These are summarized as follows:

Phase 1: *Familiarization*: That is the process of immersing oneself in your data, so that you become intimately familiar it. What this practically involves is reading and re-reading all data items, and making notes about what interests you. The aim is to get to really 'know' the data set and to engage with the data as data rather than as information. By this Braun et al. mean that the researcher reads the data analytically, looking for ideas and concepts that can help address the research question, and reading it in a curious and questioning way.

Phase 2: *Coding*: This phase turns familiarization into a systematic and thorough process. A code identifies and labels something of interest in the data – at a semantic and/or a latent level – that is of potential relevance to the research question (although it needs noting that in qualitative research the research question can evolve and be refined throughout the analytic process). The practical process of coding involves closely reading the data, and 'tagging' with a code each piece that has some relevance to the research question. That can be done in various ways (e.g. pen and paper, using a computer programme). Text can be tagged with one or more codes or it can be left untagged if irrelevant. The researcher systematically works through each data item and each new relevant extract of text is coded. It is important to keep coding flexible, open and inclusive, as the themes that might finally be are not yet known. An example of coding using physical activity data can be found in Braun et al.[19]

Phase 3: *Theme development*: This process is about clustering codes to identify 'higher level' patterns, which refers to meanings that are broader and capture more than one very specific idea. Here a theme is more than just some coherent, patterned meaning across a data set. A theme also describes something important about the data, relevant to the research question. Start the theme development process first with just the codes. This active process involves the researcher identifying ways to cluster the codes together around some (bigger) meaning or concept each all share. Not all codes need to be included in these clusters; some will not fit. Once you have some provisional or candidate themes (there is no right or wrong number, but generally you want more than one, and probably less than six), you start a process of review. An example from physical activity of theme development can be found in Braun *et al.*[19]

Phase 4: *Review themes*: Reviewing involves working with the coded data, and then going back to the whole data set. The process is about checking whether your analysis 'fits well' with the data. Revision can range from small tweaks to a complete restart of the analysis if the review raises problems. In reviewing a researcher needs to consider: (a) Does each theme have a central organizing concept so that all the data and codes cohere around a single important analytic point? (b) Is the concept of each theme distinct? (c) What are the relationships, interconnections and boundaries between the themes? and (d) Do the themes together tell a coherent and compelling story of the data, which addresses the research question? To help with reviewing and exploring and revising the relationships between candidate themes, the researcher might use visual tools like a thematic map. An example of a thematic map can be found in Braun et al.[19]

Phase 5: *Naming themes*: Once the researcher is confident that the analysis captures the data content well, addresses the research question, and is well mapped out, the themes need defining and a rich analytic narrative built. A theme definition is a brief description (a paragraph or two), which succinctly captures the 'essence' of each theme (its central organizing concept), and its scope and boundaries. Creating an analytic narrative involves not just producing a description of the theme, but also an interpretative commentary that is presented to the reader.

Phase 6: *Writing the report*: It first needs recognizing that writing in qualitative research does not happen after the analysis; it is not a 'mopping up' activity. In qualitative research writing is a form of analysis and occurs throughout the research. With that in mind, the last analytical phase involves compiling, developing, and editing existing analytic writing, and situating it within an overall report. It also involves determining a good balance between data extracts and analytic commentary. Too much data in the final report will mean the analysis is likely to be thin and confined to the most obvious observations. Good data extracts are ones that clearly and compellingly demonstrate the relevant analytic point or feature. The analytic commentary avoids summarizing the theme/data. It tells an interpretative story about the data and what it means, often in critical ways, by drawing on different theories, and in a compelling manner. Qualitative researchers, partly because of their commitment to a constructionist epistemology, are also happy to write in the 'first person'. They believe that attempts to write the researcher out of the final report is rhetorical strategy to create the illusion of objectivity.

Judging the quality of qualitative research

With regard to seeking reliability, qualitative research on health and physical activity has most often employed the technique known as inter-rater reliability. That method first involves two or more capable researchers operating in isolation from each other to independently code data without negotiation. It then involves the same researchers coming together to compare codes and reconciling through discussion whatever coding discrepancies they may have for the same unit of text. When a high level of agreement/consensus is demonstrated at the end of this process, the coding is deemed reliable. Despite being widely used, inter-rater reliability is however ineffective for reliability purposes. In their review of rigour, and drawing on numerous scholars, Smith and McGannon highlight why this is the case and why inter-rater reliability as traditionally used cannot work. It is therefore strongly recommended that this technique be dropped within physical activity and health research.[12] Following numerous other scholars, Smith and McGannon also highlighted that, for very good reasons they outline in detail, researchers doing qualitative research drop a concern with reliability and move instead toward developing rigour via, for instance, critical friends.[12]

Whilst for qualitative researchers reliability is not a relevant concern, generalizability is often of relevance. However, rather aiming to make *statistical* generalizations, what qualitative researchers often seek are different forms of generalizability. For example, given the aims, epistemology, ontology, and research methods used, qualitative researchers tend to work with *naturalistic* generalizations, whereby personal experience is presented in a way that readers are able to empathize or resonate with that experience. Here, the researcher is required to provide readers with rich, thick-descriptions of the case under study so that *the readers themselves* can reflect upon it and make connections to their own situations, or one's they have witnessed. Other types of generalizability that researchers might seek include *analytical* generalization, *transferability*, and/or *generativity* (see Sparkes & Smith, 2014).[3]

Just as generalizability means something different in qualitative research when compared to quantitative research, validity also means something different. What qualitative researchers ask is "How can a researcher distinguish a 'good' study from a 'bad' one?" and "What counts as quality research?"[20] A common response within the context of physical activity and health response is to adopt what has been variously described as a foundational, universal or criteriology approach via the criteria proposed by Lincoln and Guba.[21] However, just like inter-rater reliability, their work has now come to be seen as deeply flawed and incompatible with the guiding assumptions of qualitative research.[22] As such, research using qualitative research methods need to move past Lincoln and Guba and adopt a different approach to validity.[21]

One useful approach to understanding validity in qualitative research is through a relativist/non-foundational approach.[20] In this approach researchers do *not* seek to propose a set of *universal* criteria that can be applied to *all* qualitative research. Rather, they develop and use *lists of criteria* when thinking about how to judge their own and others' research.[3,9] This list is ongoing. It can be added to, subtracted from, and modified in light of what specific research one is doing or judging. For example, depending on the purpose of the research, researchers – including reviewers – might decide to use the following list of criteria to judge the quality of the research: substantive contribution (what the research offers); the time spent with participants (credibility); the comprehensiveness of evidence (the data offered); the way different parts of the interpretation create a complete and meaningful picture (coherence); and impact (did the research generate new questions or make a difference in society). That list is not, we should repeat, set in stone nor should be applied to all qualitative research. A list can be changed and modified within the context of actual practices/applications. Thus, as Sparkes and Smith note,[22] it is vitally important that researchers undertaking qualitative research, or judging it, take the responsibility to appreciate the growing lists of criteria being created within the field of qualitative research if qualitative research is to be judged fairly and standards remain high.

Conclusion

This chapter has provided a flavour of what qualitative research looks like and how it might be done. Whilst brief, and mindful that we could not cover all developments in the field, like how qualitative research is generating impact,[23,24] and how knowledge is effectively being translated to diverse audiences,[7,24] we have offered a contemporary resource for readers to consider using when thinking about doing qualitative research. Rather than simply borrowing by default what researchers have done in the past, and too often perpetuating problems with certain methods,[12] we also hope that readers might delve into new books dedicated to qualitative research as well as the international journals devoted to the topic, like *Qualitative Research, Qualitative Inquiry,* and *Qualitative Research in Sport, Exercise and Health.* There is much exciting work being done! We hope you might be part of the exciting future of qualitative research.

References

1 Fullagar S. Post-qualitative inquiry and the new materialist turn: implications for sport, health and physical culture research. *Qual Res Sport, Exerc Health.* 2017; **9**:247–57.

2 Smith B, Sparkes AC, editors. *Routledge handbook of qualitative research methods in sport and exercise.* London: Routledge; 2016.

3 Sparkes AC, Smith B. *Qualitative research methods in sport, exercise and health. From Process to product.* London: Routledge; 2014.

4 Holt NL. Doing grounded theory in sport and exercise. In: Smith B, Sparkes AC, editors. *Routledge handbook of qualitative research in sport and exercise.* London: Routledge; 2016. pp. 24–36.

5 Weed M. Capturing the essence of grounded theory: the importance of understanding commonalities and variants. *Qual Res Sport Exerc Health.* 2017; **9**:149–56.

6 Smith J. Interpretative phenomenological analysis in sport and exercise: getting at experience. In: Smith B, Sparkes AC, editors. *Routledge handbook of qualitative research methods in sport and exercise.* London: Routledge; 2016. pp. 219–29.

7 Smith B, Tomasone J, Latimer-Cheung A, Martin Gins K. Narrative as a knowledge translation tool for facilitating impact: translating physical activity knowledge to disabled people and health professionals. *Health Psychol.* 2015; **34**:303–13.

8   Schinke RJ, Blodgett AT. Embarking on community based participatory action research: a methodology that emerges from (and in) communities. In: Smith B, Sparkes AC, editors. *Routledge handbook of qualitative research in sport and exercise.* London: Routledge; 2016.

9   Schinke R, Smith B, McGannon KR. Pathways for community research in sport and physical activity: criteria for consideration. *Qual Res Sport Exerc Health.* 2013; **5**:460–8.

10 Robertson S, Zwolinsky S, Pringle A, McKenna J, Daly-Smith A, White A. 'It is fun, fitness and football really': a process evaluation of a football-based health intervention for men. *Qual Res Sport Exerc Health.* 2013; **5**: 419–39. (pp. 88–99). London: Routledge.

11 Smith B, Sparkes AC. Interviews: qualitative interviewing in the sport and exercise sciences. In: Smith B, Sparkes AC, editors. *Routledge handbook of qualitative research methods in sport and exercise.* London: Routledge; 2016. pp. 103–23.

12 Smith B, McGannon KR. Developing rigor in qualitative research: problems and opportunities within sport and exercise psychology. *Int Rev Sport Exerc Psychol.* 11(1), 101–121. DOI: 10.1080/1750984X.2017.1317357

13 Phoenix C, Rich E. Visual research methods. In: Smith B, Sparkes AC, editors. *Routledge handbook of qualitative research methods in sport and exercise.* London: Routledge; 2016. pp. 139–51.

14 Bundon A. The web and digital qualitative methods: researching online and researching the online in sport and exercise studies. In: Smith B, Sparkes AC, editors. *Routledge handbook of qualitative research in sport and exercise.* London: Routledge; 2016. pp. 355–67.

15 Bundon A, Smith B. From inspired to inspiring: community-based research, digital storytelling, and a networked Paralympic Movement. In: Gair S, van Luyn A, editors. *Sharing qualitative research: showing lived experiences and community narratives.* London: Routledge; 2017. pp. 10–24.

16 Smith B, Bundon A, Best M. Disability sport and activist identities: a qualitative study of narratives of activism among elite athletes with impairment. *Psychol Sport Exerc.* 2016; **26**:139–48.

17 Bell SL, Phoenix C, Lovell R, Wheeler BW. Using GPS and geo-narratives: a methodological approach for understanding and situating everyday green space encounters. *Area.* 2015; **47**:88–96.

18 Phoenix C, Orr N. Analysing *exceptions* within qualitative data: promoting analytical diversity to advance knowledge of ageing and physical activity. *Qual Res Sport Exerc Health.* 2017; **9**:271–84.

19 Braun V, Clarke V, Weate P. Using thematic analysis in sport and exercise research. In: Smith B, Sparkes AC, editors. *Routledge handbook of qualitative research in sport and exercise.* London: Routledge; 2016. pp. 191–205.

20 Burke S. Rethinking 'validity' and 'trustworthiness' in qualitative inquiry: how might we judge the quality of qualitative research in sport and exercise sciences? In: Smith B, Sparkes AC, editors. *Routledge handbook of qualitative research in sport and exercise.* London: Routledge; 2016. pp. 330–39.

21 Lincoln YS, Guba EG. *Naturalistic inquiry.* Beverly Hills, CA: Sage; 1985. Kay T. Knowledge, not numbers: qualitative research and impact in sport, exercise and health. In: Smith B, Sparkes AC, editors. *Routledge handbook of qualitative research in sport and exercise.* London: Routledge; 2016. pp. 424–37.

22 Sparkes AC, Smith B. Judging the quality of qualitative inquiry: criteriology and relativism in action. *Psychol Sport Exerc.* 2009; **10**:491–7.

23 Kay T. Knowledge, not numbers: qualitative research and impact in sport, exercise and health. In: Smith B, Sparkes AC, editors. *Routledge handbook of qualitative research methods in sport and exercise.* London: Routledge; 2016. pp. 424–37.

24 Smith, B. Sporting spinal cord injuries, social relations, and rehabilitation narratives: an ethnographic creative non-fiction of becoming disabled through sport. *Sociol Sport J.* 2013; **30**:132–52.

13 Intervention studies, training studies and determining the acute responses to bouts of exercise

Stephen R. Bird and Catherine Woods

Aims of the chapter

- To introduce research methods that may be used to assess the impact of exercise/ physical activity interventions, including those seeking behaviour change.
- To outline the methods used to determine the effects of exercise training on indicators of health.
- To describe the research designs that may be used to assess the acute short-term responses and effects of a single bout of exercise.
- To provide an insight into the factors that need to be considered when designing such studies and how to ensure the attainment of valid, reliable and high-quality data.

Introduction

Whereas observational and cross-sectional studies that compare participants following different lifestyles can identify an association between health and physical activity (PA), as well as factors that are linked to PA participation, they do not provide direct evidence of proof that a particular factor 'causes' greater PA participation, or it was the PA that caused any of the observed difference in health. This is because there may be other factors linked to PA participation, and it could be these rather than the PA that result in improved health. For example, it could be that healthy people are more likely to have a healthy diet and it's the healthy diet that is important for health, with physical activity having no effect, but being associated with health through its association with healthy eating. Similarly, cross-sectional studies do not prove the direction of cause and effect, for example, it could be that healthy people are more likely to exercise, rather than physical activity participation improving health. Consequently, whilst observational and cross-sectional studies are valuable in identifying aspects of interest and potential health factors, it is necessary to undertake physical activity intervention studies to establish cause and effect, as these will identify which factors cause changes in PA participations, and likewise training studies are needed to identify which indicators of health change when a person participates in regular exercise. Examples of these could be assessing whether the use of 'activity monitors, increases PA participation', or whether regular walking sessions improve insulin sensitivity, muscle strength, cholesterol concentrations or self-efficacy.

Terminology used in this chapter

In this chapter we will include examples of research study designs that may be used to investigate: (i) how to increase participation in physical activity; (ii) the effects of a prescribed exercise programme and (iii) the acute effects of a single bout of exercise. For clarity we will use the following terminology. The term 'intervention study' will be used to describe interventions that investigate how to increase the amount of physical activity undertaken by participants. There are many forms of intervention study, but in the context of physical activity research, this could be in the form of receiving guidance, encouragement, assessment or support that is intended to increase the level of physical activity. The term 'training study' will be used when referring to studies that are investigating the effects of undertaking a prescribed and specified programme of regular exercise, such as a walking or gym-based programs, and the term 'acute study' will be used when investigating the effects of a single bout of exercise. We recognize that these terms are not exclusive and some research may include components of each, also that other terms may be used elsewhere in the literature, and we emphasize that our choice of terms and their use here is for the purpose of clarity within this chapter.

Designing an intervention, training or acute study

The process of undertaking an intervention, training or acute study will follow the general scheme of: (i) identifying the research question to be addressed; (ii) formulating the research and null hypothesis; (iii) designing the study; (iv) gaining ethical approval; (v) recruiting participants and collecting the data; (vi) analysing the data; (vii) submitting the findings for peer-review, in the form of a manuscript, poster or oral presentation and (viii) presenting/publishing the research. This chapter will focus on the design of the study, while other chapters within this text deal with the other stages of the process.

Having identified the research question to be addressed and stated the research and null hypotheses, the researcher(s) has to design a study that will test these hypotheses in an unbiased and scientific manner. In doing so the research questions will be used to inform the design, but may also be revisited and amended if required. Throughout the study it is useful for the researcher(s) to refer back to the hypotheses at various times to ensure that the research remains targeted on addressing the key questions. For reporting your intervention description and development you may wish to consult 'TiDier', this template for intervention description and replication provides a checklist for researchers.[1,2]

Acute, intervention and training study designs

Acute study designs

The optimal design of studies assessing acute responses to single bouts of exercise is likely to differ from those investigating the effects of behavioural interventions or exercise training. This is because in acute studies involving a single bout of exercise, the effects are likely to last for a relatively short duration, and with the inclusion of a 'wash-out' period of a few days, any short-term effects are likely to have been fully reversed and the participant returned to their baseline values. For example the effects of a single bout of exercise on insulin sensitivity, which may increase for 48 hours after the bout of exercise, but typically returns to baseline within a week. In these circumstances it may be possible to use a cross-over design (Figure 13.1), in which the individual acts as their own control, thereby strengthening the statistical analyses and

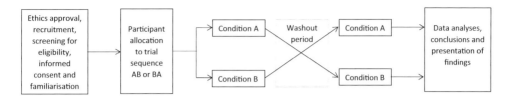

Figure 13.1 Possible design for an acute study (cross-over design).

reducing the number of participants needed to meet the required statistical power (see Chapter 17). In this design a 'control' trial is included for comparison with the exercise trial. In the above example the control trial may require the participants to go to the same location as the exercise trial, complete all pre-exercise assessments and then sit and relax for the same duration as the exercise bout, before undergoing all post-exercise assessments. This design enables any changes that occur in the exercise trial to be compared with any changes that may occur in the non-exercise control trial. Without the control trial data it is not possible to conclusively say that changes that occurred during the exercise trial were due to the exercise. For example the changes could have been due to the time elapsed since the participants' last meal. In which case, any differences between the pre-exercise and post-exercise data should be evident in both the exercise trial and the non-exercise control trial. Whereas changes that are only evident in the pre v post data of the exercise trial, and not evident in the control trial, can be attributed to the bout of exercise. The same principles would apply if only small changes in a factor such as blood pressure were seen in the non-exercise trial but significantly larger changes in blood pressure were evident in the exercise trial. Whereby the magnitude of the change could be attributed to the exercise bout.

The cross-over design is a strong design as it enables a participant's data from the exercise intervention trial to be compared with their own data from the non-exercise control trial, using statistical tests such as 'paired *t* tests' or 'Repeated measures ANOVA', see Chapter 17. In doing so it ameliorates many of the effects of individual differences and individual variability from the analyses, and reduces the number of participants that would be needed in the study if participants only undertook either the exercise or the non-exercise control condition.

Intervention and training study designs

Depending on the research question a researcher may wish to develop an intervention to increase minutes of moderate or vigorous intensity physical activity in a specific population, such as older adults or young children. This intervention will require a theoretical framework, a mode of delivery and detailed baseline and follow-up measures to determine the effectiveness of the intervention, but also to explore change in the factors responsible for any change in behaviour. For example, it may be theorized that an individual's minutes of moderate to vigorous physical activity will increase as a result of being exposed to an intervention, and it might be hypothesized that this is because the intervention participants had higher exercise self-efficacy than those who did not receive the intervention. Therefore, measures of exercise self-efficacy as well as physical activity will need to be included in the study. There are several stages to intervention design, ideally these include a literature review followed by formative research where the theoretically informed intervention ideas are tested with the target group. Following analysis of this data, the participant feedback can be used to improve the final intervention design. Depending on the time and resources available, the complexity of interventions designed to meet the same outcome, such as 'increase in minutes of moderate to vigorous physical activity (MVPA)', varies enormously, see Walsh et al., 2018[3] and Mutrie et al., 2012[4] for examples. Alternatively the researcher may wish to design a training study to assess the impact of increasing the frequency, intensity, duration or type of exercise over a period of hours, days or weeks. Here again, the design of the study will need to be informed from a review of the literature that provides the rationale for the likely efficacy of the training, along with insights into the target population.

In intervention and chronic training studies that aim to produce behaviour change and/or exercise-induced health benefits, any effects are liable to remain evident for a prolonged duration of weeks or months. Consequently, a cross-over design is not possible without a very prolonged wash-out, possibly lasting months, which makes it unpractical. Also, in an intervention study designed to change physical activity behaviour we need to limit the likelihood that factors outside of the intervention are responsible for behaviour change and with a long 'wash-out' period the risk of other factors contaminating the research increases. For example if during your intervention the Department of Health ran a public education campaign encouraging people to become more active. Consequently, since a cross-over design is usually impractical, the research design for intervention and training studies usually entails the inclusion of a separate control group (Figure 13.2). As a consequence it is common for a greater number of participants to be required, although this would also depend on the factor being assessed, how variable it is and the likely magnitude of change. The same would apply to studies in which different exercise regimens are being compared. A calculation of the number of participants that need to be recruited can be undertaken in the form of a statistical power analyses, which is undertaken once the study design has been outlined; for details see Chapter 17.

Some aspects of health, such as insulin sensitivity exhibit both acute short-term responses to a bout of exercise as well as chronic training effects. So when analysing the effects of training it is necessary to exclude any acute effects from the last exercise bout, before attributing the magnitude of any change to a training effect. This may be achieved by asking the participants to refrain from exercise for a few days prior to their post-training assessments.

Factors to consider and control when designing acute, intervention and training studies

Inclusion and exclusion criteria, recruitment, group allocation and matching

Inclusion and exclusion criteria

The type of participants recruited into a study will be determined by the topic being investigated. As a consequence the inclusion/exclusion criteria may include factors such as age, sex, health status or pre-existing disease and current levels of physical activity. All of which may be assessed via a questionnaire that's administered as part

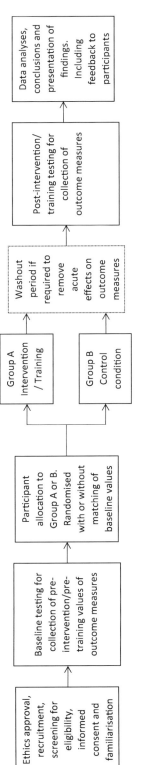

Figure 13.2 Possible design for an intervention or training study – Randomized Controlled Trial (RCT). Where Group A and B undergo different interventions. For example, A could be an intervention to improve physical activity or a prescribed exercise programme, whilst B could be the 'control' condition, which could be no exercise programme or 'normal care' in a health context. Alternatively in studies that are comparing different interventions Group A and Group B would experience different interventions. Other research designs may compare more intervention variations and thereby require additional groups (C, D, etc) at the 'intervention or training stage'.

122 *Stephen R. Bird and Catherine Woods*

of the recruitment process, and/or confirmed by some other data, such as blood test results or accelerometer data. These are important, since for example, a study investigating the potential effects of becoming less sedentary requires participants who are sedentary at the commencement of the study. If such studies were to include non-sedentary individuals, much if not all of the potential changes to health would already exist in these participants at the time of their recruitment and hence the intervention is unlikely to induce much, if any further change, thus falsely giving the impression of the activity being of no benefit to sedentary individuals. Alternatively the presence of pre-existing injury or illness could be an inclusion requirement, or an exclusion factor, depending on the nature of the study and the research question under investigation. So a person may be excluded if they have an existing injury that prevents them from completing the prescribed exercise regimen or alternatively it could be an essential inclusion criterion if the research is investigating the effects of a particular exercise rehabilitation programme or exercise programme for secondary prevention. For an example of this process see Table 13.1.

The recruitment process

The process of recruitment will need to be approved by the relevant ethics committee, and may involve posters, newspaper advertisements, television, radio, phone calls, letters or social media. In some cases these advertisements will reach many members of society, with only some being eligible to participate. Alternatively the recruitment process may be more targeted and use existing databases, such as those kept by hospitals or other organizations involved with health and specific diseases. Again, ethical

Table 13.1 Examples of inclusion and exclusion criteria that may be applied for an exercise training study to improve muscle strength and power in adults aged over 60 years

Inclusion criteria	Exclusion criteria

• Men and women aged > 60 years
• Ability to understand verbal instructions in English
• Ability to understand the concept of written informed consent – could be through an interpreter
• Able to attend exercise facility 3 times a week for 12 weeks
• Able to participate in ambulatory strength training programme
• Perceived good general health or stable medicated control of condition, includes diabetes
	• Musculoskeletal injury that would prevent participation in the prescribed strength training programme
	• Disease that would limit exercise tolerance or present more than negligible risk to participating in exercise programme
	  ○ Severe chronic obstructive pulmonary disease
	  ○ Severe cardiac disease
	• Recent (4 weeks) severe illness
	• Mental illness that would limit ability to participate in prescribed exercise programme
	• Currently taking medication that would limit exercise participation and/or adaptations to exercise training
	• Undertaken a strength training programme in the past 12 months

approval is essential since there are issues of privacy associated with such databases, some of which will have built in checks about whether a person is willing to be contacted by researchers.

If expressing an interest and meeting the criteria for participation in the study, the participant will need to be fully informed of the aims of the study, what's expected of them, and any potential risks or discomfort they may experience. If in agreement, they will then sign the form, as will the researchers: this may also need to be witnessed, and both the participant and researcher(s) will retain a copy of the signed form. At this point it is also important to remember that anyone volunteering to participate in the study will have been interested in the work and may be disappointed if not included, whether due to the inclusion/exclusion criteria or the required number of participants already being achieved. Hence the researchers need to sensitively respond to those who are not enrolled in the study and thank them for their interest.

Deception, such as concealing the true nature of the study, is rarely used, but if it is included within the design, its necessity would have been judged by the relevant ethics committee, and approval will only be given if the value of the study was deemed sufficient to warrant its use.

The required number of recruited participants

The number of participants recruited into a study will depend upon the outcome measures, variability within the population, the magnitude of any expected change induced by the intervention and the precise design of the study, all of which can be factored into a statistical power analyses, which is covered in Chapter 17. A factor to be considered when recruiting and later when analysing the data is the potential for change to occur. For example, participants with existing good healthy blood lipid profiles at the commencement of the study may have less capacity to change than those who commence the study with poor lipid profiles. When calculating the number of participants required, the researcher(s) will also need to factor in the likelihood that some will 'drop out' before the end of the study, and as a consequence the researchers will need to recruit additional participants, so that the required number complete the study and it's not left statistically underpowered. The exact number likely to drop out will depend on the type of participants, what's expected of them and the duration of the study, with training interventions likely to incur greater drop out than short-term acute studies that require less commitment from the participants. Common reasons for drop out include: ill-health of self or others, and a lack of time due to other commitments or a change in circumstances. Some studies will utilize an ongoing recruitment process, which may span many months, until the desired number of participants has been achieved. Upon completion of the study, publications may require the inclusion of details concerning how many participants completed, screening, allocation to groups, completion of the study and drop out. This may be in the form of a 'Consolidated Standards of Reporting Trials' (CONSORT) statement,[5] an example of which is presented in Figure 13.3. The details presented in this example are illustrative and the exact points in each box will vary depending on the nature of the study and the occurrences at each stage.

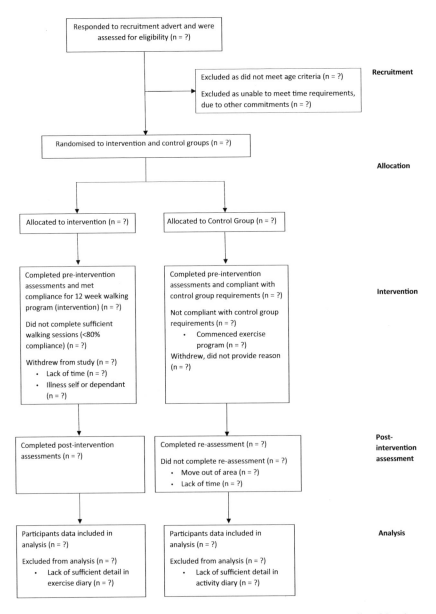

Figure 13.3 Example of a CONSORT diagram for a walking programme 5 × 30 minutes per week.

Control trials, randomization and the sequence of trials in acute studies

In acute studies, in which the single bout of exercise is unlikely to have any lasting effect, it is possible to use a design whereby all participants experience the control condition and one or more exercise bout conditions: provided sufficient 'wash-out' time is allocated between trials in order to prevent one condition contaminating the results of the subsequent condition (Figure 13.1). In these situations the study design should mix up the sequence in which the participants experience the control and exercise bout condition(s). Otherwise if all the participants experience the exercise bout after the control, any observed differences may be due to an 'order effect', which could be caused by familiarity, improved environmental conditions or any number of other factors, rather than the exercise being assessed. Mixing up the sequence should ameliorate the order effect on these factors as both the control and exercise condition(s) should be affected equally by the order. Deciding the sequence undertaken by each individual participant should be determined through a process involving randomization to prevent bias. This may be achieved through the use of sealed identical envelopes that are chosen by the participant or an independent person, with the envelopes containing details of the sequence or an equivalent digitally generated randomization process.

Control groups in intervention and exercise training studies

A control group is often essential in most intervention and training studies, since if there's only an intervention or training group, then any changes to exercise behaviour or indicators of health seen over time cannot be unequivocally attributed to the physical activity intervention. For example, changes over time could be due to other factors, such as seasonal changes in the weather, the participants becoming more familiar with the assessment protocols, dietary changes within the year or an independent national exercise promotion campaign that was not part of the study. Ideally a randomized matched control group enables the aforementioned to be accounted for, as the control group's behaviour should be affected to the same extent as the intervention/training group, and hence any effects of these extraneous variables will affect both the intervention/training and control group: meaning that any differences between the intervention/training and control groups that are identified at the end of the study can be attributed to the PA intervention or training. In intervention and exercise training studies it's rarely possible for a participant to be their own control, as the wash-out between the intervention/training and returning to baseline values is likely to be too long, as the effects may persist for weeks or months and may never be fully achieved. Which is why a cross-over design (Figure 13.1) can rarely be used, but instead a parallel control group is included in the study design (Figure 13.2). Hence at the start of an intervention or training study the participants will need to be allocated to either the control group or the intervention/exercise training group(s).

In studies where the intervention or exercise training is comparing the effectiveness of different interventions or exercise training regimens, it is possible to not include a control group since the findings and conclusions will relate to the relative efficacy of the different interventions or exercise training regimens. However, this can still mean that in the findings of the study there remains a lurking concern about the cause and effect, and whether the observed changes would have been evident over the timespan without any intervention or exercise training. Hence even in these studies the inclusion of a control group would strengthen the findings, and the researcher(s) need to assess the benefits of including a control group against the additional work and commitment cost of including one.

The role of the control group is often essential for scientific rigour, but from a pragmatic perspective, volunteers allocated to the control group may be disappointed, since having volunteered, they are likely to be in a frame of mind of 'wanting to do something', such as to do more exercise, and probably have a personal interest in getting fitter and/or healthier in the case of training studies. So if allocated to the non-exercise, non-intervention or 'usual care' control group, this may result in them dropping out, or perhaps commencing exercise under their own volition and thereby excluding themselves from the control group. To overcome this a wait-list control group may be included in the design. This is where the participants allocated to the control group agree to comply with the requirements of the control group for the required duration of the intervention, thereby providing control group data, but then commence the exercise intervention after this time, thus getting the opportunity to participate in the intervention and reduce disappointment. Whether to include this group's intervention data as well as their control data in the final analyses needs to be carefully considered and arguments can be made either way. In addition to the risk of dropping out, to be exposed to baseline and follow-up assessments as part of a control group, may for some, be sufficient to lead to change in behaviour and resultant change in an outcome measure. Therefore, your research design must include measures that can identify any changes in outcome of interest, but also data on factors potentially associated with these changes for both control and intervention conditions. This may provide relevant information in relation to understanding a low level of difference between the groups, but a significant change between baseline and follow-up for each group.

Matching of groups, allocation of participants to groups and the risk of contamination between groups in intervention and training studies

To optimize the design of intervention and exercise training studies the participants allocated to the different groups should be matched as closely as possible. This is often checked as part of the statistical analyses and reported as 'baseline data' in the findings of the study in order to provide reassurance that differences between groups at the end of the study or differences in the amount of change were not due to differences that were present before the intervention or exercise training. Attaining balanced groups can be left to chance, with participants being allocated to control or intervention/exercise group(s) completely at random, or alternatively groups can be deliberately matched based on their pre-intervention data. In the case of the latter, two participants may be determined as having the 'same' lipid profile, and then one of them randomly allocated to the control group whilst the other would be allocated to the intervention group. When undertaking this matching, the researcher needs to identify the key factors to be matched, since no two participants are likely to be matched on all factors. In studies where there is more than one intervention group, the participants would have to be matched in threes, fours or however many groups there are in the design. Such matching does of course require that a pool of participant pre-intervention/exercise training data be available to undertake the matching.

Whilst randomization and balanced randomization of participants to groups helps to prevent bias, it should be noted that given the voluntary nature of participating in intervention and exercise studies, there is always a risk of bias. This is because those who are aware of the importance of health are more likely to volunteer to participate in health interventions, whereas those who are less interested or have less time to commit to being involved in a study are less likely to volunteer.

In intervention studies there may also be a risk of contamination between groups, with the effects of one aspect of the intervention leaking from one group to another. For example, a study may be designed to determine the best way to attain compliance with an exercise regimen, with one group receiving regular telephone or email support, whilst another does not. However, if members of the supported group were more motivated by the support, but also in contact with members of the no-support group, as friends, colleagues or partners, then those from the supported group could inadvertently encourage the others to comply with the exercise regimen through exercising together or discussing how their exercise plan was going. This could result in some blurring between the supported and no-support conditions, hence the magnitude of any difference caused by the support could be masked. Researchers should be aware of this risk, which may be present when recruiting from a single location, such as a workplace. Conversely, if the two groups are from two different locations, then whilst the risk of 'contamination' is less, the group allocations would not be fully randomized, which presents other risks of bias due to differences between the locations.

Placebos, blind and double-blind data collection

If participants are aware of the aims of the study there is always a risk that they may consciously or subconsciously influence their results, a phenomena commonly referred to as the 'Hawthorne effect' and if they expect an intervention to improve their performance or results they may indeed do so, even if the substance is completely inert, a phenomena commonly known as the placebo effect. For example, thinking that a particular nutrient or intervention may improve their physical capacity may induce them to try a little harder in that trial and hence attain a better result. Hence whenever possible a placebo is used and the participant should in the case of cross-over designs be unaware of when they are taking the placebo and when they are taking the experimental substance. Likewise in intervention or exercise training studies comparing different interventions or exercise programmes, if the participant has preconceived ideas about which may be more effective this may affect their commitment and the results.

In an ideal design it is also be preferable for the researcher collecting the data to be unaware of whether a participant in an acute study is currently undergoing the experimental or placebo trial and/or to which group the participant has been allocated in an intervention or training study. This is termed as a 'double-blind' design and means that the researcher(s) cannot exhibit conscious or unconscious bias by offering more or less encouragement during particular trials, or in the way that they collect the data. The double-blind design represents a 'Gold Standard', but in reality it's not always possible given the nature of the study. For example, to achieve a double-blind design, the participant would need to be allocated their experimental substance/placebo or allocated to the intervention/control group by an independent person who is not involved with data collection in the trials. In the case of intervention and training studies the participants would also be instructed to not discuss the study with the researcher during any 'post-intervention'/'post-training' data collection session.

Furthermore, in an ideal situation the researcher undertaking the data analyses should also be blind to which trial or group that data is from. This requires each trial or group to be given a neutral code designation throughout the analyses. Then once all the analyses have been completed and any differences or effects identified, such as "Group A improved their exercise participation more than Group B", then the features of Group A and Group B can be revealed, such as which was the intervention group and which was the control. This thereby helps to ensure that there is no bias when the data are checked and cleaned. For example if a participant wasn't feeling at their best prior to one of the trials, the researcher needs to decide to remove their data if they feel that the test lacked validity under those conditions, and they need to make that decision without the knowledge of whether that was the participant's experimental or placebo trial. Likewise if the person's compliance with an intervention or exercise training programme was not 100%, decisions to include or exclude the participant's data need to be made without the knowledge of which group they were in. Hence factors such as the level at which compliance is deemed to have been sufficient should be determined before the data are analysed. For example, stating that 80% of the prescribed sessions must be completed in order for the person to have been deemed to be compliant with the intervention or exercise programme. Without the application of these rigorous and unbiased processes the data may be compromised. For example, if the researcher making the decisions to include or exclude a participant's data has prior knowledge of which trial the data is from, or to which group the participant had been allocated in an intervention or training study, there is a risk that they may decide to exclude the data if it doesn't fit their preconceived or desired outcome, yet retain the data if it does.

Repeatability, reliability and minimizing unwanted variation

An acute, intervention or exercise training study will involve the assessment of a number of key outcome measures that will provide the evidence for whether the factor, intervention or exercise training has had an effect. Typically these will be key indicators of behaviour change or health. For example: minutes of moderate intensity physical activity per week, high-density lipoprotein cholesterol concentration, percentage body fat, diastolic blood pressure, quality of life score, self-efficacy or aerobic capacity ($\dot{V}O_{2max}$). Any measurement will have some level of precision and variability, some of which will be due to limitations on the accuracy with which a factor can be measured. For example, a person's stature (height) would normally be measured to the nearest 1mm, and not to 0.1mm, since the latter is impractical. So all measurements need to be reported with a sensible level of precision, and not an excessive number of decimal places, even if that's what's produced by the computer. So rounding to a sensible level of precision is important.

Furthermore, when repeating a measurement, it may not be identical to one taken earlier, even if nothing appears to have changed. For example, blood pressure can vary from minute to minute, and body fat estimations can vary from one recording to another without the person changing in the few minutes between recordings. These differences may be due to changes in the person being measured, the way the assessor took the measurement or sample, or technical aspects of the equipment or instrumentation. From a research perspective, knowing by how much these measurements can vary is important as it tells the researcher how large any change needs to be for it to be detectable in their study. For example, if a person's aerobic capacity measurement is found to vary by ±5% on a daily basis, simply due to individual fluctuations, machine error and differences in measurement, then an intervention study will need to produce changes that are somewhat greater than 5% in order for the difference to be detected, anything less is liable to be masked by the natural daily variation and limitations on measurement reliability. There are a number of statistical methods for calculating this variation and producing a reportable measure of reliability or repeatability. They include: standard error of measurement, coefficient of variation and limits of agreement. For further details see the articles by Atkinson and Nevill.[6,7]

So to maximize the possibility of detecting effects and changes, should they exist between conditions or pre- and post-intervention/exercise training measurements, the researcher has to minimize any unwanted variability that's not caused by the factors they are assessing. The factors that the researcher will be seeking to keep consistent may be grouped under the headings of: the participant, the researcher and the environment.

(i)   Minimizing variability in the participant and researcher through familiarization sessions

With practice the researcher will become more familiar with a protocol, the equipment they are using and the best technique. This will help to reduce variability, in for example, collecting blood samples for lactate analysis. Similarly the participant may need to be familiarized with the assessment they are undertaking, the protocol and the environment. In many performance tests the participant will improve with practice as they become more familiar with the assessment, know what is required of them and how to produce their best results. This can be a problem in a study where for example a training intervention was being used to try and increase muscle power in older people. In such situations there is a risk that any improvement between the pre- and post-training tests could simply be due to practice and familiarity, rather than exercise training induced changes in muscle power. So to reduce the risk of this occurring, familiarization sessions may be incorporated into the design of the study, whereby the participant is able to practice the muscle power assessment until they produce consistent results.[8] To some extent the risk of improvements between two tests due to familiarity is partially accounted for through the inclusion of a control group, who have the same exposure to the power tests and hence familiarity, but don't undertake the training intervention. However, even with the inclusion of a control group it is desirable to minimize unwanted variation within the performance of the participants, in order to increase the likelihood of real differences being detected, rather than having them masked by the unwanted and preventable variation.

(ii)   Controlling for the condition of the participant

Since there are many factors that can affect the precise value of many indicators of health, these should be controlled for in the design. For example, recently ingested food will affect blood glucose and cholesterol levels, hence it may be necessary to require the participants to fast overnight prior to the collection of blood samples for analyses. It may also be necessary to prescribe the participants' diet in the 48 hours preceding any testing, as differences in muscle glycogen concentrations or hydration will affect exercise performance. Likewise, refraining from vigorous exercise in the 48 hours prior to assessment may be a requirement if the study design expects the participants to be fully rested and recovered. Furthermore, since a number of health and performance variables are affected by the time of day, all testing should be undertaken at the same time of day.

(iii)   Controlling for the testing environment

Since testing outcomes can be affected by the environmental conditions these need to be kept consistent. For example, the temperature of the laboratory in which the assessments or interviews are being conducted, or weather conditions if assessments are being performed outside. Likewise accurate calibration of equipment and if possible, use of exactly the same equipment items is preferable, to avoid other sources of variation.

Assessing compliance and adherence

Prior to undertaking assessments of outcome variables it is important for the researcher to be assured that the participants have complied with the pre-assessment behaviours, such as being rested, fasted, etc. This should be ascertained via a questionnaire or other data, prior to any post-intervention/training programme assessments. Also, if the study involves an intervention or regular exercise training programme, the researchers need to be assured that the participants have met the requirements, which could include the number of sessions they have completed, the duration and intensity of sessions, and in the scenario of resistance training the weights or loads they have used. These details may be attained via self-report questionnaires, the detailed recording of each session in a training diary, and with current technology may be objectively recorded through accelerometers or similar devices, which help to overcome some aspects of subjectivity and self-report (see Chapter 18).

Process evaluation

Process evaluation seeks to assess if the intervention was delivered as intended i.e. fidelity, and if the quantity of the intervention was achieved i.e. dose. Both are important as complex interventions usually involve some form of tailoring as they are adjusted to allow their implementation in different settings. Researchers need to capture what is delivered in practice, especially in relation to meeting the dose of the intervention as per the theoretical framework. Adaptations to the intervention to fit different contexts as opposed to changes that undermine the intervention fidelity need to be recorded. Methods of process evaluation include detailed training and support to intervention implementers, independent observation and documentation of adherence to protocols. For more details see the Medical Research Councils process evaluation framework,[9] or the guidelines for assessing, monitoring and enhancement of treatment fidelity in public health clinical trials.[10]

Data analyses

The analyses of data collected in intervention studies will be determined by the aims of the study and any hypotheses that are being tested. Details of the possible statistical approaches are covered in Chapter 17, so only a brief mention will be included here. Typically, data will be summarized in the form of descriptive statistics, such as means, standard errors, standard deviations and ranges, with the exact choice of statistical analyses being determined by the nature of the data and whether it meets the criteria for normality, sphericity and others. Transformations such as log or inverse may be applied if the researcher(s) wish to attain normality so that parametric statistics may be used. Alternatively if the data set continues to violate the requirements for parametric statistics even after transformations, then non-parametric statistics will need to be used. Common statistical tests used in acute, intervention and exercise training studies include: student '*t*' tests, paired '*t*' tests (if the participant's intervention results can be paired against their own results in another condition or control) and various forms of Analysis of Variance (ANOVA). Another common statistical technique is to calculate an 'Effect size', which as the name indicates is a measure of the magnitude of the effect of the intervention on the outcome measure – details of which are presented in Chapter 17. Another consideration is how the analyses deals with participants who drop out or fail to meet the compliance and adherence criteria. There are a number of approaches to this, one of which is the 'intention to treat' basis.[11]

Other considerations

Responders and non-responders

It is apparent that even when undertaking the same acute exercise bout, intervention or exercise training, not all participants will respond to the same extent. Some will display large changes, others change to a lesser degree, and some may even appear to respond adversely.[12-14] So researchers must be aware that within a study any changes may not be homogeneous, and this is also likely to be the case in the wider population, if the exercise intervention were to be adopted in a widespread manner. The issue of non-responders and adverse responders will need to be addressed within the results, interpretation and reporting of the data.

Reporting of adverse incidents

If any adverse events do occur within the study these will need to be reported to the relevant ethics committee and other authorities. Examples could include a participant becoming ill during an intervention, or their participation causing some psychological distress.

Limitations on generalizability

Researchers should be aware that the results and findings of their study may not be generalizable from one group to another. For example the responses or changes observed in a fit group may not occur in a less fit group, or the changes seen in a young group may not occur in an older group. Hence caution is needed when reporting the findings and across the field of research there is a need to ascertain whether different groups do respond in a similar manner. A fact that often forms the basis for further studies on the topic.

Reporting back to the participants

Once a study has been completed, it is desirable for the participants to be provided with feedback on the outcomes. Participants volunteer for a study due to an active interest in the topic, they commit time and effort through their participation and may experience some discomfort or inconvenience. So the researchers may be deemed to have a moral obligation to let them know how their efforts have contributed to new knowledge on the topic as well as any impact on the health of the individual. Such feedback may be in the form of a presentation evening, personalized report, a summary of the findings in lay language and perhaps a copy of the scientific paper if appropriate.

Conclusion

Acute, intervention and training studies provide an important means for gaining knowledge on how to improve exercise participation and the potential effects of exercise upon the health of the individual. The study designs here, and the principles outlined for the attainment of high-quality and meaningful data may be applied to many groups within our populations. However, in addition to these general principles and guidelines, there may be specific issues and considerations that need to be made when researching with particular groups or individuals. These are outlined in chapters 21–29 and provide further insight for researchers intending to work with these groups.

References

1 Available from: www.equator-network.org/reporting-guidelines/tidier/
2 Hoffmann TC, Glasziou PP, Boutron I, Milne R, Perera R, Moher D, et al. Better reporting of interventions: template for intervention description and replication (TIDieR) checklist and guide. *BMJ.* 2014; **348**:g1687. DOI: 10.1136/bmj.g1687
3 Walsh D, Moran K, Cornelissen V, Buys R, Claes J, Zampognaro P, et al. The development and codesign of the PATHway intervention: a theory-driven eHealth platform for the self-management of cardiovascular disease. *Transl Behav Med.* (15 Mar 2018). DOI: 10.1093/tbm/iby017. [Epub ahead of print]
4 Mutrie N, Doolin O, Fitzsimons C, Grant M, Granat M, Grealy M, et al. Increasing older adults' walking through primary care: results of a pilot randomized controlled trial. *Fam Pract.*, 2012; **29**(6):633–42.
5 Moher D, Hopewell S, Schulz KF, et al. CONSORT 2010 explanation and elaboration: updated guidelines for reporting parallel group randomised trials. *BMJ.* 2010; **340**:c869.
6 Atkinson G, Nevill AM. Statistical methods for assessing measurement error (reliability) in variables relevant to sports medicine. *Sports Med.* 1998;**26**(4):217–38.
7 Atkinson G, Nevill AM. Typical error versus limits of agreement. *Sports Med.* 2000; **30**(5):375–81.
8 Raj IS, Bird SR, Westfold BA, Shield AJ. Determining criteria to predict repeatability of performance in older adults: using coefficients of variation for strength and functional measures. *J Aging Phys Act.* 2017; **25**:94–8.
9 Moore G, Audrey S, Barker M, Bond L, Bonell C, Hardeman W, et al. Process evaluation of complex interventions: medical research council guidance. *BMJ.* 2015; **350**:h1258 DOI: 10.1136/bmj.h1258
10 Borelli B. The assessment, monitoring, and enhancement of treatment fidelity in public health clinical trials. *J Public Health Dent.* 2011; **71**(Suppl 1):S52–S63. DOI: 10.1111/j.1752-7325.2011.00233.x
11 Diggle PJ, Heagerty PJ, Kung-Yee L, Zeger SI. *Analysis of longitudinal data.* Oxford, USA: Oxford University Press; 2002.

12 Winett RA, Davy BM, Savla J, et al. Using response variation to develop more effective, personalized behavioural medicine?: evidence from the resist diabetes study. *Transl Behav Med.* 2014; **4**:333–8.

13 Pandey A, Swify DL, McGuire DK, et al. Metabolic effects of exercise training among fitness-nonresponsive patients with type 2 diabetes: the HART-D study. *Diabetes Care.* 2015; **38**:1494–501.

14 Bouchard C, Blair SN, Church TS, et al. Adverse metabolic response to regular exercise: is it a rare or common occurrence? *PLoS One.* 2012; **7**:e37887.

14 An introduction to research methods in the epidemiology of health and physical activity

Trine Moholdt and Bjarne M. Nes

Aims of the chapter

This chapter introduces some of the key methods used in epidemiologic research. We also provide some examples of epidemiological research and present research questions in health and physical activity.

What is epidemiologic research in health and physical activity?

In epidemiologic research in health and physical activity, we consider the relationships between physical activity and various health outcomes in a population. Modern epidemiologic research in this field started in the 1950s with Professor Jerry Morris's pioneering work on occupational activity and coronary heart disease[1-3], followed by the initiation of the Harvard Alumni Health Study in the early 1960s by Professor Ralph Paffenbarger Jr. At that time, public health researchers were seeking a reason for the increasing prevalence of chronic diseases, such as coronary heart disease, seen in parallel with the Industrial Revolution and its labour-saving modern technology.[4] The hypothesis was that lack of physical activity would be associated with chronic disease incidence. Since occupational physical activity was already decreasing back then, Paffenbarger established the Harvard Alumni Health Study to investigate the association between *leisure-time* physical activity and coronary heart disease. These initial studies, together with many later epidemiologic studies, provide a large body of evidence for the association between physical activity and chronic disease risk reduction.

Broadly, epidemiologic research is categorized into *descriptive epidemiology*, describing distributions of physical activity or health by time, place and person, and *analytic epidemiology*, focusing on determinants of health and physical activity variables with the goal to establish aetiology and causal associations between health outcomes and physical activity. Depending on the research question, physical activity can be either the exposure variable (an *independent variable*) or the outcome variable (a *dependent variable*). For a broad classification of study designs, see Figure 14.1.

Design of epidemiologic research studies

Descriptive studies

Descriptive epidemiologic research within health and physical activity describes the distribution of variables related to diseases, health or physical activity, in relation to person, place and time. Descriptive data provides valuable information about how

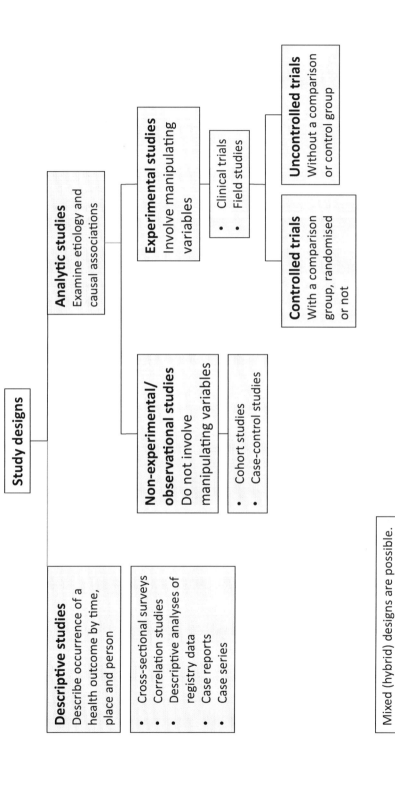

Figure 14.1 Simplified study design classification. Qualitative studies, systematic reviews and meta-analyses are not included.

different physical activity indices relate to various health outcomes. A major advantage with descriptive studies is that the information needed is often readily available and that the studies can be done easily. However, as descriptive studies only describe associations, their inherent limitation is that we cannot use a descriptive design to test for 'cause and effect', but we can use the findings to generate hypotheses for subsequent analytic studies. For example, by using data on physical activity levels, physical environment (like walkability of neighbourhoods), policy (like time of physical education in schools), throughout different European countries, you can generate hypotheses on approaches that may promote and increase physical activity, and then test these with subsequent intervention studies.[5]

A *correlational* study typically uses data from an entire population and compares outcomes (e.g. physical activity levels) between different groups or between different points in time. Bucksch and colleagues assessed the time spent on moderate-to-vigorous physical activity, television time and PC use in German adolescents between 2002 and 2010.[6] Despite a slight increase in physical activity levels over time, they observed that only 14% of 11- to 15-year-old girls and 20% of their male counterparts met the Physical Activity (PA) guidelines. Notably there was also an increase in screen time during the same time. Such studies can for example give valuable information about how well public health interventions promoting physical activity at population levels have worked.

In *cross-sectional surveys*, different exposures and health outcomes are assessed at a single point in time. Such studies are typically useful for determining whether an association is present or not rather than for testing a causal hypothesis. The main limitation of cross-sectional studies is that they cannot establish a temporal relationship between an exposure and an outcome. Cross-sectional data from the US National Health and Nutrition Examination Survey (NHANES 2005–2006) showed an inverse association between moderate-to-vigorous-intensity physical activity and depression, with an odds ratio of 0.37 in the most active compared to the least active.[7] As these data only provide a 'snapshot', we do not know whether those who were depressed reduced their physical activity due to the depression, or whether the depression was, at least in part, caused by lack of physical activity. Also, there could be another factor (e.g. pain) causing both the reduced activity level and the depression (acting as a confounder as detailed below).

Analytic studies

In an analytic study, the researchers assess whether a specific exposure or a set of exposures, such as physical activity level, determines an outcome (e.g. mortality or incidence of type 2 diabetes). By the use of an appropriate comparison, you can test epidemiologic hypotheses. Broadly, we can categorize analytic studies as observational studies, with no manipulation of variables, or intervention studies, where the researchers manipulate one or more variables to assess effects (Figure 14.1).

In *cohort studies*, a well-defined group of individuals is included and classified according to exposure status. These are then followed up over time to ascertain the outcome. Cohort studies can be either *prospective* or *retrospective*. In prospective cohort studies, the participants are grouped according to an exposure and then followed up into the future to determine whether an outcome occurs, while in retrospective cohort studies both the exposure and the outcome have already occurred at the time of the study (Figures 14.2 and 14.3).

Prospective Cohort Study

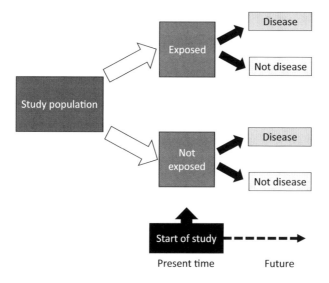

Figure 14.2 Prospective cohort studies.

Retrospective Cohort Study

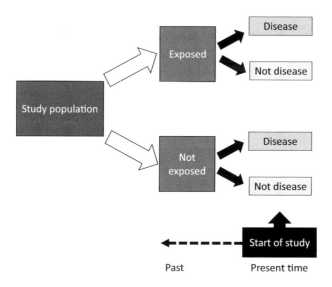

Figure 14.3 Retrospective cohort studies.

Data collection – how do we measure physical activity in epidemiologic studies?

Physical activity is a complicated behaviour with many dimensions. When we want to examine the relationship between physical activity and a health outcome, we need to concentrate on the part of physical activity that we think is most relevant for the outcome of interest. Although physical activity and exercise are related terms, physical activity includes *all* bodily movement produced by skeletal muscles that results in increased energy expenditure.[8] Therefore, when we assess physical activity in large populations, we need to specify what kind of physical activity we are measuring. We can, for example, collect data on leisure-time physical activity, occupational activity or more unstructured activities, such as housework and activities of daily living.

Traditional measures of physical activity used in epidemiologic research

Self-reported physical activity using questionnaires has been the most frequently used method of collecting data on physical activity in large populations. There is a myriad of available questionnaires, with no consensus on which is the best one and with a lack of standardization.[9] Some questionnaires aim to provide a crude classification of individuals into 'active' or 'inactive', and are typically used mainly when you need to adjust for physical activity level in determining an association among other variables.[10] Other questionnaires are more complex and aim at providing detailed information about the type of activity, frequency, duration and intensity over a specified time period by having the individuals report their habitual activity level during a specified recall period.[11] The first physical activity epidemiologic studies assessed activity at work, and its association with disease. In fact, in the legendary studies from Morris and colleagues in the 1950s, they typically classified activity levels based solely on the participants' job title.[1,2] Today we most often assess leisure-time physical activity as we can assume that in most industrialized countries this is the dimension of physical activity that accounts for the greatest part of our total physical activity.[11]

Data analysis, interpretation and presentation

Epidemiologic research typically involves collecting data on a large number of variables in many participants. All this data has to be summarized in order to make it possible to interpret the results. Different methods are used to present and summarize the data. The data collected is generally either *discrete* or *continuous*. Discrete variables have a limited number of categories while continuous variables can assume values along a continuum (often within a specified range). Discrete variables are again sub-grouped into *dichotomous* (where there are two alternative categories, with sex as a typical example, although more categories may be recognized in some studies (see Chapter 25, for further discussion) and 'non-disclosure' may be an option on some forms) or *multichotomuous* (which have several alternatives, for example ethnicity). Discrete variables are named *nominal* when there is no order of the different categories (as in the examples with sex or cultural group) and the category is merely a 'name' of the category. Sometimes, however, there is a natural order of the different categories, for example in categories of physical activity levels (inactive, low physical activity, moderate physical activity, high physical activity). Physical activity levels can, however, also be measured as a continuous variable, if you for example use number of steps or energy expenditure.

How to interpret an association

An association between an exposure and an outcome can be due to:

- A true association (causality)
- Random errors (by chance)
- Systematic errors (bias and confounding)

It can be difficult to evaluate whether an observed association between two variables is due to a causal association (i.e. that an exposure variable affects the outcome variable). We always have to consider if an association could be caused by bias in the data collection or analysis, confounding or merely the role of chance. Below we summarize some criteria for causality and different sources of bias that should be taken into account when designing a study and interpreting results. A discussion of more complex factors that influence the relationship between physical activity and health can be found elsewhere.[12]

Criteria for causality in epidemiologic studies

In 1965, the English epidemiologist Sir Austin Bradford Hill established a set of principles to help in deciding whether an observed association is a causal relationship, often referred to as the Bradford Hill criteria.[13] Although debated whether to call these principles 'criteria' for causation or just 'considerations'[14], these nine principles (Table 14.1) have been widely accepted in modern epidemiology as useful guidelines for investigating causality.

Bias

Any systematic error in an epidemiologic study that leads to an incorrect estimate of the true association between an exposure and the outcome is commonly referred to as *bias*. Bias can be subdivided based on how it may occur in the study, with the most common subcategories being: (1) Information bias, (2) Selection bias and (3) Confounding.

Information bias

Information bias in epidemiology arises from systematic errors in the collected information, leading to incorrect categorization (misclassification) of either the exposure status or the outcome of interest. Such misclassification can be either *non-differential* or *differential*. Non-differential misclassification occurs if the inaccuracy in the measurement of the exposure or outcome variable is *unrelated* to the other variable. For example, if exposure status is equally misclassified in those who get a disease and those who do not. A non-differential misclassification typically leads to weakened association between the exposure and the outcome (bias towards the null value).

Table 14.1 Criteria for causality in epidemiologic studies

Criterion	
1 Strength	The larger an association is, the more likely that it is causal. However, we cannot dismiss a cause-and-effect hypothesis merely on a small observed association.
2 Consistency	Similar results across multiple studies, with different circumstances (like places, times or participants), support a cause-effect interpretation.
3 Specificity	If an outcome is observed only in association with a single exposure, this strengthens the causal inference. If such specificity exists, we may be able to draw conclusions without hesitation. However, one-to-one relationships are not common, and most health outcomes show multi-causation.
4 Temporality	The effect generally has to occur after the cause. This is sometimes difficult to determine because early stages of a disease might cause changes in a habit (e.g. physical activity).
5 Biological gradient	A strong dose-response relationship contributes to cause-effect interpretation. This relationship is sometimes more complicated, and not always linear.
6 Plausibility	A biologically plausible mechanism linking the cause to the effect supports causality. However, what is biologically plausible depends on the biological knowledge, and absence of a known mechanism does not rule out a causal relationship.
7 Coherence	This point is linked to the plausibility criterion. Coherence between laboratory findings and epidemiological data. Lack of laboratory evidence should not be taken as an absolute criterion for no causality.
8 Experiment	To do a study where you experimentally intervene (by modifying the exposure) to determine if this changes the outcome.
9 Analogy	The effect of similar factors. If we get the same effect by slightly modifying the exposure, this will strengthen a causal interpretation of an association.

A differential bias, however, is more problematic and occurs when the misclassification of an exposure or outcome variable is not equal across groups, but *related* to the status of the other. Differential misclassification may lead to a biased association either away from or towards the null value.

A common information bias in physical activity epidemiology arises when using self-reported questionnaires to measure activity levels. People might not be able to accurately remember their activity level or may systematically over- or under-report their activity. In prospective study designs, misclassification may also arise because exposure status changes during long follow-up periods. This is typical for physical activity where the baseline status is commonly measured for a short timeframe such as a week, while you have no information on the activity level in the period until the outcome occurs. If the misclassification of physical activity is equally distributed among the different outcome categories, for example among individuals who get or do not get coronary heart disease (CHD) you have a non-differential misclassification and might not be able to detect a true association between physical activity and CHD incidence. Differential misclassification is common in case-control studies or retrospective studies, where the outcome is already known at the time of exposure or vice versa. Two typical examples of differential bias in this situation are *recall bias* and *social desirability bias*. For example, people doing high amounts of unstructured light intensity physical activity may have more problems accurately recalling their activity level compared to people doing structured vigorous activity. A comparison between self-report vigorous and light intensity activity, respectively, and CHD may therefore be prone to differential recall bias. Similarly, people may over-report their activity level because they perceive a higher activity level as more socially acceptable. If people with CHD are more likely to over-report, the results are prone to a differential social desirability bias.

Selection bias

Even in a large epidemiological study, it is usually not possible to include every person with a particular exposure or outcome. Selection bias may occur when there is a systematic difference between the characteristics of those included in a study, and those not included. Hence, the study subjects are not necessarily representative of the source population you want to draw conclusions about. In this case, the selection process weakens the external validity or *generalizability*. The major problem with selection bias occurs if the inclusion of participants based on either exposure or outcome is, somehow, related to the other variable. In retrospective studies or case-control studies, participants have already experienced the outcome and may be more likely to participate if they are also exposed. Selection bias is, however, less likely to occur in *prospective* cohort studies, because both exposed and unexposed participants are enrolled before they have experienced the outcome. Selection bias in prospective studies may still occur if the retention of participants during follow-up differs between exposed and unexposed depending on the outcome. For example, if inactive people who later got CHD were more likely to withdraw from the study than inactive people who stayed healthy, you will underestimate a true causal association. This is commonly referred to as a *loss to follow-up bias*.

Another common example of selection bias is the *healthy worker effect*. This term relates to studies that recruit people based on occupation, which makes it difficult to generalize findings because people who work are generally healthier than unemployed individuals. Similarly, since participation in a study most often is voluntary, those who volunteer may also be healthier than those who decline to take part. The results will, however, only be biased in the case of the comparison group being from the general population.

Confounding

An observed association can be due to a mixing of effects between the exposure, the outcome and another variable that is independently associated with both the exposure and the outcome variable. For example, physically active people are more likely to be non-smokers than those who are inactive. Both smoking and physical inactivity are (independently) associated with coronary heart disease. If we observe an increased risk of coronary heart disease associated with physical inactivity, this could, at least in part, be due to the confounding effect of smoking (Figure 14.4). To be a confounder, the variable has to vary between those exposed and not exposed, or those with and without the outcome. In this example, smoking status has to be different between the inactive and the active, or else there is no confounding by smoking.

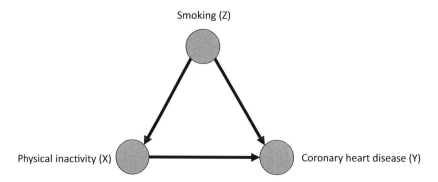

Figure 14.4 Example of confounding. Smoking (Z) is independently associated with both physical inactivity (X) and coronary heart disease (Y). An observed association between physical inactivity and coronary heart disease could therefore be confounded by smoking.

Effect modification

Effect modification occurs when the effect of an exposure variable on the outcome variable is different depending on the level of a third variable. For example, obesity is associated with increased risk of myocardial infarction (MI) in the general population, but the effect may vary considerably across subgroups with different fitness levels. Several studies have shown that overweight or obese people who have a high fitness level have lower risk of MI compared to overweight/obese people who are low fit. Hence, fitness level acts as an effect modifier of the association between body composition status and MI. While confounding is a distortion of the effect that we want to eliminate, effect modification is a biological phenomenon that should not be controlled or adjusted for, but described and reported in order to give further insight into the association. Biological effect modification can be examined by stratifying the analysis by the level of the potential effect modifier.

How to control for bias and confounding in design and analysis

Bias in epidemiological studies can be minimized by appropriate design of the study, accurate measurement methods and careful selection procedures in accordance with your research questions. As outlined above, selection bias and information bias are less likely in prospective cohort studies compared to retrospective, case-control or cross-sectional studies.

Confounding, however, is a potential problem in all epidemiological studies aiming to make causal inferences. In clinical trials, the most common way to deal with the problem of confounding is randomization of participants. A successful randomization process ensures that baseline values for all variables, except the exposure variable, are evenly distributed across groups. In observational studies, potential confounders can be dealt with before analysing the data, by restricting the study sample to certain levels of a potential confounder, or during analysis, by stratification into subgroups based on level of a confounder or by statistical adjustments. Multivariate analysis is the most common solution if confounders are present in cohort studies. A large number of confounders can then be handled simultaneously and controlled for. A premise for statistical adjustment for confounders is that data is available for each potential confounding variable. This is, however, not always the case and researchers should take into account the possibility of unmeasured (residual) confounding when interpreting the results. Another potential pitfall when evaluating cause-effect relationships in epidemiological studies is the possibility of reverse causation. Reverse causation means that instead of an exposure or risk factor *causing* disease it might be the other way around, the disease itself or unmeasured markers of disease causes the exposure or risk factor. For example people with severe angina may be less likely to be physically active and also have a higher risk of more severe CHD such as myocardial infarction. Hence, an interpretation that inactivity causes myocardial infarction might be partly biased since in fact the unmeasured underlying disease (angina) is causing the inactivity. The problem of reverse causation in prospective studies can be dealt with by excluding events during the first years of follow-up and hence reduce the impact of unmeasured underlying disease. It is usually difficult to eliminate all sources of bias in epidemiological studies. Researchers should, however, aim to minimize them, and at least identify those that cannot be avoided, so the reader is able to take them into account when interpreting the results.

Current topics in physical activity epidemiology

Dose response

Today we have clear evidence that physical inactivity is an important cause of at least 35 chronic conditions.[15] Therefore, the present focus of epidemiologic research within the field of physical activity and health is not so much on *whether* physical activity reduces the risk of poor health outcomes, but rather on the details of the type of activity and dose needed. This can then be used to refine the recommendations for physical activity for promoting and maintaining health using the latest epidemiological evidence. However, as we know that the majority of the population does not fulfil the recommended activity level[16], we also need to find a minimum level of physical activity associated with health benefits. Some recent studies indicate that even very small amounts of activity, for example breaking up prolonged sitting with low intensity walking every 30 minutes, or by climbing stairs for some seconds repeatedly throughout the day, can improve glucose tolerance and cardiorespiratory fitness.[17,18] In a detailed pooled analysis of the dose-response relationship between leisure-time physical activity and mortality, with a total of more 660,000 participants, Arem and colleagues[19] observed a 20% risk reduction associated with those who performed some physical activity, compared to inactive individuals, albeit that the amount of physical activity was less than the recommended level of physical activity. In line with this, a study including 416,000 Taiwanese men and women showed a three-year longer life expectancy for individuals who walked briskly for 15 minutes each day.[20] Currently, the exact shape of the dose-response curve is not known and probably differs between various health outcomes. Other areas of research interest include the intensity of the physical activity and its timing within the day, particularly in relation to food intake.

Sedentary behaviour

Research on sedentary behaviour as a potential risk factor for many chronic diseases and mortality has emerged in the last decade, and increased dramatically, albeit with a slight decline in the last few years (Figure 14.5).[12]

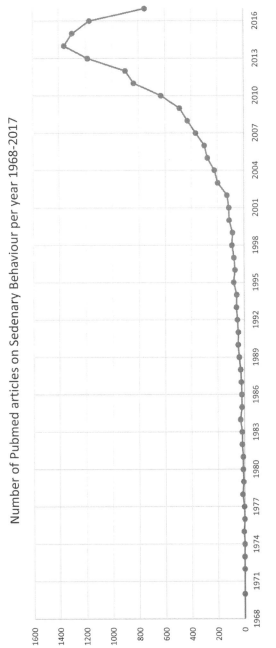

Figure 14.5 Number of articles retained in Pubmed when using 'Sedentary behaviour' as search term.

High amounts of sedentary behaviour (often measured by proxy measures like television-viewing time) associates with increased risk for several chronic conditions and mortality.[21-23] A highly relevant question is whether sedentary behaviour is an *independent* risk factor, regardless of physical activity, in other words: if a person is physically active, will this attenuate or eliminate the detrimental effects of sedentary time? Ekelund and co-workers[24] examined this question in a meta-analysis including more than 1 million men and women. They found that high levels (60–75 min per day) of moderate intensity physical activity eliminated the increased risk of death associated with many hours of sitting. However, they observed only an attenuation of the increased risk associated with many hours of daily television-viewing time by high levels of physical activity. Such examinations of the joint effects of physical activity and sedentary behaviour is important for public health guidelines since many individuals sit for a prolonged period every day. For further details on research into sedentary behaviour see Chapter 15.

References

1   Morris JN, Heady JA, Raffle PA, Roberts CG, Parks JW. Coronary heart-disease and physical activity of work. *Lancet (London, England)*. 1953; **265**(6796):1111–20; concl.
2   Morris JN, Crawford MD. Coronary heart disease and physical activity of work; evidence of a national necropsy survey. *Br Med J*. 1958; **2**(5111):1485–96.
3   Morris JN, Kagan A, Pattison DC, Gardner MJ. Incidence and prediction of ischaemic heart-disease in London busmen. *Lancet (London, England)*. 1966; **2**(7463):553–9.
4   Lee IM, editor. *Epidemiologic methods in physical activity studies*. New York, NY: Oxford University Press; 2008.
5   Gerovasili V, Agaku IT, Vardavas CI, Filippidis FT. Levels of physical activity among adults 18–64 years old in 28 European countries. *Prev Med*. 2015; **81**:87–91.
6   Bucksch J, Inchley J, Hamrik Z, Finne E, Kolip P. Trends in television time, non-gaming PC use and moderate-to-vigorous physical activity among German adolescents 2002–2010. *BMC Public Health*. 2014; **14**: 351.
7   Vallance JK, Winkler EA, Gardiner PA, Healy GN, Lynch BM, Owen N. Associations of objectively-assessed physical activity and sedentary time with depression: NHANES (2005–2006). *Prev Med*. 2011; **53**(4–5):284–8.
8   Caspersen CJ, Powell KE, Christenson GM. Physical activity, exercise, and physical fitness: definitions and distinctions for health-related research. *Public Health Rep*. 1985; **100**(2):126–31.
9   van Poppel MN, Chinapaw MJ, Mokkink LB, van Mechelen W, Terwee CB. Physical activity questionnaires for adults: a systematic review of measurement properties. *Sports Med (Auckland, NZ)*. 2010; **40**(7):565–600.
10 Caspersen CJ. Physical activity epidemiology: concepts, methods, and applications to exercise science. *Exerc Sport Sci Rev*. 1989; **17**:423–73.
11 Pettee KK, Storti, KL, Ainsworth BE, Kriska AM. Measurement of physical activity and inactivity in epidemiologic studies. In: Lee IM, Blair SN, Manson J, Paffenbarger RS, editors. *Epidemiologic mehtods in physical activity studies*. New York: Oxford University Press; 2009.
12 Bauman AE, Sallis JF, Dzewaltowski DA, Owen N. Toward a better understanding of the influences on physical activity: the role of determinants, correlates, causal variables, mediators, moderators, and confounders. *Am J Prev Med*. 2002; **23**(2 Suppl):5–14.
13 Hill AB. The environment and disease: association or causation? *Proc Roy Soc Med*. 1965; **58**:295–300.
14 Phillips CV, Goodman KJ. Causal criteria and counterfactuals; nothing more (or less) than scientific common sense. *Emerg Themes Epidemiol*. 2006; **3**: 5.

15 Booth FW, Roberts CK, Laye MJ. Lack of exercise is a major cause of chronic diseases. *Compr Physiol.* 2012; **2**(2):1143–211.

16 Loyen A, Clarke-Cornwell AM, Anderssen SA, et al. Sedentary time and physical activity surveillance through accelerometer pooling in four European countries. *Sports Med.* 2017; **47**(7):1421–35.

17 Allison MK, Baglole JH, Martin BJ, Macinnis MJ, Gurd BJ, Gibala MJ. Brief intense stair climbing improves cardiorespiratory fitness. *Med Sci Sports Exerc.* 2017; **49**(2):298–307.

18 Henson J, Davies MJ, Bodicoat DH, et al. Breaking up prolonged sitting with standing or walking attenuates the postprandial metabolic response in postmenopausal women: a randomized acute study. *Diabetes Care.* 2016; **39**(1):130–8.

19 Arem H, Moore SC, Patel A, et al. Leisure time physical activity and mortality: a detailed pooled analysis of the dose-response relationship. *JAMA Intern Med.* 2015; **175**(6):959–67.

20 Wen CP, Wai JP, Tsai MK, et al. Minimum amount of physical activity for reduced mortality and extended life expectancy: a prospective cohort study. *Lancet (London, England).* 2011; **378**(9798):1244–53.

21 Liu M, Wu L, Yao S. Dose-response association of screen time-based sedentary behaviour in children and adolescents and depression: a meta-analysis of observational studies. *Br J Sports Med.* 2016; **50**(20):1252–8.

22 Biswas A, Oh PI, Faulkner GE, et al. Sedentary time and its association with risk for disease incidence, mortality, and hospitalization in adults: a systematic review and meta-analysis. *Ann Intern Med.* 2015; **162**(2):123–32.

23 Shen D, Mao W, Liu T, et al. Sedentary behavior and incident cancer: a meta-analysis of prospective studies. *PloS One.* 2014; **9**(8):e105709.

24 Ekelund U, Steene-Johannessen J, Brown WJ, et al. Does physical activity attenuate, or even eliminate, the detrimental association of sitting time with mortality? A harmonised meta-analysis of data from more than 1 million men and women. *Lancet (London, England).* 2016; **388**(10051):1302–10.

15 Research into sedentary behaviour

Nicola D. Ridgers and Simone J.J.M. Verswijveren

Aims of the chapter

This chapter will provide an overview of the definition of sedentary behaviour, the techniques used to measure sedentary behaviour, the prevalence of sedentary behaviour, and associations between sedentary behaviour and health in children and adults. Key points from this chapter will then be demonstrated using two case studies. This chapter aims to serve as an initial introduction to sedentary behaviour research.

Introduction

In the past 15–20 years, there has been a significant increase in research focusing on sedentary behaviour.[1] This body of research can be broadly categorized into six main areas based on the behavioural epidemiology framework.[1] These categories are: (1) the effects of sedentary behaviour on health, (2) measurement, (3) prevalence, (4) correlates and determinants, (5) interventions, and (6) policy and practice.[1-3]

Understanding physical inactivity and sedentary behaviour

The terms 'physical inactivity', 'sedentary' and 'sedentary behaviour' have all been used within the human movement and physical activity literature. However, there have been inconsistencies in the terminology used within different studies, creating considerable confusion for researchers, practitioners and policy makers.[4-5] These inconsistencies can be attributed to the evolution of physical activity epidemiology over the past 50 years.[6] The term 'sedentary' had been used to define individuals who engaged in too little exercise, which is a subset of physical activity that is characterized by its planned, structured and repetitive nature.[7] With the increase in research that documented the health benefits of individuals engaging in regular physical activities, not just exercise, public health guidelines were developed that highlighted the importance of physical activity accumulation throughout the day.[6] This resulted in individuals being classified as sedentary if they did not engage in enough moderate-to-vigorous physical activity (MVPA) to be classed as active based on these guidelines.[6] The use of the term 'sedentary' here was based on a lack of activity above a certain threshold (e.g. 3 or 4 metabolic equivalent tasks (METs) for adults and children, respectively), rather than assessing the actual behaviours someone may engage in that could be classed as sedentary (e.g. computer use). It also meant that someone who engaged in high levels of light physical activity (LPA), which has been shown to confer health benefits,[8,9] was also considered sedentary.[1]

In 2000, Owen and colleagues highlighted that sedentary behaviour is a construct in its own right and distinct from physical activity.[10] It was proposed that it was a class of behaviours that can coexist alongside and compete with physical activity, and they stated that research was required to understand the potential health impacts of engaging in sedentary behaviours.[10] Derived from the Latin word 'sedere' ('to sit'), sedentary behaviours include those that involve low energy expenditure and high sitting: such as television viewing, computer use, car travel.[10] However, despite the growth in research focusing on sedentary behaviours in the ensuing years, confusion remained over the definitions being used.[6] As a consequence, in 2017, Tremblay and colleagues proposed the following standardised definition:[11] Sedentary behaviour was defined as "any waking behavior characterized by an energy expenditure ≤ 1.5 metabolic equivalents (METs), while in a sitting, reclining or lying posture" (p. 540).[4] This is distinct from physical inactivity,[4] which has been defined as "an insufficient physical activity level to meet present physical activity guidelines" (p. 9).[11] In contrast, physical inactivity is a criterion-referenced definition that identifies those who are insufficiently active to benefit their health, but does not quantify how much sedentary behaviour they engage in.[12] Based on these definitions, it is possible for someone to be physically inactive but to engage in few sedentary behaviours, or to engage in high levels of both sedentary behaviour and physical activity (see case study 1 below).[12]

Measurement of sedentary behaviour

The definition of sedentary behaviour includes a postural component (i.e. sitting/reclining/lying) and an energy expenditure component (i.e. ≤ 1.5 METs). Historically, sedentary behaviour measures used in research have assessed time spent engaged in specific behaviours (using subjective measures) or low energy expenditure (using objective measures). To date, no field-based tools directly measure both components of the definition.[13] Whilst a number of different techniques have been used to assess sedentary behaviour, the more frequently used measures will be summarized below.

Self-report measures

Subjective measures, such as self-report questionnaires, checklists and time use diaries, enable researchers to determine time spent in sedentary behaviours. These are practical and useful methods for collecting information on actual behaviours in large samples. Self-report measures usually require an individual to recall or estimate specific behaviours such as television viewing, computer use and sitting time at work over a typical week, for example.[14,15] Whilst the advantages of self-report measures include lower participant burden, lower administration costs and ease of use in population-level studies, they are limited by social desirability (i.e. tendency for respondents to provide favourable responses), and the ability of the participant to comprehend the questions being asked and remember behaviours.[16,17] This latter point is particularly relevant for children, who have lower cognitive functioning than adults, which reduces their ability to accurately recall both physical activity and sedentary behaviours.[17] Indeed, this is likely to explain the lower validity and reliability found for self-reports used with children.[14] In adolescents and adults, the validity and reliability of self-report measures varies dependent on the tool being assessed,[14,18,19] so it is important to consider this in the selection of questionnaires, for example.

As an individual can engage in many sedentary behaviours in a varied and sporadic manner across the day, it is unsurprising that self-report measures often measure sedentary behaviour more globally. Indeed, as sitting time is ubiquitous, self-report measures tend to focus on behaviours that involve sitting/reclining postures and screen use, which may be easier to recall than sitting time per se.[1,2] Most measures do not capture multiple behaviours,[14] and are unlikely to be representative of the many sedentary behaviours that could have been engaged in throughout the day.[20] Further problems are also evident when considering the evolution of screen use in recent years. For example, it is possible to watch television programmes on a smartphone, which raises questions of how best to categorize such behaviours (i.e. television viewing or phone use), and read a book on an e-reader (i.e. screen use or reading). Furthermore, individuals may use multiple screens at the same time.[21] Consequently, current self-report measures may not be accurately capturing time spent engaged in sedentary behaviours in such cases, highlighting a need to continue to develop and validate appropriate measures as technology evolves.

Accelerometers

Rapid technological advances in objective measures have enabled researchers to measure free-living behaviours over a period of time (e.g. multiple consecutive days) and quantify time spent in different activity intensities.[22] Accelerometers, which are small motion sensors typically worn on the hip, are the most commonly used objective device. Accelerometers (e.g. ActiGraph, Actical) detect accelerations produced by human movement,[23] which are then often converted to counts for analysis. These counts are then used to determine the amount of time per day that someone engages in different activity intensities by applying cut-points or threshold values to the data. Cut-points have been developed based on energy expenditure prediction equations, and have been validated for use in different populations.[22,24] It is also possible to analyse accelerometer data to obtain detailed information about how activity is accumulated (e.g. patterns of movement, sustained bouts of activity).[2,25] The limitation of using cut-points is that this approach does not accurately predict physical activity intensity across a range of behaviours;[26] consequently techniques for analysing raw data have also been more widely used in recent years.[26]

Hip-mounted accelerometers estimate sedentary time based on a lack of movement.[14,27,28] This means that standing as opposed to sitting may also be recorded as low movement or a lack of movement, as the data falls below the cut-point used to distinguish between sedentary time and LPA.[27,28] Standing has been shown to be a LPA behaviour, as it requires isometric contraction of the postural muscles and greater energy expenditure than sitting still.[29] As accelerometer-derived sedentary time may include both sedentary behaviours and standing time, this may have implications for research examining associations between sedentary time and health.[2,27] A second issue relating to the use of accelerometers is that if an individual does not wear the device, it is hard to distinguish periods of sedentary time from non-wear as the data will look alike. This means that long periods of unbroken sedentary time may be removed as non-wear, but shorter periods of non-wear may be included as sedentary time, based on the decisions used to process the data.[30–32] This can result in increased or decreased estimates of sedentary time volume, which may also influence associations with health.[31,32]

More recently, accelerometers have been developed to assess posture. The activPAL is the most commonly used accelerometer to measure posture, which is estimated through the measurement of the longitudinal acceleration and inclination of the thigh.[5,33] The main strength of the activPAL is the ability to distinguish between time spent sitting, standing and stepping.[34] Moreover, it is possible to assess postural transitions, namely the number of times a person goes from sitting to being upright and vice versa.[13] This provides insights into how frequently sitting time is interrupted, which may be more accurate than breaks in sedentary time as classified by accelerometers, as it is not reliant on data exceeding a cut-point,[35] and marks the start and end of a sitting bout.[13] The validity of the activPAL for assessing sitting and standing time has been examined in a number of populations. In general, acceptable validity has been demonstrated in children and adults for sitting and standing,[28,34,36,37] though irregular sitting styles have been shown to impact on the ability of the activPAL to accurately classify sitting time, especially in children.[28,38]

Prevalence of sedentary behaviours and sedentary time

Children and adults spend a significant proportion of their day being sedentary.[39] Typically, adults and adolescents (i.e. ≥ 13 years old) engage in ≥ 8 hours, and children engage in ≥ 6 hours of sedentary time per day.[39] This total is accumulated throughout the day within different settings, particularly at work/school and at home.[3,39,40] The following sections will provide a summary in relation to these different settings and corresponding sedentary behaviours.

Work/School

Since the rise of the internet and evolution of computers, a shift in the workforce has occurred from traditionally physically demanding occupations towards sedentary occupations.[25,41] Research has shown that office workers spend $\geq 80\%$ of their work hours sedentary,[42] which equates to approximately 7 hours per day based on self-reported work hours.[42,43] Notably, occupational sedentary time is often accumulated in long bouts with few breaks.[42–44] This highlights that for adults working in office-based settings, occupational sedentary time is a major contributor to adults' total daily sedentary time. Similarly, children spend up to two-thirds of their school day sedentary, largely attributable to time spent sitting in class.[27,45,46] Given that both adults and children spend most their waking hours at work and school, respectively, it is not surprising that efforts to reduce sedentary time in these settings are the focus of interventions.[3,40,47]

Home

Previous studies have shown that television viewing is a prevalent behaviour and a significant contributor to the amount of time that adults and children spend sedentary.[48,49] For example, studies have found that adults spend up to ~2 hours a day watching television on average.[20,50] Similar findings have been reported for children and adolescents.[3,49,51] However, other types of sedentary behaviours also occur at home, that include leisure-time computer usage, reading and listening to music.[52,53] Whilst it has been shown that television viewing can account for 45% of leisure-time sedentary behaviours,[54] it is important that researchers are aware of other behaviours that contribute to the amount of time individuals spend sedentary per day and consider these in the design of interventions.

Sedentary behaviour and health

Whilst knowledge concerning the effects of sedentary behaviour and prolonged periods of sitting time on health is in its relative infancy,[25] the first evidence suggesting that sitting has a negative effect on health was reported in 1953 by Morris and colleagues.[55] This research showed that the seated drivers of London's double-decker buses were more likely to die suddenly from coronary thrombosis than the conductors who usually stood up. More recently, a body of research has emerged that has investigated the implications that engaging in high levels of sedentary behaviour (i.e. overall sedentary time, sitting time, television or screen time and leisure sitting time, dependent on the measures used) may have for people's health.

Systematic reviews have reported that adults' sedentary time is associated with a greater risk for all-cause mortality, cardiovascular disease incidence or mortality, cancer incidence or mortality and type 2 diabetes in adults.[56,57] These findings are mostly independent of physical activity.[56] Similar results have been observed for television viewing and the prevalence of metabolic syndrome and increased risk of being overweight.[48,58] Interestingly, research suggests that high levels of moderate intensity physical activity (i.e., about 60–75 min per day) could eliminate the increase in risk of death associated with sitting time, but not for television viewing (>5 hours or more a day).[59] This might be explained by measurement issues associated with self-reporting these behaviours, snacking behaviours that accompany television viewing or prolonged sedentary time after eating.[59] However, it should be noted that the high levels of activity that eliminated this risk equate to twice the adult recommendations, which may be difficult to achieve for physically inactive adults.

In children and adolescents, research has shown that screen time and television viewing are associated with unfavourable body composition, higher clustered cardio-metabolic risk scores, as well as poorer behavioural and psychological health.[3,60,61] In contrast, several reviews have noted that there is little available evidence to suggest that objectively measured daily sedentary time is associated with children and adolescents' health, independent of physical activity.[62,63] However, it is possible that since children have had lower exposure to the effects of sedentary time this may potentially reduce its measurable impact on their health.[62]

Case study 1: is it possible to be physically active and sedentary?

It was noted that it is possible for someone to be highly sedentary and still meet physical activity guidelines. This is known as the active couch potato phenomenon.[1] For example, consider a child (Child 1) who is active during recess, lunchtime and after school, but who is driven to school and sits for long periods during class time. It is possible that this child meets current physical activity guidelines for children (i.e. engage in MVPA every day for at least an hour)[64] but can still also accumulate a high volume of sedentary time on the same day (see Figure 15.1). Alternatively, consider a child (Child 2) who engages in some physical activity during recess and lunchtime, but has the option of standing during class time (i.e. engages in LPA). This child is physically inactive (i.e. not meeting guidelines), but is not sedentary (see Figure 15.1). This

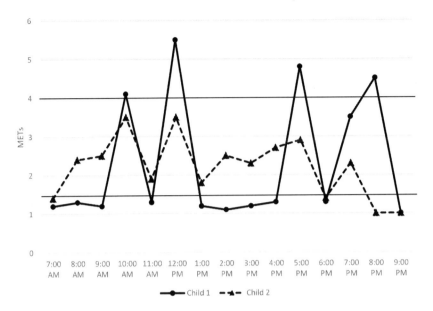

Figure 15.1 The active couch potato and inactive non-sedentary phenomena.

highlights that how activity and sedentary time is accumulated throughout the day (i.e. activity patterns) can differ between children. This should be considered when designing strategies to increase activity levels and decrease sedentary time.

The lines on Figure 15.1 indicate the thresholds used to determine the time sedentary time (≤ 1.5 METs), LPA (1.5–3.99 METs) and MVPA (≥ 4 METs). These thresholds are based on energy expenditure prediction equations (see *Accelerometers* section).

Case study 2: where should we focus our efforts to reduce sedentary behaviours?

Television viewing has been found to have a detrimental effect on children and adolescent's cardio-metabolic risk factors, independent of physical activity.[63,65] Early studies implemented interventions that were relatively successful in reducing television viewing in youth.[3,60] However, focusing on television viewing (or screen time more broadly) only targets one form of sedentary behaviour time that typically accounts for approximately half of a child's total daily sedentary time.[2,40] To illustrate this, consider a child who watches television for 101.5 minutes per day.[51] This does not include the 45 minutes per day they also spend playing computer games and using the computer for leisure.[51] Television viewing and total screen time accounts for approximately 25% and 36%, respectively, of their daily sedentary time based on data from the same larger study.[66] Similar estimates of television and screen use have been reported in other studies.[65] This means that up to 75% of their daily sedentary time is being accumulated elsewhere, including at school (e.g. sitting in class) and passive travel. This example highlights that intervening in a range of settings and targeting different sedentary behaviours are needed to benefit health.[40]

Summary

This chapter has presented a summary of research conducted with a focus on sedentary behaviour. With standardized definitions of sedentary behaviour and physical inactivity now available and being used more widely, along with emerging new technologies for data collection greater insights into the risk that too much sitting and high engagement in sedentary behaviour poses to health will continue to emerge. This will inform future research that will focus on how to effectively decrease the amount of time that children, adolescents and adults spend sedentary each day.

References

1 Owen N, Healy GN, Matthews CE, Dunstan DW. Too much sitting: the population health science of sedentary behavior. *Exerc Sports Sci Rev.* 2010; **38**(3):105–13.

2 Tremblay MS, Colley RC, Saunders TJ, Healy GN, Owen N. Physiological and health implications of a sedentary lifestyle. *Appl Physiol Nutr Metab.* 2010; **35**:725–40.

3 Salmon J, Tremblay MS, Marshall SJ, Hume C. Health risks, correlates, and interventions to reduce sedentary behavior in young people. *Am J Prev Med.* 2011; **41**(2):197–206.

4 Sedentary Behaviour Research Network Letter to the editor: standardized use of the terms sedentary and sedentary behavioiurs. *Appl Physiol Nutr Metab.* 2012; **37**(3):540–2.

5 Chastin SFM, Granat MH. Methods for objective measure, quantification and analysis of sedentary behaviour and inactivity. *Gait Posture.* 2010; **31**(1):82–6.

6 Pate RR, O'Neill JR, Lobelo F. The evolving definition of "sedentary". *Exerc Sports Sci Rev.* 2008; **36**(4):173–8.

7 Caspersen CJ, Powell KE, Christenson GM. Physical activity, exercise, and physical fitness: definition and distinctions for health-related research. *Public Health Reports.* 1985; **100**(2):126–31.

8 Carson V, Ridgers ND, Howard BJ, Winkler EAH, Healy GN, Owen N, et al. Light-intensity physical activity and cardiometabolic biomarkers in US adolescents. *PloS One.* 2013; **8**:e71417.

9 Howard B, Winkler EA, Sethi P, Carson V, Ridgers ND, Salmon J, et al. Associations of low- and high-intensity light physical activity with cardiometabolic biomarkers. *Med Sci Sports Exerc.* 2015; **47**(10):2093–101.

10 Owen N, Leslie E, Salmon J, Fotheringham MJ. Environmental determinants of physical activity and sedentary behavior. *Exerc Sports Sci Rev.* 2000; **28**(4):153–8.

11 Tremblay MS, Aubert S, Barnes JD, Saunders TJ, Carson V, Latimer-Cheung AE, et al. Sedentary Behavior Research Network (SBRN) – Terminology consensus project process and outcome. *Int J Behav Nutr Phys Act.* 2017; **14**:75.

12 van der Ploeg HP, Hillsdon M. Is sedentary behaviour just physical inactivity by another name? *Int J Behav Nutr Phys Act.* 2017; **14**:142.

13 Edwardson CL, Winkler EAH, Bodicoat DH, Yates T, Davies MJ, Dunstan DW, et al. Considerations when using the activPAL monitor in field-based research with adult populations. *J Sport Health Sci.* 2017; **6**(2):162–78.

14 Lubans DR, Hesketh K, Cliff DP, Barnett LM, Salmon J, Dollman J, et al. A systematic review of the validity and reliability of sedentary behaviour measures used with children and adolescents. *Obes Rev.* 2011; **12**:781–99.

15 Hart TL, Ainsworth BE, Tudor-Locke C. Objective and subjective measures of sedentary behavior and physical activity. *Med Sci Sports Exerc.* 2011; **43**(3):449–56.

16 Prince SA, Adamo KB, Hamel ME, Hardt J, Connor Gorber S, Tremblay M. A comparison of direct versus self-report measures for assessing physical activity in adults: a systematic review. *Int J Behav Nutr Phys Act.* 2008; **5**:56.

17   Sirard JR, Pate RR. Physical activity assessment in children and adolescents. *Sports Med.* 2001; **31**(6):439–54.

18   Jefferis BJ, Sartini C, Ash S, Lennon LT, Wannamethee SG, Whincup PH. Validity of questionnaire-based assessment of sedentary behaviour and physical activity in a population-based cohort of older men; comparisons with objectively measured physical activity data. *Int J Behav Nutr Phys Act.* 2016; **13**:14.

19   Prince SA, LeBlanc AG, Colley RC, Saunders TJ. Measurement of sedentary behaviour in population health surveys: a review and recommendations. *PeerJ.* 2017; **5**:e4130.

20   Sugiyama T, Healy GN, Dunstan DW, Salmon J, Owen N. Is television viewing time a marker of a broader pattern of sedentary behaviour? *Ann Behav Med.* 2008; **35**(2):245–50.

21   Jago R, Sebire S, Gorely T, Cillero IH, Biddle SJ. "I'm on it 24/7 at the moment": a qualitative examination of multi-screen viewing behaviours among UK 10–11 year olds. *Int J Behav Nutr Phys Act.* 2011; **8**:85.

22   Trost SG, Loprinzi PD, Moore R, Pfeiffer KA. Comparison of accelerometer cut-points for predicting activity intensity in youth. *Med Sci Sports Exerc.* 2011; **43**(7):1360–8.

23   Welk GJ. Principles of design and analyses for the calibration of accelerometry-based activity monitors. *Med Sci Sports Exerc.* 2005; **11**(Supplement):S501–S11.

24   Evenson KR, Catellier DJ, Gill K, Ondrak KS, McMurray RG. Calibration of two objective measures of physical activity for children. *J Sports Sci.* 2008; **26**(14):1557–65.

25   Dunstan DW, Healy GN, Sugiyama T, Owen N. 'Too much sitting' and metabolic risk – Has modern technology caught up with us? *Eur Endocrinol.* 2010; **6**:19–23.

26   Bassett DRJ, Rowlands A, Trost SG. Calibration and validation of wearable monitors *Med Sci Sports Exerc.* 2012; **44**(Supplement 1):S32–S8.

27   Ridgers ND, Salmon J, Ridley K, O'Connell E, Arundell L, Timperio A. Agreement between activPAL and ActiGraph for assessing children's sedentary time. *Int J Behav Nutr Phys Act.* 2012; **9**:15.

28   Ridley K, Ridgers ND, Salmon J. Criterion validity of the activPALTM and ActiGraph for assessing children's sitting and standing time in a school classroom setting. *Int J Behav Nutr Phys Act.* 2016; **13**:75.

29   Hamilton MT, Hamilton DG, Zderic TW. Role of low energy expenditure and sitting in obesity, metabolic syndrome, type 2 diabetes, and cardiovascular disease. *Diabetes.* 2007; **56**(11):2655–67.

30   Ridgers ND, Fairclough SJ. Assessing free-living physical activity using accelerometry: practical issues for researchers and practitioners. *Eur J Sports Sci.* 2011; **11**(3):205–13.

31   Evenson KR, Terry JJW. Assessment of differing definitions of accelerometer nonwear time. *Res Quar Exerc Sport.* 2009; **80**(2):355–62.

32   Chinapaw MJ, de Niet M, Verloigne M, De Bourdeaudhuij I, Brug J, Altenberg TM. From sedentary time to sedentary patterns: accelerometer data reduction decisions in youth. *PLoS One.* 2014; **9**(11):e111205.

33   Dowd KP, Harrington DM, Bourke AK, Nelson J, Donnelly AE. The measurement of sedentary patterns and behaviors using the activPALTM Professional physical activity monitor. *Physiol Meas.* 2012; **33**(11):1887–99.

34   Grant PM, Ryan CG, Tigbe WW, Granant MH. The validation of a novel activity monitor in the measurement of posture and motion during everyday activities. *Br J Sports Med.* 2006; **40**:992–7.

35   Lyden K, Kozey Keadle SL, Staudenmayer JW, Freedson PS. Validity of two wearable monitors to estimate breaks from sedentary time. *Med Sci Sports Exerc.* 2012; **44**(11):2243–52.

36   Dowd KP, Harrington DM, Donnelly AE. Criterion and concurrent validity of the activPAL™ Professional physical activity monitor in adolescent females. *PLoS One.* 2012; **7**(10):e47633.

37   Aminian S, Hinckson EA. Examining the validity of the ActivPAL monitor in measuring posture and ambulatory movement in children. *Int J Behav Nutr Phys Act.* 2012; **9**:119.

38   Davies G, Reilly JJ, Paton JY. Objective assessment of posture and posture transitions in the pre-school child. *Physiol Meas.* 2012; **33**(11):1913–21.

39   Owen N, Salmon J, Koohsari MJ, Turrell G, Giles-Corti B. Sedentary behaviour and health: mapping environmental and social contexts to underpin chronic disease prevention. *Br J Sports Med.* 2014; **48**(3):174–7.

40   Salmon J. Novel strategies to promote children's physical activities and reduce sedentary behavior. *J Phys Act Health.* 2010; **7**(Suppl 3):S299–S306.

41   Straker L, Mathiassen SE. Increased physical work loads in modern work – a necessity for better health and performance? *Ergonomics.* 2009; **52**(10):1215–25.

42   Parry L, Straker L. The contribution of office work to sedentary behaviour associated risk. *BMC Public Health.* 2013; **13**:296.

43   Thorp AA, Healy GN, Winkler E, Clark BK, Gardiner PA, Owen N, et al. Prolonged sedentary time and physical activity in workplace and non-work contexts: a cross-sectional study of office, customer service and call centre employees. *Int J Behav Nutr Phys Act.* 2012; **26**:9.

44   Sudholz B, Ridgers ND, Mussap A, Bennie J, Timperio A, Salmon J. Reliability and validity of self-reported sitting and breaks from sitting in the workplace. *J Sci Med Sport,* (In press, e-pub ahead of print). DOI: 10.1016/j.jsams.2017.10.030

45   Abbott RA, Straker LM, Mathiassen SE. Patterning of children's sedentary time at and away from school. *Obesity* (Silver Spring). 2013; **21**(1):E131–3.

46   Bailey DP, Fairclough SJ, Savory LA, Denton SJ, Pang D, Deane CS, et al. Accelerometry-assessed sedentary behaviour and physical activity levels during the segmented school day in 10–14-year-old children: the HAPPY study. *Eur J Pediatr.* 2012; **171**(12):1805–13.

47   Stephens SK, Winkler EAH, Trost SG, Dunstan DW, Eakin EG, Chastin SFM, et al. Intervening to reduce workplace sitting time: how and when do changes to sitting time occur? *Br J Sports Med.* 2014; **48**(13):1037–42.

48   Thorp AA, Owen N, Neuhas M, Dunstan DW. Sedentary behaviors and subsequent health outcomes in adults: a systematic review of longitudinal studies, 1996–2011. *Am J Prev Med.* 2011; **41**(2):207–15.

49   Gorely T, Biddle SJ, Marshall SJ, Cameron N. The prevalence of leisure time sedentary behaviour and physical activity in adolescent boys: an ecological momentary assessment approach. *Int J Pediatr Obes.* 2009; **4**(4):289–98.

50   Dunstan DW, Barr EL, Healy GN, Salmon J, Shaw JE, Balkau B, et al. Television viewing time and mortality: the Australian diabetes, obesity and lifestyle study (AusDiab). *Circulation.* 2010; **121**(3):384–91.

51   Robinson S, Daly RM, Ridgers ND, Salmon J. Children's screen-based behaviors and associations with cardiovascular risk factors. *J Pediatr.* 2015; **167**:1239–45.

52   Ridley K, Ainsworth BE, Olds TS. Development of a compendium of energy expenditures for youth. *Int J Behav Nutr Phys Act.* 2008; **5**:45.

53   Ainsworth BE, Haskell WL, Leon AS, Jacobs DRJ, Montoye HJ, Sallis JF, et al. Compendium of physical activities: classification of energy costs of human physical activities. *Med Sci Sports Exerc.* 1993; **25**(1):71–80.

54   Sugiyama T, Healy GN, Dunstan DW, Salmon J, Owen N. Joint associations of multiple leisure-time sedentary behaviours and physical activity with obesity in Australian adults. *Int J Behav Nutr Phys Act.* 2008; **5**:35.

55   Morris JN, Heady JA, Raffle PAB, Roberts CG, Parks JW. Coronary heart disease and physical activity of work. *Lancet.* 1953; **265**(6795):1111–20.

56   Biswas A, Oh PI, Faulkner GE, Bajaj RR, Silver MA, Mitchell MS, et al. Sedentary time and its association with risk for disease incidence, mortality, and hospitalization in adults: a systematic review and meta-analysis. *Ann Int Med.* 2015; **162**(2):123–32.

57   Wilmot EG, Edwardson CL, Achana FA, Davies MJ, Gorely T, Gray LJ, et al. Sedentary time in adults and the association with diabetes, cardiovascular disease and death: systematic review and meta-analysis. *Diabetologia.* 2012; **55**(11):2895–905.

58   Williams DM, Raynor HA, Ciccolo JT. A review of TV viewing and its association with health outcomes in adults. *Am J Lifestyle Med.* 2008; **2**(3):250–9.

59   Ekelund U, Steene-Johannessen J, Brown WJ, Fagerland MW, Owen N, Powell KE, et al. Does physical activity attenuate, or even eliminate, the detrimental association of sitting

time with mortality? A harmonised meta-analysis of data from more than 1 million men and women. *Lancet.* 2016; **388**(10051):1302–10.

60   Tremblay MS, LeBlanc AG, Kho ME, Saunders TJ, Larouche R, Colley RC, et al. Systematic review of sedentary behaviour and health indicators in school-aged children and youth. *Int J Behav Nutr Phys Act.* 2011; **8**:98.

61   Carson V, Hunter S, Kuzik N, Gray CE, Poitras VJ, Chaput JP, et al. Systematic review of sedentary behaviour and health indicators in school-aged children and youth: an update. *Appl Physiol Nutr Metab.* 2016; **41**(6 Suppl 3):S240–S65.

62   Cliff DP, Hesketh KD, Vella S, Hinkley T, Tsiros MD, Ridgers ND, et al. Objectively measured sedentary behaviour and health and development in children and adolescents: systematic review and meta-analysis. *Obes Rev.* 2016; **17**:330–44.

63   Biddle SJH, García Bengoechea E, Wiesner G. Sedentary behaviour and adiposity in youth: a systematic review of reviews and analysis of causality. *Int J Behav Nutr Phys Act.* 2017; **14**:43.

64   Department of Health. Australia's physical activity and sedentary behaviour guidelines for children (5–12 years) [Internet]. Canberra: Department of Health; 2014 Jun. [cited 2017 Nov 6]. Available from: www.health.gov.au/internet/main/publishing.nsf/content/health-pubhlth-strateg-phys-act-guidelines

65   Carson V, Janssen I. Volume, patterns, and types of sedentary behavior and cardio-metabolic health in children and adolescents: a cross-sectional study. *BMC Public Health.* 2011; **11**:274.

66   Gabel L, Ridgers ND, Della Gatta PA, Arundell L, Cerin E, Robinson S, et al. Associations of sedentary time patterns and TV viewing time with inflammatory and endothelial function biomarkers in children. *Pediatr Obes.* 2016; **11**:194–201.

16 Ensuring quality data
Validity, reliability and error

Damian A. Coleman and Jonathan D. Wiles

Aims of the chapter

Meaningful research findings can only be attained through the collection of valid and reliable data. The aims of this chapter are therefore to provide an understanding of the various forms of validity and reliability, and how they may be assessed and reported. It will also provide guidelines for maximizing validity, reliability and accuracy of measurements.

Ensuring quality data

Exercise science is rapidly evolving, with new ideas, concepts, equipment and techniques improving our insight into the interactions between health, disease progression and exercise intervention. Part of this forward momentum is linked to scientists being able to effectively utilize techniques and equipment to derive data which clearly informs decision making; this is often referred to as 'clean data'. Theoretically, critical evaluation of each new generation of data should allow us to collect data that is even cleaner, and thus has increased value in the process of interpretation.

So what is clean data?

Normally when we set out to evaluate a client in a clinic setting, or begin steps for data collection on a research project we will have established clear aims (and objectives). This could involve measuring blood markers that then may lead to an intervention, or exploring relationships between physical activity and health related risk factors. Only by collecting precise data, or data that is free from errors can we achieve those aims. The monitoring of resting blood pressure within a clinical environment provides us with a good example of how important clean data is. A client could come to an open clinic and have their resting blood pressure measured for diagnostic purposes. We know resting blood pressure has some biological variability and we are aware of factors (stress, minor illness, exercise responses, diet) that might contribute to this variability, potentially resulting in a distorted blood pressure reading which could easily be misinterpreted. As such, we try to minimize the impact of these factors prior to the assessment to obtain a 'true' reading. Therefore, the committed practitioner and researcher will have reviewed previous work for information on how to collect precise blood pressure data and they will try to control as many of the factors listed above as possible to ensure that the data generated is effective for making the correct decision.

In fact collecting clean data for a client or research participant should be considered an ethical requirement. Codes of conduct for most accrediting organizations typically specify that the consenting patient has the right to expect that procedures and practices are effective, and part of this is to ensure that these measures are error free in their collection and subsequent interpretation.

So how do you collect clean data?

Having alluded to this already, a key factor is to scour the available literature on a particular method or technique that you intend to use so that you can fully reference and support your actions in the data preparation and collection process. Additionally, referring to the manufacturer instructions in the early stages of designing your procedures is always a useful exercise. Engaging with other practitioners and/ or researchers about the pragmatics of using the equipment and techniques will also help to guide your decision making during the planning phase. Indeed, one benefit of conference and workshop engagement for your personal Continuing Professional Development (CPD) is the opportunity to engage with presenters and other attendees utilizing similar techniques and equipment. Whilst the value of this is obvious when using relatively new equipment or techniques, it is worth bearing in mind that there may still be problems with established technology (which could easily invalidate results) that never make it to the methods sections of academic papers. For example, the panic in our laboratory when the 'gold standard' lactate and glucose analyser went into auto calibration at an inconvenient time was probably echoed in hundreds of labs around the world in the 1990s, but the process associated with dealing with this problem we have never seen published in any academic paper or user manual. This experiential knowledge is most easily accessed through interaction with other clinicians and researchers.

Another key factor to consider is that a potential source of imprecision in data collection lies with the clinician. Therefore, it is very important that techniques are practiced prior to data collection and there is no assumption on the part of the team collecting data that all experimenters or clinicians would get identical results with their data collection techniques. Indeed, this general appreciation that quantitative data collection error can vary between people has led to institutions such as the International Society for the Advancement of Kinanthropometry (ISAK) requiring practitioners to be aware of the error in their measurements as part of their accreditation.

Why is all of this so important?

All scientific research produced, whether it be an undergraduate dissertation or a clinical trial destined for publication in a top medical journal, is subject to academic scrutiny. One of the first things a reviewer of an academic paper or report will consider is the credibility of your data. They will look at the absolute measurement scores and relate them to industry normative data. You may have an exceptional intervention study that altered maximal oxygen uptake by 25%, but if the initial estimate was exceptionally high or low you would struggle to convince reviewers that your data is credible. Precise data collection can also enable you to conclude from the data in a more cost-effective manner. For experimental studies, precision of measurement allows us to identify statistically significant trends with smaller populations of participants (this can save substantial hours in the laboratory and save valuable resources).

Precise data also allows for explicit interpretation of individual changes to an intervention, which is very useful if there are responders and non-responders to interventions that warrant further interrogation.

Defining validity and reliability

Previously we have discussed precise data collection and the benefits of this process. We generally refer to this as the validity of measurement. Sometimes valid (error free) measurement is achievable, but sometimes we have to accept that measurement has a degree of inaccuracy. However, where we do have inaccuracies, it is critical that repeat measurements are consistent (or reliable). To illustrate this example, if we obtained a packaged blood sample that we knew contained 4.00 mmol·l^{-1} of glucose, we could use this sample to check commercially available blood glucose monitors to assess their validity. It is highly unlikely that each glucose monitor would give an identical 4.00 mmol·l^{-1} result when the blood was processed. Monitor A might give a value of 3.7 mmol·l^{-1} and Monitor B might read 4.3 mmol·l^{-1} etc. However, the point here is that we could still work with these pieces of equipment if the repeat measurements presented similar numbers. If we ran repeated samples through Monitor A and they were consistently 0.3 mmol·l^{-1} lower than the 4.0 mmol·l^{-1} true value, then we could slightly adjust the numbers or inform the client to add ~0.3 mmol·l^{-1} to every measurement that they take. Monitor A would not be a valid monitor, but the repeat measurements are consistent so we could consider this to be reliable and we can henceforth adjust our interpretations accordingly. On the other hand, if we assessed Monitor B and found that some samples came out higher than 4.0 mmol·l^{-1} and some samples came out lower than 4.0 mmol·l^{-1} the client or practitioner would have much more difficulty in the interpretation of the data. Using Monitor B we would find it impossible to interpret if a client was hypoglycemic (blood glucose less than 4.0 mmol·l^{-1}) from a single measure because the measure is not valid (i.e. it does not replicate the true value) and it is not reliable because the values obtained by repeated sampling keep changing. With Monitor A and our adjustments we could confidently ascertain if a client was hypoglycemic; even though ideally we would be using a tool and practice that gave us values of 4.0 mmol·l^{-1} every single time with repeated measurements.

Whilst the broad definition of validity refers to the precision and accuracy of measurement it is important to be aware that there are different types of validity that are relevant to the researcher or clinician based on the experimental tools that they are using.

For most of the work that we conduct, the following forms of validity are likely to be the most important to consider.

Ecological validity

Ecological validity refers to the ability to apply the findings beyond the clinic and research setting. Our investigative work in the field of isometric exercise and reducing blood pressure began initially utilizing a £65,000 isokinetic dynamometer to prescribe precise exercise intensities, clearly not ecologically valid (how many hypertensive individuals can afford that equipment?). Subsequent work has moved on to utilizing more accessible exercise protocols that can take place in the home in an attempt to make this work more ecologically valid.

Internal validity

Internal validity refers to the extent to which we employ a strong 'evidence-based' approach to link the relationships that are evident in our conclusions. This often requires some substantial control of 'confounding' variables that also exert an influence upon the variables under investigation. Imagine that we wanted to investigate the exercise adherence patterns in a group of patients who were categorized as 'pre-diabetic' compared to a group of participants who exhibited a normal blood glucose response during monitoring (our control group). If we provided an exercise plan to all participants that walked through the door of the clinic, it would be likely that there would be a variety of random differences between the pre-diabetic and control group. Some of these differences may be irrelevant to our study (e.g. hair colour or height), however some variables may influence exercise adherence patterns (employment hours, previous history of exercise, body mass, age, motivation, previous history of intervention, etc.). For internal validity we try and control many of these variables so that we can clearly make judgements and conclusions about the relationship between our status (normal or pre-diabetic) and exercise adherence.

External validity

External validity is a third form of validity that is very important to consider, and to some extent is at odds with internal validity. If we have tightly controlled many variables during participant selection for internal validity, the question then arises "can we then generalize finding beyond these participant types?" This is very important in terms of your interpretation of data because it simply refers to how broadly your findings can be generalized. As scientists we have to be extremely careful in extrapolating beyond our sample of data (because we could be making rather large assumptions). Thus, during the process of 'sample selection' for experimental studies you must make a clear decision about who your findings may be applicable to. Therefore, if you want to extrapolate findings to a broad population then sample a broad population, and if you want to apply your work to both male and female patients, then include both sexes in your sample. This means your inclusion criteria is very important in this process to ensure that you are thinking about the implications of your data during the experimental design phase.

All we need then is very precise (usually very expensive) kit, thousands of participants, and to take all measures in a real-world situation. However unfortunately, there are never opportunities that encompass all of these factors, the resources and costs of including broad (all encompassing) studies are often prohibitive from the outset, and normally (for the sake of internal validity) we are much more specific with our inclusion criteria. But, with an understanding of external validity the scientist will be extremely careful with any speculation around their data (to other participant groups for example), and this will often be presented as a 'direction for future research' near the end of a research paper.

Construct validity

Construct validity is the broad concept that the measure utilized in your study is actually measuring what you claim it is measuring. There are many questionnaires developed to try and gain information from participants, some of these questionnaires are extremely well known and utilized in the exercise field (e.g. the Exercise Self-Efficacy Scale),[1] which have been designed and assessed to ensure the measure is clearly informing the researcher about the parameter under investigation. However, there are many other forms of questionnaire that fail at a really simple level in terms of construct validity. For example, cross-sectional or longitudinal studies into physical activity and health status commonly ask questions about the number of hours of activity you regularly complete on a weekly basis. The validity issue here is that if it's only the amount of hours that's asked for, and there is a complete disregard for exercise intensity, which is known to be a factor in health outcomes, then the question will fail to provide key information and a clear picture on the topic of physical activity and health outcomes. Questions on exercise intensity may be less commonly included compared to those about hours of activity, probably because exercise intensity is relatively more difficult to accurately assess, in comparison to counting hours of activity, and thus the construct validity of the tool is very limited in giving us a clear picture of physical activity and outcomes. In this instance the questionnaire and data would simply tell us about the duration of exercise, and for 'duration of exercise' this questionnaire would be valid in this context.

Content validity

Content validity considers if the measure adopted covers a representative sample of the variable under investigation. For example, a questionnaire or interview to provide the patient view of a clinical practice must allow the participants the opportunity to represent their views of the clinical practice. The value of the data depends upon the content validity; so a simple question such as "are the practices at the clinic performed in a professional manner?", could be presented so that the patient has just a 'yes or no' option. This has poor content validity because it does not give us much detail in the process of interpreting the data. Further probing questions allowing open and unrestricted detail to be extracted on the personal experiences of the patient would allow for the full represented sample of patient views (and content) to be presented, but obviously this would then require significant time in analysis compared to the yes/no answer format.

Criterion validity

Criterion validity is the extent to which a measure is related to an outcome of another measure, and these outcomes could be linked to an outcome in the future (often referred to as predictive validity) or at the same moment in time (concurrent validity). An example of concurrent validity in our field would be the exploration of the question "do our current physical activity patterns inform us about our current health status"? To determine predictive validity, we would need longitudinal data to then make decisions based on whether the physical activity data collected today allows us to predict future health outcomes.

Assessing validity and reliability

Good research process should include an assessment of validity and reliability as part of routine processes. Assessment of these factors can dramatically reduce problems in the future by informing practitioners if equipment and procedures are providing accurate results, and/or how confident the practitioner can be in the interpretation and feedback to clients.

Assessing validity

There are a number of steps to assessing the validity of data. Whilst some of these steps are very simple, do not overlook or fail to report/interpret these stages, because all stages are very important in the evaluation of validity. The ideal situation is that you have identified a 'gold standard' or true measure to compare your tools/procedures against. This could be a comparison of readings on your blood glucose analyser to a sample of 'known' concentrations (the previous 4.0 mmol·l⁻¹ example), or very basically the use of calibrated weights placed on the laboratory scales. The known concentrations of glucose and the calibrated weights would both be considered our 'gold standard' and our comparison of other techniques to these would give us an indication of how close we are to these true measures. Before comparing your data to gold standard measures or techniques it is recommended that you read the seminal paper by Martin Bland and Douglas Altman,[2] which has close to 40,000 citations at the point of writing this chapter.

Working example

Imagine the scenario where we are interested in the heart rate response to a treatment. A 12 lead ECG assessment requires nursing staff to prepare the patient, take the measures and a consultant to confirm the heart rate recording, and thus this is an expensive assessment to conduct. A cheap heart rate monitor also claims to assess heart rate accurately, but our first steps must be to ascertain if this cheaper piece of equipment is valid when compared to the gold standard ECG system. The ideal scenario is that when cross comparing data, the data is collected at an identical time point (rather than in two separate assessments). This cannot always be the case, for example predictors of maximal oxygen uptake would require multiple visits to a laboratory because a participant could not undertake two tests at one time point. With heart rate monitoring however it is possible to record using both systems at the same time point, and Table 16.1 presents the data on 10 participants who were assessed during this comparison study.

Step 1

The first step is simply to look at the data. Bearing in mind we should always report the data to the resolution that we measure the data (in this case to whole beats per minute) the 12 lead and the heart rate monitor give us mean values of 68 b·min⁻¹. These are very similar, likewise the standard deviation values are 12 b·min⁻¹ for the ECG system compared to 14 b·min⁻¹ for the heart rate monitor. Despite these similarities, you can see from the difference score column in Table 16.1 that there is some variability in the scores obtained on our heart rate monitor compared to the 12 lead ECG system.

Step 2

The second step is to ascertain if there is a significant difference between the two measurement types. A basic paired *t*-test (if the data are parametric) will tell you if

Table 16.1 Raw data comparing two methods of heart rate assessment

Participant	12 Lead ECG	Heart Rate Monitor (HRM)	Difference (12 lead minus HRM)
1	65 b·min⁻¹	68 b·min⁻¹	−3
2	66 b·min⁻¹	71 b·min⁻¹	−5
3	58 b·min⁻¹	56 b·min⁻¹	2
4	78 b·min⁻¹	81 b·min⁻¹	−3
5	75 b·min⁻¹	74 b·min⁻¹	1
6	81 b·min⁻¹	92 b·min⁻¹	−11
7	85 b·min⁻¹	78 b·min⁻¹	7
8	49 b·min⁻¹	51 b·min⁻¹	−2
9	55 b·min⁻¹	51 b·min⁻¹	4
10	66 b·min⁻¹	59 b·min⁻¹	7
Mean	67.8 b·min⁻¹	68.1 b·min⁻¹	−0.3
Standard Deviation	11.8 b·min⁻¹	13.7 b·min⁻¹	5.6

there is a significant trend indicating one piece of equipment is reading higher than the other piece of equipment. In the example above there is no significant difference, you may have guessed this with the raw mean scores being only 0.3 b·min⁻¹ different between pieces of equipment (in this example the p-value is 0.87).

Step 3

The next question relates to the relationship between the two pieces of kit. Do high readings on the 12 lead ECG also lead to high readings on the heart rate monitor? And likewise for low readings? A simple Pearson's correlation will help to answer this question. Figure 16.1 below indicates the relationship between the 12 lead system and the heart rate monitor, this yields a strong positive relationship between the two systems, the correlation coefficient (r) is 0.94. Looking at Figure 16.1 and the trendline we can see that not all data sit on the trendline and that if we used the equation of the line to predict the heart rate value on the heart rate monitor from ECG or vice versa then there would be some error in the predictions. Again the key to interpreting the data is to spend some time looking at the figure. At the mid-range point of 65–67 b·min⁻¹ on the ECG system there are 3 data points, these are presented in a lighter gray. You can clearly see that for these similar readings on the ECG system these values range between 59 and 71 b·min⁻¹ on the heart rate monitor. This provides clear indication that there is error between these systems and that the error is not consistent. A consistent error would result in an identical standard deviation between assessments (in step 1), a statistically significant difference in step 2 and a perfect correlation between the two pieces of equipment (Pearson's correlation of $r = 1.00$).

So we have error between the two systems which is not consistent, and again you may have ascertained this from Table 16.1 with the difference scores being quite variable between participants.

Step 4

This is the slightly more complex part of assessing validity (or agreement) between methods. We can calculate 95% limits of agreement between these two methods. The data from this analysis can then be used to make a judgement by the practitioner

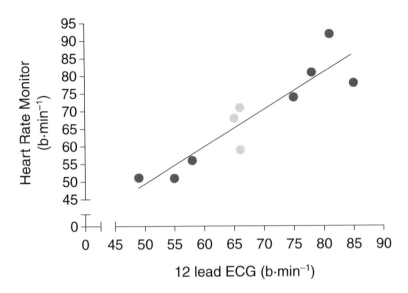

Figure 16.1 The relationship between two methods of heart rate assessment.

whether the agreement is close enough to make clinical decisions. We actually use some of the data from step 1 in the process of generating limits of agreement. Firstly we calculate the difference between the two measurements and the standard deviation of these differences. From the raw data we have a mean difference of –0.3 b·min⁻¹ and a SD of individual differences of 5.6 b·min⁻¹ values noted in Table 16.1. Based on the relationship between the distribution of data and our standard deviation we would expect most (95%) of the difference scores to lie between ±1.96 standard deviations of the mean difference. Working with our numbers, this would give us 95% limits of agreement of

$$- 0.3 + (1.96 \times 5.6) = 10.7 \text{ b·min}^{-1}$$
$$- 0.3 - (1.96 \times 5.6) = -11.3 \text{ b·min}^{-1}$$

Thus for any measure taken with the 12 lead ECG system, the cheaper heart rate monitor may be approximately 11 beats higher, or 11 beats lower for heart rate measurement. Whether this is problematic would now be a clinical decision, but if a change in resting heart rate of 5 b·min⁻¹ was clinically important or relevant, then the heart rate monitor clearly cannot detect such a small change. In fact a true recording in resting heart rate from the ECG system of 65 b·min⁻¹ could yield scores of 54 to 76 b·min⁻¹ at the start of a study using the heart rate monitor, and a change measured at the end of a study or intervention on the ECG system to 60 b·min⁻¹ could return values of 49 to 71 b·min⁻¹ using the cheaper tool. Or put another way, a true reduction in heart rate *could* appear as a rise in heart rate if the heart rate monitor was adopted in this study or intervention.

    Bland and Altman warn about only engaging the more basic analysis (steps 1–3) in the process of ascertaining if gold standard equipment agrees with other measurement tools,[2] and they also clearly identify that the clinical relevance of the limits calculated is a key part of the judgement in terms of utilizing equipment or techniques once they have been assessed in this manner.

Assessing reliability

Consistency of measurement is a further consideration, and often at the outset of an investigation repeated assessments using a particular tool or technique are used to assess if consistent measures can be taken. Consistency is vital if changes in scores pre and post an intervention are going to be detected for participants in a study or for a single patient in returning to the clinic to assess changes in health parameters.

Working example

Assessing reliability requires duplicate measures where you are confident no changes have taken place. If a group of clients came to the laboratory at 10 am and 12 pm, and on each occasion they had a sum of 7-sites skinfold assessment undertaken, it would be highly unlikely that these values would deviate in this period and thus we could undertake an objective assessment of how much variation occurs in our ability to take these measures. Table 16.2 shows the data from these two assessments, and you will probably realize this data set-up looks similar to the data Table 16.1 used to assess validity. However Table 16.2 is constructed on repeated measures using the same equipment, rather than comparing a piece of equipment to a gold standard measure.

The steps described above in terms of validity are still relevant here. Firstly look at the data (mean scores and the standard deviations, there are only very small differences between the mean data, and slightly more variability in the second sample of skinfold measures (see the standard deviation scores). Secondly ascertain if there are significant differences between the data sets (in this example a paired *t*-test yields a *p*-value of 0.81), and thirdly ascertain if the scores are ordered correctly, are high skinfold scores at 10 am corresponding with high skinfold scores at 12 pm? In this instance these two assessments are significantly related with a Pearson's *r* of 0.96.

Table 16.2 Raw data comparing two 7-site skinfold assessments

Participant	10 am sample	12.00 pm sample	Difference (10 am minus 12 pm sample)
1	47 mm	52 mm	−5 mm
2	66 mm	65 mm	1 mm
3	44 mm	35 mm	9 mm
4	82 mm	88 mm	−6 mm
5	77 mm	74 mm	3 mm
6	59 mm	52 mm	7 mm
7	47 mm	49 mm	−2 mm
8	59 mm	60 mm	−1 mm
9	87 mm	85 mm	2 mm
10	66 mm	70 mm	−4 mm
Mean	63.4 mm	63 mm	0.4 mm
Standard Deviation	15.1 mm	16.7 mm	5.0 mm

Using the data in this format we can calculate a statistic called the 'typical error', which is reviewed in detail by Hopkins.[3] This statistic gives us the test-retest error for ~52% of the population. The calculation is simple, we use the standard deviation of the difference scores (in this instance 5.0 mm) divided by the square root of 2 (1.4142). The square root of 2 is used in this calculation simply based on the mathematical relationship between the variance (inconsistencies) in the difference scores being equivalent to the sum of the variance of the two trials. Variance is equivalent to the standard deviation squared, thus because this statistic is calculated from the analysis of two trials the standard deviation of the difference is divided by the square root of 2. In this example the typical error of measurement is 5.0 / 1.4142 = 3.5 mm.

So how can we utilize the typical error in our experimental design or protocols for patient assessment? The first piece of information that is easily obtained is to identify if you become more reliable when you repeatedly assess your participants (maybe in planning the reliability study add further trials at 2 pm and 4 pm). If typical error drops, then you have less error in your measures as you become more familiar with the technique or client. If your scores do reduce, then this can inform the number of trials of familiarization that are required to minimize measurement error in your data collection. Mean values or median values across multiple assessments also reduce the measurement error, any fluctuations in error in those process are somewhat smoothed before going into the analysis. Typical error can be used in the estimation of sample sizes for experimental studies, and if the error is low we can use fewer participants, which can be of real benefit and cost. However, if in exploring the reliability of your measurement you require each participant to have five or six visits to derive the reliable measures with low error scores, this may not be possible. You may have to accept a higher error rate from one or two visits and recruit more participants because of this error. For single measures on an individual the measurement error should be used to interpret if changes have occurred with any reassessment. In the current example, if a client returned and had reduced their sum of skinfolds by 3 mm, you could not be confident that a true change has taken place because the number falls within the typical error of measurement for 52% of cases. If you wanted to be more stringent with confidence of 95%, multiplying the typical error by 2.77 (this number is the square root of 2 multiplied by 1.96) and a change of >9.7 mm (3.5 mm × 2.77) would be required on an individual basis to be more fully confident that the change that occurred is not simply due to measurement error. The review by Hopkins provides a detailed insight into the use of this statistic, and the coefficient of variation statistic which presents the typical error as a percentage error score in its calculation.[3] In using this process however, there is the temptation to set a percentage threshold and grade reliability accordingly. For example, variation of 5% or less is acceptable, and above 5% is unacceptable. The threshold set for reliability measures should simply reflect the measure you are taking, and having high variability is not a problem if the changes you are looking for are also large, thus making interpretation of the data relatively straightforward.

In the context of data interpretation plotting the error around all individual change scores in a study will also allow the researcher to interpret if there is true individual responses to a treatment. Studies often report individual variation around change scores to interventions, however many of these variations are simply a manifestation of error within the measurement. For a detailed review of this material visit Atkinson and Batterham.[4]

Conclusion

In summary, a consideration of the validity and reliability of measurement from the outset of a study is vital to avoid the more costly process of data clean-up at a later stage of the investigation and/or potentially a significant waste of resources. From a practitioner's perspective the techniques and issues raised in this chapter should be regularly revisited to ensure data collected can be interpreted in a meaningful manner for the client, and should be an integral part of routine laboratory practices for the same reasons.

References

1   McAuley E. Self-efficacy and the maintenance of exercise participation in older adults. *J Behav Med.* 1993; **16**:103–13.
2   Bland JM, Altman DG. Statistical methods for assessing agreement between two methods of clinical measurement. *Lancet.* 1986; **327**:307–10.
3   Hopkins W. Measures of reliability in sports medicine and science. *Sports Med.* 2000; **30**:1–15.
4   Atkinson G, Batterham A. True and false interindividual differences in the physiological response to an intervention. *Exp Phys.* 2015; **100**:577–88.

17 Quantitative data analyses

R.C. Richard Davison and Paul M. Smith

Introduction and chapter aims

Ideally, prior to collecting any data, a researcher should have considered the type of data analysis that would be most appropriate, and any study design should be influenced by the proposed data analysis methodology. Without this prior consideration there is a risk that the researcher may collect a considerable amount of data that cannot be analysed in a way that enables them to answer the original research question: this is frankly an unethical approach to research, as a considerable amount of time, effort and resources could be used and wasted.

Furthermore, even when more complex statistical processes have been appropriately selected for the main analysis, it is still advisable and necessary to complete a range of basic descriptive (or simple) statistics to get a full understanding of the data set that you are dealing with, before proceeding with any further analysis. The outcomes from these fairly simple tests can, and should guide or confirm the most suitable follow-up analysis. In some cases, it will alert you to the unsuitability of some more complex statistical tests as this analysis will reveal that the data set is not compatible with that method. Most common is the realization that the data are not 'normally distributed' (see below).

The aims of this chapter are to provide the novice researcher with an understanding of basic preliminary data evaluation, descriptive statistics, hypothesis testing and alternative means for assessing data that are typically used in physical activity and health research. This chapter will provide some insight into how to approach your data analysis and the options available to you. Beyond this, it is intended that the reader should pursue available options in greater depth through established texts on statistical analyses, as well as related digital resources and software.

Types (typology) of numerical data

Before undertaking even the most basic of simple statistics, it is important to evaluate the nature of the numerical data that you will, or have collected. This starts with classifying the data, and a suggested typology is outlined below.[1]

Nominal data

This is where data are categorized by name or classification, for example gender, physical activity type or disease. A nominal categorization gives no indication of scale or size.

Ordinal data

You have ordinal data when a variable has some order to it. For example, a ranking of physical activity levels (low-active, moderately active, very active) or exercise intensity (moderate, heavy, extreme). However, it does not imply that there is a consistent gap between positions on this scale. In other words, the difference between 1st and 2nd on an ordinal ranking scale could be quite small whereas the difference between 2nd and 3rd could be quite large.

Interval data

With interval data, there is a scale where the gaps between points on the scale are equal. In this situation, zero does not indicate the absence of the variable, but simply represents another point on the scale, so this scale can also include negative numbers or values. An example of this is temperature, whereby 0°C does not mean 'no temperature', it just represents the temperature at which water freezes. Likewise ratios are meaningless, for example 40°C cannot be described as 'twice as hot as 20°C'. To illustrate this, just convert the values to degrees Fahrenheit to see what happens to the zero value – it is no longer zero, and as for the ratio, it does not remain as a ratio of 2:1.

Ratio data

A ratio scale also has equal gaps between points, but in this case, the value zero means zero, i.e. nothing. For example, with a measure of distance, zero means no distance. Further, with ratio data, you can have a meaningful ratio, 2 km is twice as far as 1 km, and these distances are always in a ratio of 2:1, even if you convert distances to miles. Similarly in the context of a change in body mass: no change in body mass is indicated by a value of 0 kg, and a 2 kg reduction in body mass is a quarter (0.25) of an 8 kg reduction in body mass. This ratio of a quarter remains, even if the weight loss is expressed in pounds.

The nature of the data you have will determine the types of statistical analyses that you are able to undertake in the context of how you may describe the data using descriptive statistics (means, standard deviations, frequencies, etc.), and compare the influence of factors within your data set. There are rules to guide you to the correct statistical analyses.[2] Some of the key considerations involved in this process are outlined here, and further details on these are presented in other statistical texts. The selection of the appropriate analyses becomes more obvious as you get to know your data, which often commences with the use of 'descriptive statistics'. Furthermore, it is easy to forget that since all statistical tests have some rules on their use, the inappropriate use of statistical tests may lead you to the wrong conclusions. So, before you commence any statistical tests, the starting point is to get a feel for the nature of the data by assessing the central tendency, variability and normality. The outcomes from this will guide you to the best follow-up test or data transformation if required.

Descriptive statistics

When faced with a set of data in the form of a spreadsheet of numbers, it's difficult to get a feel for the data, and even more difficult to effectively compare two sets of data. To enable a better understanding of the data they are summarized using descriptive statistics, such as frequencies in the case of nominal data, or averages for interval or ratio data. To get an even better appreciation of an interval or ratio data set, the average is usually presented with a measure that indicates the spread of the data around that average, such as the range or standard deviation. Information about these descriptive statistics and their use is outlined below.

Measures of central tendency and variability

The term 'central tendency' arises from the tendency for quantitative data to cluster around a central value, as in a normal distribution. The key measures of central tendency are the arithmetic mean, median and mode, the characteristics of which are described in Table 17.1. Generally, these only give you a partial picture of the characteristics of your data set and thus you also need to understand the variability of that data around these measures of central tendency. With the addition of range, interquartile range and standard deviation, you will gain a much better basic analysis and understanding of the shape of your data set. All statistical software will give you some or all of the following measures of central tendency and variability.

Normality of data

If we were to measure the systolic blood pressure of 500 patients, we would expect this data set to be fairly normally distributed: that is, most patients would have a systolic blood pressure close to the mean value and only a few patients would have either a much lower or much higher systolic blood pressure. No 'real' data are ever fully normally distributed but if we plotted this data in the form of a histogram it would make what is called a bell-shaped curve, as presented in Figure 17.1. If the data were perfectly normal then the mean = median = mode. Additionally, the distribution of the data around the mean can be described by calculating the 'Standard Deviation' (SD) of the data, as:

68.27 % of the data would fall between mean ±1 SD;
95.45 % of the data would fall between mean ±2 SD;
99.73 % of the data would fall between mean ±3 SD.

How do you test for normality?

Plotting a simple histogram of your data immediately tells you if it clearly lacks normality. Then, in a statistical package you can produce a skewness score, where zero represents perfectly normal. In addition there are the Kolmogorov-Smirnov test (K-S) and Shapiro-Wilk (S-W) tests, which determine if the data is significantly non-normal. However the K-S test is susceptible to extreme values and thus the S-W test is more commonly recommended, particularly for sample sizes of <50. If your data is not normal, this finding can rule out a number of further statistical tests. In this situation you then have two options, either:

- use a statistical test that does not require normality (usually a form of non-parametric test); or
- transform your data, which can produce a normal distribution, thereby enabling you to use a test that does require the data to be normally distributed (usually a form of parametric test). In this case, we suggest you take professional advice on the best type of transformation, but it most commonly involves log transformation of your data.

Table 17.1 Measures of central tendency and variability

Measure	Description	Advantages	Disadvantages
Mean (μ)	Average value for all of your data.	Easily understood. Used in many statistical procedures.	May not be a real value (e.g. 2.4 cardiac episodes per year). Can be affected by extreme values.
Median	Middle value in a data set.	Easy to understand, not influenced by outliers.	Data must be in rank order. Not used in further statistical tests. Not particularly good at comparing different data sets.
Mode	Most frequent/ common value.	Easily understood, not affected by outliers. Good for nominal data.	It may not exist in data where there is only one of each value.
Range	The difference between the largest and smallest value in your data.	Easy to compute and understand. Gives you a guide to the potential values for your variable.	Does not use all of the data thus very influenced by outliers. No indication of the spread of the data.
Interquartile range	The range of the middle 50% of the scores.	Not affected by outliers as it focuses on the middle 50%.	Not easy to calculate or understand. Does not use all of the data.
Standard Deviation (SD or σ)	Basically describes the average deviation from the mean.	Uses all of the data. Used in a number of other statistical procedures. In normally distributed data it is reasonable to expect a known percentage of the data to fall within ±1, ±2 and ±3 SD of the mean (68%, 95% and 99%, respectively). Researchers know this and at a glance can gain a feel for the data from your presentation of just the mean and SD (see below).	Hard to calculate manually. Distorted by extreme values.

As indicated above, for most sets of normally distributed data you should quote the 'mean ± standard deviation (±SD)' as this gives the reader a feeling for the average value and spread of the data. If you are comparing between groups, the SD value gives you an idea of how different the spread is within each group, and whether further data manipulation is required to correct these differences to make a meaningful comparison (e.g. the use of a log or rank transformation procedure). Also, when comparing across groups, the use of a pooled SD (the weighted average SD of the groups)[3] enables you to calculate the effect size which in itself is an important measure in order to interpret your findings (see later in this chapter). Note that the SD of a sample should not change as the sample size increases, provided that the original sample was normally distributed and was a representative sample of the larger population.

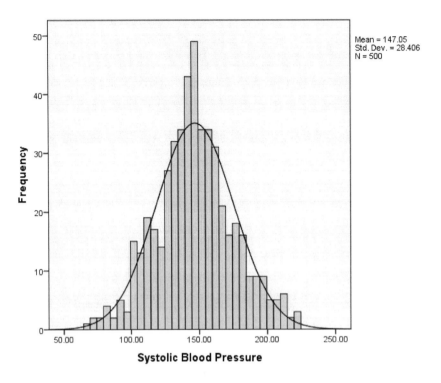

Figure 17.1 Normal distribution curve.

Confidence Interval (CI) and Standard Error of the Mean (SEM)

Other useful descriptive statistics are the standard error of the mean (SEM) and 95% Confidence Interval (95% CI). SEM is a measure of the error or variability of repeated sample means taken from the same population. In other words the standard deviation of their sample means and thus represents the error in one sample mean in predicting the population mean. Unlike standard deviation, SEM will decrease with sample size as gaining more information about a population will lower the error in the prediction of the population mean. The SEM value is calculated by dividing the sample SD by the square route of the sample size (*n*).

In most research studies you are unlikely to be able to collect data on every member of a targeted population, in which case the data you collect will be from a 'sample' of that population. Since it is rarely possible to measure every person (case), there is always a degree of uncertainty of how representative your sample is of the overall population. However, it is possible to describe (statistically) this degree of uncertainty. One way is to compute a confidence interval (CI), which is a method of describing the likelihood of the true population mean being included within a specific range of values. Usually described as a 95% CI, this provides a range of values within which you can be 95% certain contains the true population mean. Most statistical software packages will calculate the 95% CI for you, as it is the product of the standard error of the sample mean (SEM) and *t*-distribution value for the sample size. As a result, one aspect of a 95% CI is that as you increase the sample size, the range of values associated with the 95% CI decreases, and the range of scores possible for the true population mean narrows. Indeed, in the extreme, if you were to measure all members of a population, the 95% CI should theoretically be the mean with no range of values around it, as your sample is the whole population and the mean of your sample is the mean of the population.

Determining associations in your data

If your research study is seeking to assess an association between factors, applying well-founded rules will guide you to the correct test, of which there are many. In the case of nominal data, where you have frequencies, a Chi-square analysis may be applicable, whereas ratio data require a different group of statistical tests and your analyses may involve some form of correlation. There are many different types of correlation and your choice will be determined by the nature of your data. To illustrate this form of analyses, here we present an example using a commonly utilized test. A Pearson Product Moment correlation coefficient (r) or inter-class correlation, involves linear regression and should only be computed using pairs of interval or ratio scale data. While an r-value cannot establish cause and effect, it can provide you with a good indication of the direction (either positive or negative) and strength of association between a pair of variables. A correlation coefficient can range from –1.00, a perfect, negative correlation, to 0.00, no correlation whatsoever, to +1.00, a perfect, positive correlation. An r-value of +0.70 would indicate a reasonably strong, but not perfect positive correlation, whereas an r-value of –0.70 would indicate a reasonably strong, but not perfect negative correlation (Figure 17.2).

By squaring the r-value, one is able to compute an associated coefficient of determination (R^2). So, for example, if one computed a correlation coefficient of $r = 0.56$ between height (m) and body mass (kg), the r^2 value would be 0.31 (to 2 decimal places). If one then multiplies this value by 100, a percentage value is derived, which provides one with an estimate of common, or shared variance between the pairs of variables. In other words, in this example variations in height account for 31% of the variations observed for body mass, and vice versa.

In the case of an inter-class correlation, two different data sets are required before they can be correlated against each other. For example, one could run a correlation analysis between height (m) and lung volume, measured as forced vital capacity (FVC; L). Typically speaking, the taller an individual is, the larger we might expect their FVC to be; therefore, we may anticipate a moderate-to-strong, positive correlation – perhaps of a magnitude range between +0.50 to +0.70. Similarly, if one were to correlate leg strength, as measured by a one repetition, maximum (1RM) leg press, and average velocity (m/s) in a 'Shuttle Walking Test' in an elderly population, a positive correlation would also be hypothesized. However, if one plotted 1RM leg press strength against time taken to complete the 'Shuttle Walking Test', one may hypothesize that a negative correlation would emerge. This hypothesis would be developed since a stronger, elderly person would have the leg power to walk faster, they would thus complete the 'Shuttle Walk Test' in less time, so the relationship between the variables becomes negative in nature, but may remain equal in magnitude, and importance.

When interpreting a correlation coefficient, it is important to note that magnitude of scores are not considered. Therefore, if one correlated the five values of 1, 2, 3, 4 and 5 against 1, 2, 3, 4 and 5, a perfect, positive correlation of $r = +1.00$ would be computed. But this is also true if one correlated 1, 2, 3, 4 and 5 against 10, 20, 30, 40 and 50, which this also results in $r = +1.00$.

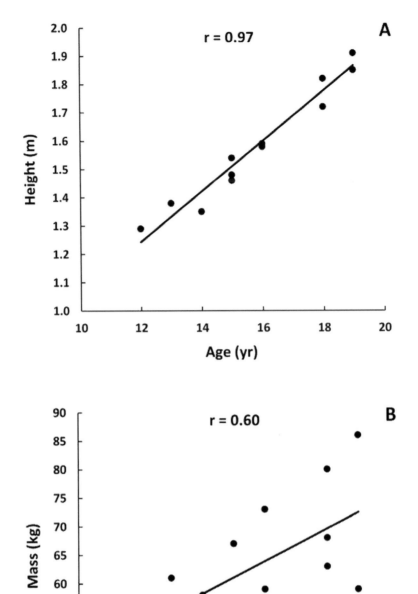

Figure 17.2 Examples of correlations coefficients depicting: panel **A** – a strong, positive relationship; panel **B** – a moderate, positive relationship; panel **C** – no relationship; and panel **D** a strong, negative relationship.

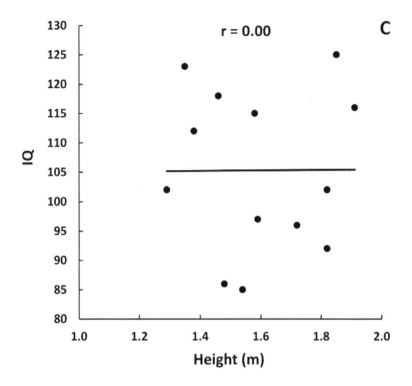

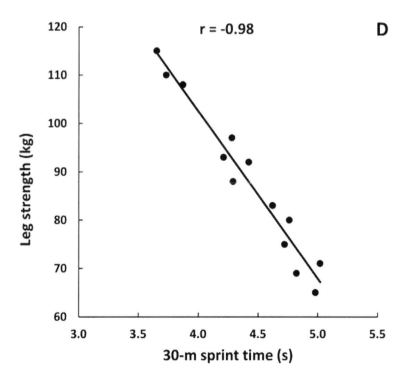

Figure 17.2 Continued

Often, correlation analyses are used in the context of criterion (predictive) validity. For example, in physical activity, one may be interested in exploring how the outcome of a standardized 6-min walk test (6MWT: distance; m) could be used to estimate values of $\dot{V}O_{2peak}$ and associated cardiopulmonary responses and functional capacity of a group of individuals with peripheral artery disease. To explore relationships between the 6MWT and other parameters, you would calculate multiple r-values, and associated regression equations could be created for pairs of variables. For example:

6MWT (m) vs. $\dot{V}O_{2peak}$ (ml·kg^{-1}·min^{-1});
6MWT (m) vs. metabolic equivalents (presented as MET multiples) at exhaustion;
6MWT (m) vs. peak heart rate (b·min^{-1}); and
6MWT (m) vs. cardiac output (l·min^{-1}).

This information, and knowledge about the association between each pair of variables could then be used to estimate (or predict) values of cardiopulmonary and functional measures in other patients with similar disease symptoms and physical characteristics, simply from the results of a simple 6MWT.

In addition to calculating each r-value and associated R^2, one could also compute an associated standard error of estimate (or regression; S). Essentially, S represents and calculates the average distance each datum (data point) lies away from the predicted, linear regression. Some statistical analysis programmes are able to automatically calculate S, which is considered by many as a useful and practical means by which to explore and interpret relationships. Here, the natural units of measurement are used, providing a more realistic, and intuitive assessment of the extent by which one variable can be used to predict another.

As a final point, when calculating r-values great care is needed to ensure that a variable does not occur on both the x- and y-axis. Surprisingly, it is relative easy to find examples of this in the published literature. For example, we might expect that there is a relationship between aerobic fitness ($\dot{V}O_{2max}$) and body mass – we could hypothesize that larger people should have a greater $\dot{V}O_{2max}$. However if we first make $\dot{V}O_{2max}$ relative to body mass i.e. expressed as ml·kg^{-1}.min^{-1} and then plot this against body mass, body mass now appears in both the x- and y-axis. The impact of this is that the relationship between these variables becomes artificially strengthened, resulting in an increase in the r-value, possibly making this relationship significant ($p < 0.05$) when in reality it is not. A more appropriate approach would be to correlate body mass (kg) against absolute $\dot{V}O_{2max}$ (l·min^{-1}), and then explore the nature and strength of the relationship.

Interventions and hypothesis testing

In our research endeavours, we each have specific areas of interest within which we can easily identify relevant research questions. At the outset of a research study we may, or may not have a view relating to the likely outcome of a research study, and researchers often set up a hypothesis for each research question developed (see following section). Within any given piece of research, there may be several (interrelated) questions, and a hypothesis should typically be developed and stated for each.

From your initial background reading and in the development of your research proposal (Chapter 6), you will have identified your research question(s), and you will be in a position where you need to develop a suitable research study design and identify all proposed procedures before an application for ethical approval can be submitted. Thereafter, you will be in a position to recruit participants and commence data collection to help test your stated hypothesis(es). Depending upon what your research intends to investigate, you will need to ensure the quality and technical specification of your research study design is sufficiently robust. In other words, your design should pay attention to your independent variable(s), those elements of the research design you have control of, and you are able to modify. Dependent variables, often referred to as outcome variables, are those that will determine the outcome of your study and any conclusions drawn. A suitable research design will allow you to explore how the manipulation of an independent variable affects dependent variables: hopefully you will be able establish cause-and-effect relationships between your variables, draw specific and objective conclusions and offer important, practical recommendations.

Research and scientific writing is very much about storytelling: once you get towards the end of your story, you have to revisit the beginning and identify how your results and conclusion relate to your initial, stated objectives. Having collected, analysed and interpreted your data, you will have developed important information and you then need to revisit your hypotheses. Depending upon the outcomes of your research study, you should either (explicitly) accept or reject each hypothesis. Furthermore, within an applied research discipline it is also important that you at least attempt to identify realistic and meaningful practical recommendations – otherwise, what would be the point in doing the research?

Developing hypotheses

Hypotheses exist in one of two forms: either as a null hypothesis (H0); or as an alternative (experimental) hypothesis (H1). If you set up a H0, you would make a statement along the lines that you would not expect to observe a difference in the outcome of a dependent variable, irrespective of an intervention employed. In contrast, a H1 states that a difference is expected, and you can develop either a generic H1, or a directional H1: in the case of the latter, not only would you state that you expect to observe a difference, but you also specify the direction in which you expect a difference to occur. If we consider an example, we may be interested in whether a physical activity intervention improved the 'Depression scores' of patients suffering from mild depression. Hypotheses we may develop and state include:

  H0: No difference in the pre- vs. post-exercise intervention mental health (depression scores) of people with mild depression;
  H1 (generic): It is anticipated there will be a difference in the pre- vs. post-exercise intervention mental health (depression scores) of people with mild depression;
  H1 (directional): It is expected that the mental health (depression scores) of people with mild depression will improve after an exercise intervention.

Using appropriate statistical tests you can then analyse your data to determine whether the null hypothesis (H0) is likely to be correct. Details of this process can be found in statistics texts, but in general, if the analysis reveals that there is less than a 5% ($p < 0.05$) chance of the null hypothesis being correct, it would be 'rejected' and one of the alternative hypotheses deemed to be correct. In the above example if $p < 0.05$ the hypothesis that "No difference in the pre- vs. post-exercise intervention mental health of people with mild depression" would be rejected. You would conclude that there was "a difference in the pre- vs. post-exercise intervention mental health of people with mild depression", the directional hypothesis that "the mental health of people with mild depression will improve after an exercise intervention" could be the conclusion drawn if your statistical analysis supported this.

The value of probability at which the null hypothesis is rejected is traditionally set at around 5% ($\alpha = 5\%$), although there is nothing sacred about 5% and other values may be argued for. Indeed α may need to be adjusted depending on statistical factors, such as how many statistical tests are being used in the analyses of the data. It is also sometimes reported that whilst $p < 0.05$ was not quite reached, it was close to that critical value, perhaps indicating that with further data, achieved by recruiting a larger sample size, there would be grounds to reject the null hypothesis. The basis of these discussions can be found in relevant statistical texts.

Type 1 and Type 2 errors

With hypothesis testing you should be aware that with a statistical outcome that gives you $p < 0.05$ you can be fairly confident of rejecting the null hypothesis (H0) and concluding that an alternative hypothesis (H1) is true; however, you can never be 100% certain. Even when $p < 0.001$, there is still a slight possibility (~1 in a thousand chance) that you may incorrectly reject the null hypothesis, and make the wrong conclusions. This relates to the concept of Type I and Type II errors. A Type 1 error, also referred to as a 'false positive', is when you reject the null hypothesis, when in reality it's correct. The probability of this is low, i.e. $< 5\%$ or whatever α was set at. Whereas a Type II error, also referred to as a 'false negative' is when you do not reject the null hypothesis, typically when $p > 5\%$, when in reality it is false. One reason for a Type II error is insufficient data, and you can assess whether this is likely to be the case in your research study by undertaking an assessment of 'statistical power'.

Statistical power

One of the dilemmas facing researchers when planning their studies is knowing how many participants to recruit and include. If you recruit too few participants, you may end up with insufficient data to generate valid and meaningful findings and a potential Type II error. This is a scenario whereby the study would be referred to as 'statistically underpowered'. Conversely, you would risk wasting precious time and resources if you recruit and assess far more participants than necessary. Undertaking a statistical power analyses is one approach for determining a statistically appropriate number of participants. A statistical power analysis requires the researcher to collect information from the literature and input into a calculation: factors such as "the amount of variability in the population of the factors being assessed", the amount of change or difference that may be expected in the factor, the degree of certainty that they want in their findings, i.e. they may want an 80% chance of detecting a statistically significant difference or change, if it exists at all.

Statistical formulae and packages for calculating the required sample size are available, and researchers should use these in the planning their research studies.[4]

Quantitative research: experimental designs, interventions and measures of control

Depending upon the area of research you are interested in, and the nature of the research question(s) you are attempting to address and answer, you will need to develop a specific research design. As mentioned above, the main objective of a quantitative piece of research is to explore, evaluate and draw conclusions about relationships between variables. To evaluate the outcome of an intervention, we would typically employ inferential statistics. Examples include the determination of a pairwise correlation coefficient (r), an evaluation of the systematic difference between means of a variable, either under different conditions or between groups (e.g. by using a *t*-test, or Analysis of Variances Test – ANOVA), or by calculating an effect size. As indicated above, with conventional, inferential (difference testing) statistics we base our interpretations and conclusions on a predetermined, a priori level of statistical significance. This expected outcome is usually set at a 95% level of probability ($p \leq 0.05$). In other words, you would conclude there to be a statistical difference if your statistics indicated you could expect to observe the same outcome at least 19 times out of 20, i.e. 95% of the time.

Experimental designs

Characteristics of a research design include the number of participants you recruit, the number of subgroups you will employ and quality control measures you put in place. It is possible that your research design will only require the use of a single participant group, employing a within, intra-participant, or repeated measures design. Statistically, this is a powerful design to employ, as you will effectively factor out individual differences: in other words, you would compare data for each participant against themselves, either under different conditions and/or over time.

However, in other examples you will need to recruit at least two or possibly more participant subgroups. In this instance, you will be using an inter-participant or between-participants design, also referred to as an independent measures design. This is a popular design and frequently used in the context of a randomised controlled trial (RCT). In this case you would recruit participants, assess their eligibility against a specific set of in-/exclusion criteria, before randomly allocating them to either: (1) an intervention group, or (2) a control group. In the context of your study, individuals in the control group would be required to continue as normal and enable you to evaluate the extent of systematic error (or bias) within your measurement(s). Within your analysis, and interpretation of your results, you would expect any change due to your intervention to be greater in magnitude than any systematic error measurement (see Chapter 16 for an assessment of random or systematic error). Alternatively, with a multiple groups design, you could separate participants based upon existing characteristics such as sex, age, body mass, body composition, socioeconomic background and so on. Inherently, a between-subject group design includes individual differences, thus, in order to achieve a similar level of statistical power you will typically need to recruit far more participants.

One of the most important characteristics of research is internal validity, which reflects the extent to which one can identify causal relationships between independent and dependent variables. The format of a research study, and associated control measures put in place as part of the research design will considerably influence the extent of internal validity one can achieve. If you have gone to lengths to ensure a robust, quality assured research design is employed, you will be able to draw specific conclusions. Indeed, the studies that are suitably designed ensure that the extent of systematic error (or bias), and the impact of extraneous and potentially confounding variables is minimized. Threats to internal validity include:

*   Extraneous and confounding variables;
*   Selection bias;
*   History – concepts of knowledge and learning/developing strategies;
*   Maturation;
*   Acute de-/training effects;

- Repeated testing – concepts of fatigue and motivation;
- Instrument change and calibration;
- Participant mortality (drop out);
- Experimenter observation and participant reactivity – also referred to as the Hawthorne effect; and finally
- Experimenter bias, *to name but a few.*

Other important forms of validity include external validity, ecological validity, content validity and construct validity. It is interesting to note, however, that if one goes to lengths to ensure a high degree of internal validity, this often reduces the extent of external validity, which relates to the extent by which your research findings can be generalized and applied to a wider population, and vice versa. Further details of which can be found in chapters 3, 13 and 16.

In order to provide assurances of quality control, thus adding to the robustness and technical specification of your study, other research design characteristics can be included. For example, using a single group, repeated measures design, you may wish to include an initial phase of familiarization and habituation for all participants. This is especially important if the task you will require your participants to complete is relatively novel task or form of assessment, in which case you might anticipate a reasonably large learning effect. Other characteristics you could employ in this instance is use of a placebo (single-blind), counter-balanced trial order design, which goes some way to protecting against such issues as learning, fatigue, variations in trial preparation, mood and motivation, which might all influence trial outcome, to some extent. Further, to ensure experimenter bias does not come into play you could use a double-blind research design. In this case, as well as participants being unaware of the trial order, the researcher(s) is (are) also unaware of trial order, therefore, they cannot meaningfully influence any aspect of testing that might bias outcome: for example, they will not be able to motivate participants more during an experimental, compared to a placebo trial. For further information see Chapter 13.

Effect size

As mentioned in the section above, researchers will typically design an experiment to test a hypothesis and achieve the all-important statistical significance ($p < 0.05$). A simple two sample comparison will result in a $p < 0.05$, if there is no overlap in the two respective 95% confidence intervals. For a paired comparison, if zero is not included in the 95% CI, it will be found to be significant. However, statistical significance is not the same as importance, and can be considerably influenced by sample size. The larger the sample size the smaller the confidence interval for a given variable. Further, there is an impression that non-significant research findings, where $p > 0.05$ are not publishable, as it is often interpreted that no effect or difference exists, but this may not be the case. It may simply be the case that observed changes are small, and the study design, perhaps due to a small sample size, is inadequately 'powered' and unable to identify effects using conventional statistical procedures, as described previously in this chapter.

An alternative approach is to calculate an effect size, for example, the standardized mean effect expresses the mean difference between two groups in standard deviation units. Effect size is a simple way of quantifying the difference between two groups that has many advantages over the use of tests of statistical significance alone. Effect size emphasizes the size of the difference rather than confounding this with sample size. Typically, you will see this reported as Cohen's *d*, or simply referred to as '*d*'. It can be used, for example, to accompany reports associated with outcomes of *t*-test and ANOVA tests. It is also widely used in the context of meta-analyses. Cohen's *d* is an appropriate effect size for the comparison between two means. Linked to an independent samples *t*-test, Cohen's *d* is determined by calculating the mean difference between two data sets, and then dividing the result by the pooled standard deviation. Most statistical packages will include the software for the calculation of effect size.

Cohen suggested that $d = 0.2$ be considered a 'small' effect size, $d = 0.5$ represents a 'medium' effect size and $d = 0.8$ a 'large' effect size. Thus, if mean values of each (independent) group do not differ by more than 0.2 standard deviations, the difference should be considered as only trivial, even if your associated parametric statistic was significant, and indicated there was a statistical difference – i.e. $p < 0.05$. As an example a group of middle-aged men ($n = 32$) enrolled on a 12-week walking programme had body mass measured before and after. The mean reduction in body mass was –0.57 ± 1.24 kg. Despite being relatively small this was a significant ($p < 0.05$) reduction with an effect size of 0.46 which would be considered just below 'medium'. In many cases in health/clinical research it is then up to the researchers to decide whether the difference or change due to treatment is of 'clinical' significance, also referred to as a threshold for a clinically important effect.[5] It is possible for your analysis to reveal a statistically significant effect from some treatment but for the magnitude of this effect to be so small as to have minimal or trivial clinical significance. Conversely it is equally possible for your statistical analyses to fail to show statistical significance ($p > 0.05$), yet for the magnitude of change or difference to be clinically important.

An effect size provides a reader of your research with a different view of your data, which is independent of sample size. It is also an additional tool in interpreting the practical or clinical significance of the results of any research study and thus, it is important and highly recommended that you consider including such information when reporting your findings.

Meta-analysis

In science it is common for a consensus to be developed from a number of published studies that have explored the same research question, and completed the same or similar study design in doing so. Individually the outcomes of these studies may not provide compelling evidence of a real effect. For example a number of 'under-powered' studies may suggest a 'trend' towards an important benefit, but individually not reach statistical significance ($p < 0.05$). However, if a sufficient number of similar studies in a given field are conducted, results can be combined in an attempt to develop a consensus of opinion, providing a more reliable and conclusive opinion that will have used a combined population, bigger than any single, prior population. This approach is known as a meta-analysis (for further information see www.cochrane.org). There are strict criteria for undertaking a meta-analyses, particularly in the inclusion/exclusion criteria that determine whether a study should be included in the meta-analysis. These criteria ensure that only high-quality, well-conducted studies are included, regardless of whether they have found statistically significant effects or not. Hence a consensus will be generated from a collection of high-quality studies.

The combination of outcomes from several studies in a meta-analysis can provide confirmation of a real significant effect. It is common for the outcomes of such an analysis to be illustrated using either a forest plot or blobbogram. The general format of these graphical displays include the details of the studies considered listed in a left hand column, with each study in a separate row and on the right-hand side is an outcome measure for each study, normally the mean with 95%CI. Other columns can be included within such graphical illustration, for example, the inclusion of associated odds ratios (OR) or relative risk (RR), which are commonly used as outcome measures in health research.

This method has become particularly popular in health-based studies where it graphically represents the meta-analysis of the results in randomized controlled trials. Unfortunately, meta-analyses are subject to two key limitations, those of heterogeneity of results due to slightly different methodologies, and a problem of pooled results by combining the outcomes of several studies. However, the forest plot quickly demonstrates to the reader the within-study variability and a comparison of the overall mean effect from each study, thus providing a very easily understood summary of the meta-analysis findings avoiding misinterpretation of combined results.

Figure 17.3 provides a typical example of a forest plot, in which the left-hand column lists the names of 3 studies, and to the right of this, each study's mean and 95% Cis are presented, and aligned with an OR scale along the base of the plot: with OR = 1.00 indicating no effect or no difference. The solid vertical line emanating from the 1.00 point on the OR scale enables an easy visualisation of where the mean for each study sits relative to an OR of 1.00, and whether the 95% CIs for each study includes an OR of 1.00. The combined OR for all the studies (Overall), as calculated from the meta-analysis is then presented in the bottom row of the plot and thereby presents a clear indication of where the combined data sits in terms of OR and 95% CI. The mean overall effect is indicated by a dotted vertical line, emanating from the mean of the combined data. The inclusion of this dotted line enables an easy visual presentation of where the mean for each study fits in terms of the overall mean, and displays the extent to which a study may have reported a mean OR value that was larger or smaller than the overall mean, along with the magnitude of this difference from the overall mean as indicated by the distance between the study mean and dotted line. The example presented in Figure 17.3 indicates a 'negative' effect, in that the mean overall effect, as represented by the dotted line, is to the right of the 1.00 point on the OR scale, and corresponds to an OR value of 1.75. Although there are different ways of describing the analysis particularly in terms of risk of developing certain pathologies, and the overall effect of 1.75 in this example would mean that the odds of developing high blood pressure are on average 75% higher in those with low physical activity. Therefore it is important when interpreting forest plots to fully understand how the research question has been framed and subsequently communicated in the particular meta-analysis.

Furthermore, in the example presented in Figure 17.3, all the studies reported a mean OR above 1.00. Two have 95% CIs that do not cross the 1.00 line, whilst one of the 95% CIs includes an OR value of 1.00 (it crosses the solid vertical line), suggesting that it would not have been statistically significant ($p > 0.05$). In many meta-analyses, many of the included studies may have this characteristic of indicating a possible difference in the mean value, but not attaining statistical significance of $p < 0.05$, perhaps due to a small sample size and inadequate statistical power. However, the value of a meta-analysis is through combining the results of these studies, and if there is a general consensus, such as when all or almost all of the mean values are to one side (right or left) of the 1.00 OR point, it is likely that the overall mean will also be on that side. With the increased amount of data, the 95% CI for the overall mean may no longer cross the 1.00 point, thereby suggesting statistical significance for the combined data. Although, as indicted previously, when interpreting such results, researchers need

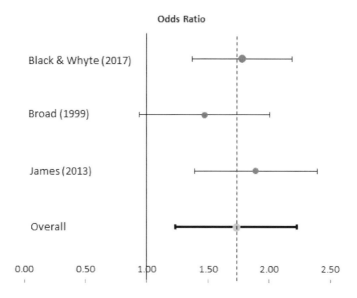

Figure 17.3 Forest plot of the Odds Ratio of individuals with low physical activity developing high blood pressure.

to give careful consideration as to whether attaining statistical significance is important or whether an effect size without statistical significance is important (where the overall 95% CI may still cross the OR 1.00 point), as well as the clinical significance of the overall effect calculated from the meta-analyses. For further information on meta-analyses, see Chapter 5.

Conclusion

This chapter has presented an overview of the essential elements that need to be considered in the analyses of quantitative data. It should be read along with other chapters (such as chapters 13 and 16) that present information on the design of studies, how to ensure that data are valid and reliable and methods used to objectively assess these issues. The information presented here should be considered as a first step in introducing the issues, and having gained an awareness of these the reader should pursue the relevant ones in greater depth through related statistical analyses texts and resources. If applied correctly and objectively the researcher can hope to avoid the concept attributed to British Prime Minister Benjamin Disraeli who is quoted as saying that there are "*Lies, Damned Lies, and Statistics*".

References

1 Stevens SS. On the theory of scales of measurement. *Science.* 1946; **103**(2684):677–80.
2 Available from: https://stats.idre.ucla.edu/other/mult-pkg/whatstat/
3 Available from: www.statisticshowto.com/pooled-standard-deviation/
4 http://powerandsamplesize.com/calculators
5 A new view of statistics. Available from: http://sportsci.org/resource/stats/

18 Measurement of physical behaviours in free-living populations

Alan E. Donnelly and Kieran P. Dowd

Chapter aims

This chapter will provide a brief overview of the techniques available for the measurement of physical behaviours, including information on how they are utilized, their validity, their practicality and issues such as the minimum duration of measurement required to gather a sample that is representative of the volunteer's normal physical behaviours.

Introduction

'Physical behaviours' is a term allocated to all behaviours undertaken during the 24-hour cycle, and includes: sleep, lying down, sitting, standing and physical activity. Broadly speaking, activities undertaken when waking are essentially either sedentary (sitting, lying down) or active (e.g. walking and running), with standing being somewhere between the two in terms of energy expenditure. 'Physical activity' is any bodily movement which requires energy expenditure, and is generally classified by intensity into bands reflecting light physical activity (less than 3 METs), moderate physical activity (3–6 METs) and vigorous physical activity (greater than 6 METs). International guidelines provide a minimum recommended daily amount of moderate-to-vigorous physical activity (MVPA) to maintain health, often 30 minutes per day for adults and 60 minutes per day for children.[1] There is widespread interest in measuring human physical behaviours, given the weight of epidemiological evidence linking physical behaviours to health.[2] This may include one or a combination of the following variables: the type of activity, the amount of activity (minutes), energy expenditure, intensity, pattern of activity or other measures. For researchers, the vast array of activity measurement methods available can be daunting, and selecting an appropriate measurement method for their population can seem highly problematic.

Indeed, one of the first things to ask when choosing a measurement technique for physical behaviours is "which outcome measure am I most interested in?" For instance, researchers with a focus on total energy expenditure alone might be happy to measure only 24-hour energy expenditure. Researchers with a different focus may ask whether a specific population is achieving the minimum recommendations for daily time spent in MVPA, or alternatively the profile of activity and sedentary behaviours across a day (see Chapter 15). Knowing and understanding the outcome measure of interest for a planned study is a key aspect of the selection process for measurement methodology. Other pragmatic factors will be important, such as how well the particular population will comply with a measure and the cost of administering the measure.

Why measure physical behaviours?

The most frequent day time behaviour in most populations is *sedentary behaviour*. Sedentary behaviour has recently been defined as "any waking behaviour characterized by an energy expenditure which is less than or equal to 1.5 metabolic equivalents (METs) while in a sitting or reclining posture".[3] There has been an increasing research focus on sedentary behaviour as evidence accumulates of its association with negative health outcomes. These include cardiovascular disease, site-specific cancers, diabetes and increased all-cause mortality.[4-6] Given the high prevalence of sedentary behaviour, particularly in developed countries (mean/median total daily sitting times in most developed countries are between 4 and 6 hr[7,8]), it has been estimated that approximately 6% of all deaths could be attributed to total sitting time.[6] There is growing evidence to suggest that both the time spent sedentary during the day and the pattern of sedentary behaviour (particularly longer bouts of sedentary time) are influencers of health outcomes.[9]

More recently there has been a growing interest in *standing time*, as some preliminary evidence has been presented from cross-sectional studies indicating a positive relationship between standing time and measured health indices.[10,11] However, there is a dearth of research of strong methodology which confirms the positive benefits of standing. Many studies of standing behaviour have used single-question recall-based methods, which are limited in terms of validity and reliability. However, the use of postural measurement devices is growing. Such devices generally use an accelerometer worn either on the hip or thigh to determine body position. Device-based measurement indicates that many populations spend a considerable amount of time standing (4–6 hours daily), with considerable variation between individuals.[12,13] Hence to gain a full appreciation of the issues associated with physical behaviours and health, it is necessary to measure the physical behaviours using valid and reliable techniques.

Assessing measurement accuracy

When selecting a measurement technique for physical behaviours, researchers and practitioners need to consider not only feasibility and practicality of the measure, but also the measurement properties, such as validity, reliability and sensitivity. *Validity* refers to the degree to which a method measures what it is intended to measure, and is most often investigated by comparing the proposed measurement method's results with another comparable measure.[14] Criterion validity is when a measure is validated against the 'gold standard' measure. Gold standard measures may include direct observation, where every activity type is noted, or energy expenditure measured by doubly labelled water. Good agreement between the proposed method and the gold standard provides some assurance that the results are an accurate reflection of physical activity behaviour. *Reliability* refers to the degree to which a test can produce consistent results on different occasions, when there is no evidence of change, while *sensitivity* is the ability of the test to detect changes in behaviours over time when a real change has occurred.[15]

The fact that volunteers are aware they are being measured can create problems with accuracy. For instance, reactivity may mean that the act of measuring physical activity may change a person's behaviour. This can occur during measurement using direct observation,[16] or when wearing an activity monitor causes the participant to alter their habitual physical behaviour.[17] When using self-report measures, social desirability may result in over-reporting of physical activity among participants keen to comply with the intervention aims or national recommendations.[18] These factors require careful consideration when selecting methods for assessing physical behaviours. Furthermore, researchers should be cognizant of the minimum sample duration necessary for their sample to be representative of the participant's long-term behaviour.

Physical behaviour measurement techniques

Metabolic measurement

Measurements made in laboratory conditions undoubtedly provide the most accurate record of energy expenditure. Lab-based measurement of physical behaviours to quantify energy expenditure is commonplace, often measuring physical activity undertaken on stationary exercise apparatus such as treadmills and cycle ergometers. Such techniques allow a high degree of accuracy in measurement of energy expenditure, via indirect calorimetry using expired gas collection and analysis.[19] Indirect calorimetry involves collecting exhaled gases via a mouthpiece, measuring the expired gas volume (corrected for temperature, air pressure and humidity) and examining the concentrations of oxygen and carbon dioxide to estimate energy expenditure. In studies focused on activities of daily living, the use of whole-room calorimetry, where the volunteer can move about within the chamber without a mouthpiece, allows for more realistic measurement but at significantly greater cost.[19] While accurate, these stationary techniques are often not suited to prolonged measurement periods due to the invasiveness and cost of such measures. Portable gas analysis systems are also available, which enable the measurement of non-stationary free-living activity behaviours. Such measures also enable outdoor measurement but their use in prolonged data collection is limited to a few hours by battery life and potential discomfort to participants.

An alternative, which is considered the gold standard measure of total daily energy expenditure, is the use of the doubly labelled water technique.[20,21] In this method, volunteers ingest a solution of a measured amount of water containing heavy isotopes of deuterium labelled water (^2H_2O) and oxygen labelled water ($H_2^{18}O$). Measurement of the relative amount of these isotopes in urine samples is then utilized to estimate the total energy expenditure from all causes over a specific period.[22] This method does not allow the measurement of energy expenditure during specific activities, requires access to specialist equipment (an isotope ratio mass spectrometer), requires specialist users with substantial expertise and is expensive.

Self-report methods – questionnaires and interviews

Self-report methods generally rely on recall, and include recalling information from different durations (i.e. the previous 24 hours, the previous week or the previous year), providing details of a typical week or inputting information into a physical activity log/diary. Such instruments have many advantages; for instance they can be employed to record the most frequent sports and recreation activities undertaken and can provide information on the location of physical activity, who the activity was completed with and on determinants of physical activity. They are simple to use, can be exceptionally cheap and can be processed and analysed extremely efficiently, particularly if they are web-based or completed on a tablet or smartphone. There are large numbers of validated questionnaires available which have been widely employed internationally, including the International Physical Activity Questionnaire, the Global Physical Activity Questionnaire and the Physical Activity Frequency Questionnaire. When selecting a measure to quantify physical behaviours, care must be taken to ensure that the behaviour of interest to the researcher is examined by the measure, and that the measure is age and culturally appropriate for their population of interest (i.e. any sports examples used should be relevant to the population of interest).[23,24] It is also imperative for researchers to consider that any self-report measure used to quantify frequency, intensity or duration of physical activity is likely to have limited reliability and validity when compared to laboratory measures.[24,25]

Values for the criterion and concurrent validity of self-reported measures of physical activity are widely available in the literature. However, the term 'validated' is often interpreted as meaning that the measure is accurate, rather than accepted as meaning that values (regardless of how good or bad) for validity are available. A recent review has reported the highly variable values for the criterion and concurrent validity of self-report measures of time spent in physical activity of different intensities,[25] suggesting significant variability in the measures. Such information casts some doubt on the use of self-report measures in research studies, particularly in studies where time spent in physical activity (and for time spent in light, moderate and vigorous physical activity bands) is a primary outcome measure. Similarly, lack of precision, large bias and low correlation with an objective measure have been reported for self-reported sedentary time.[17] There is no doubt that questionnaires and diaries are easy to implement, are a cost-effective tool and provide valuable detail of context, environment and determinants of physical activity for researchers. However, their ability to quantify time spent in physical activity as a primary outcome measure is questionable,[26] and findings from such measures should be interpreted with caution. In recent decades, other more valid measurement methods of physical behaviours in free-living settings have been developed.

Pedometers

Standard pedometers record step count, usually with a high degree of accuracy. These devices provide information on daily step count and are generally simple to use and understand. Pedometer-determined step count is generally slightly lower when compared to direct observation.[25] Despite this, pedometers have relatively high levels of accuracy across all speeds, but appear to be more accurate at determining step count at higher walking speeds compared to lower walking speed.[25] Pedometers do not detect upper body movements, while they can struggle to detect some lower-body movement, such as shuffling and stair climbing.[27] The loss of validity at low walking speeds may be an important issue for researchers working with an elderly population, clinical population or people with a disability, as such speeds will dominate their physical behaviour profile. Overall, pedometers are a cheap, relatively valid and well-tolerated method of determining step count, but they are limited in their ability to quantify activity patterns, intensity and duration.

Accelerometers

Accelerometer-based activity monitors have become the most commonly used objective measurement system for the quantification of frequency, intensity and duration of free-living physical behaviours. Accelerometer devices are small, and are usually worn on the body, attached to a belt at the hip, worn on a wrist or adhered to the skin on the thigh, the chest or elsewhere. They record acceleration, either in a single plane (uniaxial) or in three planes (tri-axial).[28]

Early accelerometer-based activity measurement devices lacked substantial memory capacity, so instead of storing the raw acceleration data, they compressed it into a single figure (called an 'accelerometer count') for a fixed time period (or 'epoch') initially 60 seconds long.[28] The use of these early devices has resulted in many researchers expressing data in counts per epoch. Published validations are available for most research-grade accelerometers which allow counts per epoch to be converted into an estimate of energy expenditure or exercise intensity via cut-points or count-to-activity thresholds (see Figure 18.1).[29] Most commonly, cut-points or thresholds are applied to the compressed acceleration data stored by the devices to determine whether the activity level during that epoch is in sedentary, light, moderate or vigorous intensity bands.[30,31] Thus the duration of each epoch is allocated to either sedentary time, or light, moderate or vigorous intensity and the time spent in each intensity on each day can be quantified by simply adding up the relevant epochs.

Although the epoch-based system enabled far longer recording periods, it has limitations. When longer epochs are used (i.e. 60 seconds), the start and end of exercise bouts may fall in the middle of an epoch, reducing accuracy.[31] Generally, shorter epochs have greater accuracy of measurement. Many recent accelerometer devices have greater data storage capacity, and store the raw acceleration signal (sampled

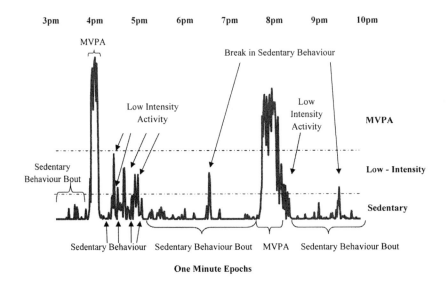

Figure 18.1 The application of intensity thresholds to accelerometer data.[16] The *x*-axis represents time in 1 minute epoch values of the accelerometry measurements. The height of the data on the *y*-axis represents the intensity of the epoch values, with higher data points equalling higher intensities.

many times per second) rather than a compressed version of the data, removing any errors resulting from the use of epochs.[32]

Accelerometer measurement is by no means perfect. Although accelerometers have better criterion validity than self-reported methods, they do not perfectly represent energy expenditure.[25] The accelerometer devices are only as good as the validation methods employed to calibrate their outputs, and many validations omit certain exercise types (such as cycling) to provide a more acceptable validation figure based on a wide range of exercise types. Moreover, accelerometers are unable to measure external resistance, and cannot distinguish between walking up and down a gradient. Other factors can influence the results; non-wear time (when the participant takes off the device and forgets to replace it) can result in gaps in the recording, differences in wear location requires different considerations for analysis, differing criteria for data inclusion (what constitutes a valid day) results in difficulties in comparison between studies, while many such devices are not waterproof, so cannot measure water-based activity. Most accelerometer devices cannot distinguish sitting and standing, and may misclassify some standing time as sedentary time and/or light physical activity,[33,34] which as indicated previously may be an important distinction to make.

An alternative approach to threshold-based accelerometer data processing is to use machine learning methods to automatically identify specific activities from the accelerometer signal, and then attribute specific energy costs to each of these activities. This methodology holds much promise, for it may be possible to reduce some of the errors (e.g. failing to provide an accurate energy cost for cycling) inherent in the use of threshold-based processing methods. This method can be used either to measure time spent in the different physical activity intensity bands, or total energy expenditure over the sample period.[32]

Heart rate monitors

Heart rate is responsive to exercise, and monitors which continually record heart rate can be used in activity measurement.[14] These are connected via electrodes, or using a simple metal contact in a wrist-worn device. The value of heart rate recording over accelerometers is that they record the physiological response to activity, rather than just movement. Heart rate can be used to classify activity as sedentary, light, moderate or vigorous physical activity using the FLEX heart rate approach.[17,35] Potential confounders to heart rate recording accuracy are fitness-related variability in the linearity of heart rate response to intensity (aerobically trained individuals will have a lower heart rate for any given intensity of activity) and problems maintaining electrode contact to the skin. Additionally, there are age-related changes in heart rate response to activity, and the possibility that medication such as beta blockers may produce a blunted heart rate response to activity. Overall, the validity and reliability of heart rate monitors as measures of physical activity is similar to that of accelerometers.[25] The choice of these devices over accelerometers would be highly dependent upon the focus of the research, in addition to practical issues such as volunteer compliance and study duration. In common with accelerometer-based measurements, researchers should be guided by published information on individual device validity, reliability and sensitivity when selecting a heart rate monitoring device.

Combined sensors

Combined sensors utilize a mix of movement and physiological responses to activity, for example acceleration and heart rate. Algorithms developed by the manufacturers are employed to produce an estimate of energy expenditure and intensity band of any activity. Combined sensors appear to be relatively accurate for the measurement of energy expenditure, though there is little data to date on their reliability and sensitivity.[24]

Postural measurement

Postural measurement devices, such as the activPAL activity monitor, focus on the measurement of body position, allowing direct measurement of sitting or lying time, and of standing time.[36] Postural devices are generally placed on the hip or on the thigh, and record the change in posture during standing and sitting using an accelerometer. Such device records the time of each sit-to-stand and stand-to-sit transition, allowing accurate measurement of time spent sedentary, and patterns of sedentary behaviour.[37] Since postural measurement devices incorporate accelerometers, it is also possible to use the same device as an activity monitor, quantifying activity data into light and MVPA using thresholding.[37] Such devices are revolutionizing the study of sedentary behaviour and patterns and can be used as 24-hour measurement devices for up to a 2-week period.

Wearable fitness devices

In the last few years, there has been dramatic growth in the use of consumer-grade accelerometer devices or 'wearables' like the Fitbit, Garmin and Polar devices. These devices are cheap to use, widely available and provide personalized feedback to the wearer. However, their use as research-grade measurement devices has been limited by the small number of published validations for the devices, and by the fact that most of the devices upload their data to a server, from which only summary data for the day or week can be obtained (though there is growing literature on their use in interventions). Some manufacturers now allow researchers to access more detailed reports on each participant's activity behaviour, but often for a significant fee. Where peer-reviewed validation papers exist and demonstrate good agreement with gold standard measurement, these devices offer a low-cost alternative measurement system for free-living physical activity.[38,39] However, users should be certain that the validation applies to their specific model of the device and is conducted in a comparable population.

Smartphones

Smartphones incorporate tri-axial accelerometers, and with around 2 billion sold at time of writing, these devices offer significant potential for activity measurement. Numerous phone applications are available which can process accelerometer data to display step count and energy expenditure. This resource may be of significant value in large-scale 'big data' studies,[40] but on an individual level, the fact that the phone is not consistently on the wearer (it can be left on a counter or desk) and that its location on the body is variable (e.g. in a jacket or trouser pocket, in a rucksack or shoulder bag) may be problematic for the measurement of energy expenditure and measurement of time spent in different physical activity intensity bands. The few studies undertaken to date have found average to excellent levels of accuracy for behavioural measurement, but more studies examining the accuracy of smartphones are required.[14]

Other methods

The field of physical behaviour measurement is constantly evolving, with continual development of techniques to overcome weaknesses in current measurement methods. Techniques abound, but two that are worth mentioning are the use of the Global Positioning System (GPS) and the use of wearable cameras. The global positioning system (GPS) is a satellite-based navigation system that is capable of providing location information at any point on the Earth's surface.[41] GPS has the potential to become a valuable tool for improving the assessment of physical activity, especially outdoors. The use of GPS can allow the distance covered outdoors to be measured, and in conjunction with mapping tools, the effects of gradient can be factored in to energy expenditure calculations.[42] However, limitations include the need for a clear line of site to the satellites, meaning that activity indoors and to some extent outdoors amongst buildings, in forests and near hills can be difficult to measure. Wearable cameras use an outward-facing camera, which collects photographs at regular intervals.[43] The photographs can be viewed by the researcher, and to some extent obvious activities (i.e. walking, driving etc.) can be categorized. This method is particularly good for recording the context of physical behaviours. Both methods require the collection of private personal data (location or photographs), so a robust ethical approach needs to be taken to protect the volunteers' privacy; in the case of wearable cameras this may require the deletion of photographs after use.

Conclusions

There are many different methods available for data collection on physical behaviours in free-living experimental participants. All have varying degrees of measurement properties, cost and practicality. The decision on which is most appropriate is dependent upon the primary outcome of the study. If it is physical activity, then a number of objective measurement systems might each be appropriate. If it is sitting time or standing time, then a postural measurement device would be best. For physical activity measurement, a key factor is whether the system has been validated for the primary outcome measure in the target population, and how valid the measure is. Reliability and sensitivity to change are also key measurement properties to be considered; however, these are not as frequently examined or reported in the literature. Pragmatic issues will play a major part in the decision; researchers are most likely to use a system they already have, while if devices are to be purchased, cost will be of major importance. Finally, researchers should be aware that recall-based instruments generally have poor validity for measuring hard outcomes like time spent in MVPA and time spent in sedentary behaviour, and it may be necessary to use more objective measurement systems for these variables.

References

1   Committee PAGA. *Physical activity guidelines advisory committee scientific report*. Washington, DC: US Department of Health and Human Services; 2018.
2   Ekelund U, Steene-Johannessen J, Brown WJ, Fagerland MW, Owen N, Powell KE, et al. Does physical activity attenuate, or even eliminate, the detrimental association of sitting time with mortality? A harmonised meta-analysis of data from more than 1 million men and women. *Lancet*. 2016; **388**(10051):1302–10.
3   Tremblay MS, Aubert S, Barnes JD, Saunders TJ, Carson V, Latimer-Cheung AE, et al. Sedentary behavior research network (SBRN) – terminology consensus project process and outcome. *Int J Behav Nutr Phys Act*. 2017; **14**(1):75.

4 Biddle SJ, Bennie JA, Bauman AE, Chau JY, Dunstan D, Owen N, et al. Too much sitting and all-cause mortality: is there a causal link? *BMC Public Health*. 2016; **16**:635.

5 Biswas A, Oh PI, Faulkner GE, Bajaj RR, Silver MA, Mitchell MS, et al. Sedentary time and its association with risk for disease incidence, mortality, and hospitalization in adults: a systematic review and meta-analysis. *Ann Int Med*. 2015; **162**(2):123–32.

6 Chau JY, Grunseit AC, Chey T, Stamatakis E, Brown WJ, Matthews CE, et al. Daily sitting time and all-cause mortality: a meta-analysis. *PloS One*. 2013; **8**(11):e80000.

7 Bauman A, Ainsworth BE, Sallis JF, Hagstromer M, Craig CL, Bull FC, et al. The descriptive epidemiology of sitting. A 20-country comparison using the International Physical Activity Questionnaire (IPAQ). *Am J Prev Med*. 2011; **41**(2):228–35.

8 Loyen A, Verloigne M, Van Hecke L, Hendriksen I, Lakerveld J, Steene-Johannessen J, et al. Variation in population levels of sedentary time in European adults according to cross-European studies: a systematic literature review within DEDIPAC. *Int J Behav Nutr Phys Act*. 2016; **13**:71.

9 Ekelund U, Steene-Johannessen J, Brown WJ, Fagerland MW, Owen N, Powell KE, et al. Does physical activity attenuate, or even eliminate, the detrimental association of sitting time with mortality? A harmonised meta-analysis of data from more than 1 million men and women. *Lancet*. 2016; **388**(10051):1302–10.

10 Healy GN, Winkler EAH, Owen N, Anuradha S, Dunstan DW. Replacing sitting time with standing or stepping: associations with cardio-metabolic risk biomarkers. *Eur Heart J*. 2015; **36**(39):2643–9.

11 Van Der Berg JD, Van Der Velde J, De Waard EA, Bosma H, Savelberg HH, Schaper NC, et al. Replacement effects of sedentary time on metabolic outcomes: the maastricht study. *Med Sci Sports Exerc*. 2017; **49**(7):1351–8.

12 Dowd KP, Harrington DM, Hannigan A, Donnelly AE. Light-intensity physical activity is associated with adiposity in adolescent females. *Med Sci Sports Exerc*. 2014; **46**(12):2295–300.

13 Smith L, Hamer M, Ucci M, Marmot A, Gardner B, Sawyer A, et al. Weekday and weekend patterns of objectively measured sitting, standing, and stepping in a sample of office-based workers: the active buildings study. *BMC Public Health*. 2015; **15**(1):9.

14 Warren JM, Ekelund U, Besson H, Mezzani A, Geladas N, Vanhees L. Assessment of physical activity – a review of methodologies with reference to epidemiological research: a report of the exercise physiology section of the European Association of Cardiovascular Prevention and Rehabilitation. *Eur J Cardiov Prev Rehab*. 2010; **17**(2):127–39.

15 Bort-Roig J, Gilson ND, Puig-Ribera A, Contreras RS, Trost SG. Measuring and influencing physical activity with smartphone technology: a systematic review. *Sports Med*. 2014; **44**(5):671–86.

16 Carson V, Janssen I. Volume, patterns, and types of sedentary behavior and cardio-metabolic health in children and adolescents: a cross-sectional study. *BMC Public Health*. 2011; **11**(1):274.

17 Ceesay SM, Prentice AM, Day KC, Murgatroyd PR, Goldberg GR, Scott W, et al. The use of heart rate monitoring in the estimation of energy expenditure: a validation study using indirect whole-body calorimetry. *Br J Nutr*. 1989; **61**(2):175–86.

18 Chastin SFM, Dontje ML, Skelton DA, Cukic I, Shaw RJ, Gill JMR, et al. Systematic comparative validation of self-report measures of sedentary time against an objective measure of postural sitting (activPAL). *Int J Behav Nutr Phys Act*. 2018; **15**:12.

19 Levine JA. Measurement of energy expenditure. *Public Health Nutr*. 2005; **8**(7a):1123–32.

20 Schoeller DA, Ravussin E, Schutz Y, Acheson KJ, Baertschi P, Jequier E. Energy expenditure by doubly labeled water: validation in humans and proposed calculation. *Am J Physiol Regul Int Comp Physiol*. 1986; **250**(5):R823–R30.

21 Westerterp KR. Assessment of physical activity: a critical appraisal. *Eur J Appl Physiol*. 2009; **105**(6):823–8.

22 Speakman J. *Doubly labelled water: theory and practice*. Chapman and Hall, London: Springer Science & Business Media; 1997.

23   Sallis JF, Saelens BE. Assessment of physical activity by self-report: status, limitations, and future directions. *Res Quar Exerc Sport.* 2000; **71**(Suppl 2):1–14.

24   Shephard RJ. Limits to the measurement of habitual physical activity by questionnaires. *Br J Sports Med.* 2003; **37**(3):197–206.

25   Dowd KP, Szeklicki R, Minetto MA, Murphy MH, Polito A, Ghigo E, et al. A systematic literature review of reviews on techniques for physical activity measurement in adults: a DEDIPAC study. *Int J Behav Nutr Phys Act.* 2018; **15**(1):15.

26   Steene-Johannessen J, Anderssen SA, Hendriksen IJ, Donnelly AE, Brage S, Ekelund U. Are self-report measures able to define individuals as physically active or inactive? *Med Sci Sports Exerc.* 2016; **48**(2):235–44.

27   Corder K, Brage S, Ekelund U. Accelerometers and pedometers: methodology and clinical application. *Curr Opin Clin Nutr Metab Care.* 2007; **10**(5):597–603.

28   Chen KY, Bassett Jr DR. The technology of accelerometry-based activity monitors: current and future. *Med Sci Sports Exerc.* 2005; **37**(11):S490–500.

29   Freedson PS, Melanson E, Sirard J. Calibration of the computer science and applications, inc. accelerometer. *Med Sci Sports Exerc.* 1998; **30**(5):777–81.

30   Orme M, Wijndaele K, Sharp SJ, Westgate K, Ekelund U, Brage S. Combined influence of epoch length, cut-point and bout duration on accelerometry-derived physical activity. *Int J Behav Nutr Phys Act.* 2014; **11**(1):34.

31   Ridgers ND, Salmon J, Ridley K, O'Connell E, Arundell L, Timperio A. Agreement between activPAL and ActiGraph for assessing children's sedentary time. *Int J Behav Nutr Phys Act.* 2012; **9**(1):15.

32   Troiano RP, McClain JJ, Brychta RJ, Chen KY. Evolution of accelerometer methods for physical activity research. *Br J Sports Med.* 2014; **48**(13):1019–23. doi: 10.1136/bjsports-2014-093546.

33   Dowd KP, Harrington DM, Donnelly AE. Criterion and concurrent validity of the activ-PAL™ professional physical activity monitor in adolescent females. *PloS One.* 2012; **7**(10):e47633.

34   Hart TL, Ainsworth BE, Tudor-Locke C. Objective and subjective measures of sedentary behavior and physical activity. *Med Sci Sports Exerc.* 2011; **43**(3):449–56.

35   Livingstone M, Prentice AM, Coward W, Ceesay SM, Strain JJ, McKenna PG, et al. Simultaneous measurement of free-living energy expenditure by the doubly labeled water method and heart-rate monitoring. *Am J Clin Nutr.* 1990; **52**(1):59–65.

36   Edwardson CL, Winkler EA, Bodicoat DH, Yates T, Davies MJ, Dunstan DW, et al. Considerations when using the activPAL monitor in field-based research with adult populations. *J Sport Health Sci.* 2017; **6**(2):162–78.

37   Dowd KP, Harrington DM, Bourke AK, Nelson J, Donnelly AE. The measurement of sedentary patterns and behaviors using the activPAL (TM) Professional physical activity monitor. *Physiol Meas.* 2012; **33**(11):1887–99.

38   Evenson KR, Goto MM, Furberg RD. Systematic review of the validity and reliability of consumer-wearable activity trackers. *Int J Behav Nutr Phys Act.* 2015; **12**(1):159.

39   Ferguson T, Rowlands AV, Olds T, Maher C. The validity of consumer-level, activity monitors in healthy adults worn in free-living conditions: a cross-sectional study. *Int J Behav Nutr Phys Act.* 2015; **12**(1):42.

40   Althoff T, Hicks JL, King AC, Delp SL, Leskovec J. Large-scale physical activity data reveal worldwide activity inequality. *Nature.* 2017; **547**(7663):336.

41   Krenn PJ, Titze S, Oja P, Jones A, Ogilvie D. Use of global positioning systems to study physical activity and the environment: a systematic review. *Am J Prev Med.* 2011; **41**(5):508–15.

42   de Müllenheim PY, Dumond R, Gernigon M, Mahé G, Lavenu A, Bickert S, et al. Predicting metabolic rate during level and uphill outdoor walking using a low-cost GPS receiver. *J Appl Phys.* 2016; **121**(2):577–88.

43   Doherty AR, Kelly P, Kerr J, Marshall S, Oliver M, Badland H, et al. Using wearable cameras to categorise type and context of accelerometer-identified episodes of physical activity. *Int J Behav Nutr Phys Act.* 2013; **10**(1):22.

19 Measurements of physical health and functional capacity

Brett Gordon, Anthony Shield, Isaac Selva Raj, and Noel Lythgo

Introduction

Exercise and physical activity are important for the development and maintenance of physical health and functional capacity. Ensuring physical health and functioning are important for the prevention of non-communicable diseases,[1-4] along with costly health and medical interventions. Reductions in muscle mass, strength, power and functional capacity with advancing age are well documented[5,6] and numerous exercise interventions, if adhered to, have the potential to slow or even partially reverse these trends.[7-10] The evaluation of physical health and function occurs in three key domains: cardiovascular health, metabolic health and musculoskeletal health. This chapter aims to describe the common physical health measures in the key domains, their validity and reliability, along with how measures of physical health respond to physical activity participation. Due to the sheer number of tests and measures available, this will not be a comprehensive examination of each available measure. For detailed procedures and instructions on how to carry out these tests, you are directed to the relevant references.

Clinical health measures

Blood pressure

Normal (healthy) blood pressure (BP) is less than 120 mmHg systolic and less than 80 mmHg diastolic,[11] however these might require adjustment when automated blood pressure devices are used.[12] Skilled individuals can easily measure BP with a sphygmomanometer (either mercury or aneroid) cuff placed over the bicep and pressure increased to occlude blood flow in the brachial artery. This manual technique has been the gold standard for measuring BP after allowing patients to rest for up to five minutes, however it is dependent upon the skill of the person examining BP.[13] The sensitivity of manual measurements conducted in the clinic is not sufficient to determine diagnosis or guide treatment,[14] with automated BP devices now the preferred method[12,15] or tending to become the preferred method[16] for measuring systolic blood pressure (SBP) and diastolic blood pressure (DBP). Automated devices typically have demonstrated validity with manual auscultation using an aneroid sphygmomanometer.[17-19] However, one-off measures taken in a clinic remain unlikely to accurately determine BP abnormalities and 24-hour ambulatory BP monitoring might be required for absolute diagnostic purposes.[14]

During exercise or activity, SBP rises in response to increased stroke volume and cardiac output to meet the oxygen demands of activity. Too great a rise however, places the individual at risk of a haemodynamic event such as myocardial infarction or stroke. Patient movement, mechanical vibration and artefact can impair auscultation during exercise.[20] Particular automated devices (SunTech Tango; CardioDyne NBP 2000)[18,21] have been proven valid for the measurement of both SBP and DBP during exercise in comparison to manual auscultation. However, others have failed to demonstrate validity.[19] A lack of validity in some cases might be due to medical conditions[22] or activity where blood volume (and therefore pressure) is constantly changing. Anxiety around the test must be considered, as SBP has been shown to reduce with subsequent exposures of a treadmill test completed with individuals naïve to using a treadmill.[23]

Transient reductions to SBP and DBP in the hours following an exercise session are in the order of 5 mmHg and 3 mmHg respectively, with little difference between aerobic and resistance modes of exercise.[24] Exercise of at least 4 weeks' duration, regardless of the mode, is likely to reduce both SBP and DBP, with greatest improvements occurring in the first six months and in people with the highest blood pressure readings.[25] When considering only aerobic exercise, three sessions a week for 16 weeks, continuous or interval-based programming equally reduces blood pressure.[26] Reductions in BP following resistance exercise in comparison to a no-exercise control begin after 3 months of training; however, individual changes might be observable with as little as 2 months of resistance training.[27] The BP effects of moderate intensity resistance exercise can persist over a 24-hour period.[28] Participating in physical activity or exercise will positively benefit blood pressure, with the magnitude and duration of the response related to the health status of the individual, along with the mode and intensity of exercise.

Heart rate

Heart rate (HR) also increases with exercise, with a pre-exercise anticipatory rise usually observed. The rise in HR is linear with oxygen consumption,[29] however it provides no additional information of individual health beyond its use in predicting maximal oxygen consumption ($\dot{V}O_{2max}$). Measurement of HR in beats per minute is standard, however there is a variation in the duration between each beat. Heart rate variability (HRV) best describes this inter-beat variation and is determined by the R-R interval measured by electrocardiogram (ECG).[30] A minimum 5-minute measurement period is required, with greater validity with increased measurement duration.[30] Some Polar™ monitors can validly measure R-R interval and provide increased participant comfort over ECG.[31,32] A longer R-R interval signifies a better health outcome, and reflects a lower overall HR, but other equations to estimate time and frequency domains of variation reflect the balance between sympathetic and parasympathetic activity on cardiac contraction.

Single sessions of aerobic exercise increase average nocturnal HR, however the variability between consecutive R waves are reduced, with a dose-response effect identified.[33] A period of adaptation to exercise is likely though, as a decrease in parasympathetic activity occurs with a single session of resistance exercise and an increase in parasympathetic activity occurring only after an extended period of resistance training.[34]

Endothelial dysfunction

Atherosclerosis occurs in response to damaged endothelial cells, which cause lipid molecules to accumulate and reduce the diameter of arteries. Atherosclerosis is measured by common carotid intima-media thickness and the response of coronary arteries to locally infused acetylcholine.[35] Atherosclerotic arteries result in increased peripheral resistance and elevated blood pressure, which is why endothelial dysfunction is a significant factor in hypertension and related organ damage. How compliant arteries are to changes in blood flow determines the degree of endothelial dysfunction. Flow-mediated dilation (FMD) is an accurate and reproducible method of assessing arterial compliance[36] and correlates well with endothelial dysfunction of coronary arteries. The accuracy of FMD though is dependent on the level of skill of the Doppler ultrasound operator to measure the diameter of the brachial artery. The same skill is not required to measure blood velocity, which changes in response to hyperaemia. Removing an occluding cuff (as in FMD) or passive motion (assessor generated knee flexion and extension – referred to as passive leg movement induced hyperaemia) induces the hyperaemia and enables the determination of endothelial function. Passive leg movement (PLM) when in a seated upright position has shown construct validity with FMD to assess the level of cardiovascular risk through atherosclerosis.[37] Alternately, measurement of aortic pulse wave velocity (PWV) and augmentation index (arterial stiffness) is accurate and reliable with a tonometry-based device (SphygmoCor Xcel),[38] although operator skill will affect the outcomes.

While continuous or interval-based aerobic exercise reduces resting blood pressure, interval-based exercise appears to also reduce arterial stiffness.[26] Although moderate intensity resistance exercise has an acute effect on brachial SBP in active men of all ages, it does not influence PWV, despite young males experiencing an acute rise in arterial stiffness (augmentation index) with resistance exercise.[39] Therefore, high-intensity exercise might be required to modulate arterial stiffness; however, observations of small or absent responses could be due to poor sensitivity of the measurement through poor operator skill.

Blood lipids

Metabolic dysfunction contributes to the development of atherosclerosis and cardiovascular disease (CVD). Blood lipids are a reliable laboratory marker to evaluate CVD risk, with the ratio of total cholesterol and high-density lipoprotein cholesterol (HDL-C) the best predictors of cardiac mortality.[40] Total cholesterol is measurable with a portable system from a capillary blood sample, providing accurate and reliable measurements that can discriminate between expected normal and high outcomes.[41] Reliability for measuring cholesterol has been established with a different point-of-care device, although accuracy remains an issue.[42]

Exercise will induce positive blood lipid adaptations,[43] although depending on the precise outcome (total cholesterol, HDL-C, low-density lipoprotein cholesterol (LDL-C), triglycerides) there is likely to be a different response to a single exercise session compared to multiple days of aerobic exercise in terms of both the nature and degree of change.[44] Diet or diet combined with exercise appear to beneficially change total cholesterol and LDL-C, although exercise on its own has minimal effect.[45] However for HDL-C, exercise alone tends to induce beneficial changes with minimal effect in response to diet only and diet combined with exercise.[45] Finally, tri-glycerides tend to be improved with both diet or exercise alone and when completed in combination.[45] Resistance training seems to be much more beneficial compared to no-exercise for reducing total cholesterol, LDL-C and triglycerides, but does not appear to influence HDL-C.[46]

Body composition

The distribution of body fat can affect the presence and degree of insulin resistance[47,48] and lipid accumulation,[48,49] potentially through the secretion of cytokines from visceral adipose tissue. A number of adipocyte-secreted cytokines are involved in the inflammatory response, hunger suppression and insulin resistance.[50] Measurement and determination of body composition, as opposed to a simple measure of body mass, is therefore important when demonstrating the effectiveness of exercise or physical activity programmes. A thorough assessment of the various methods of body composition measurement is available and highlights limitations of inherent errors in equipment, standard equations, patient characteristics and observers.[51] The use of bioelectrical impedance analysis (BIA) for estimating body composition is limited by poor validity and large measurement error.[52] Measurement errors are also common when using dual-energy X-ray absorptiometry (DXA), however standardizing the protocol provides acceptable accuracy for measuring whole-body fat mass and fat-free mass.[53] When considering the quality of fat-free mass, ultrasound is suitable to reliably measure muscle cross-sectional area.[54] Readily available and inexpensive options for assessing overweight and obesity (as opposed to body composition) exist and include body mass index (BMI), waist circumference and skinfold thickness. There is good agreement between BMI and waist circumference, however skinfolds do not tend to agree with any method.[55] Waist circumference, while correlated with fat mass, has a moderate relationship to proportion of body fat, fat mass index and a fat-free mass index.[56] Therefore, while they are appropriate measures to indicate an effect from exercise training, they cannot indicate changes in fat mass or fat-free mass and their reliability is also low.

Aerobic exercise might best facilitate reduced body mass, which will benefit total cholesterol and LDL-C.[57] However, reduced body mass is mostly related to dietary restriction. Higher-intensity exercise (including resistance training) has a strong likelihood of a beneficial response for reduced body mass through increased energy expenditure, but the evidence is not consistent.[58] Exercise is also important to minimize the amount of muscle mass loss when body mass is reduced following energy restriction.[59] Reduction in muscle mass can have important implications for functional capacity and musculoskeletal health, which make strategies and interventions for minimizing such losses of key importance.

Glycaemic control and insulin sensitivity

Point-of-care devices can reliably measure blood glucose, but issues of accuracy remain.[41] Blood glucose can be measured using laboratory devices, but the techniques for collecting, storing and analysing samples are critical for accurate outcomes.[60] Capillary blood samples are also likely to produce lower glucose concentrations, with reduced accuracy around the hypoglycaemic range.[61] Glucose is an important initial indicator of metabolic health, with values considered normal or unexpected depending on whether the individual is in a fasted or fed state. Due to the previously mentioned factors surrounding accuracy of measuring glucose, repeat measures of glucose are required to confirm diagnoses or changes in response to treatment. In addition to collection techniques, continuous glucose monitoring systems (CGMS) have confirmed large day-to-day variations in glucoses, despite no difference in daily mean glucose concentrations.[62] Accuracy of CGMS is approximately 65% or within ~1.0 mmol·l[-1], although accuracy declines under hypoglycaemic conditions.[63–65] Importantly though, the accuracy of CGMS has improved over time.[63] Glycated haemoglobin (HbA1c: the amount of glucose bound to a haemoglobin protein molecule) is now the preferred method to diagnose diabetes mellitus.[66,67] Because haemoglobin molecules are turned over approximately every 12 weeks, the HbA1C concentration is very stable.[68] Point-of-care testing to assess HbA1c has produced accurate and reliable outcomes in comparison to laboratory methods.[69]

Insulin regulates the blood glucose concentration, and muscles' sensitivity to insulin is improved by exercise.[70] Estimates of insulin sensitivity are provided by a ratio of glucose and insulin concentrations during fasting conditions and/or in response to an oral glucose tolerance test (OGTT). These estimations of insulin sensitivity or insulin resistance have established accuracy (by correlating with direct invasive measurements) but lack absolute reference values, therefore diminishing their clinical value.[71] OGTT derived estimates of insulin sensitivity are highly reproducible,[72] which make them appropriate to measure the effect of interventions designed to improve glucose metabolism. However, intravenous glucose tolerance testing (IVGTT) might have better reproducibility than the OGTT.[73]

Although exercise as typically prescribed to patient populations has minimal direct influence on body mass, it is beneficial for glycaemic control[74] and reducing the risk of developing diabetes.[75] The absolute glucose response to a single session of exercise is not clear, with reports of benefits[76] and no benefits,[77] although it is likely there is little difference between aerobic and resistance exercise modes. Particularly in people with diabetes, improved glycaemic control occurs with exercise participation.[78,79] Improved insulin sensitivity also occurs.[78,80] Although resistance training has not received as much focus, it too results in improved glycaemic control.[81,82] Glycaemic control improves with enhanced body composition (increased fat-free mass),[83] which occurs with exercise independently of changes in body mass.[84,85]

Strength and functional capacity measures

Muscle strength

The most common strength measurement techniques include isokinetic and isometric dynamometry, hand-held dynamometry, 1 repetition maximum (1RM) tests of weight-lifting performance and submaximal lifting tests (3–6RM tests). Isokinetic dynamometry has good to excellent reliability,[86 87] allows the measurement of concentric, eccentric and isometric strength and is considered the gold standard amongst strength tests. However, dynamometers are expensive and their use is time consuming. Hand-held dynamometers offer a relatively inexpensive means of measuring isometric strength and have modest to excellent reliability,[88] which likely depends heavily on the experience of the operator. Assessment of weight-lifting ability via 1–6RM maximum tests is also reliable and relatively inexpensive.[89–91] Assessing strength via 3–6RM maximum tests is a commonly employed alternative to 1RM tests when elderly participants are recruited,[92,93] although the rationale for this is not clear. In young adults, elevations in blood pressure and other indices of cardiac stress are no larger and are sometimes smaller in 1RM than in 3–6RM tests,[94] so it is incorrect to assume that 3–6RM tests protect against high cardiovascular loads. Obviously, 3–6RM loads are lighter but it is not clear whether this protects against musculoskeletal injury by comparison with 1RM tests.

Tests of muscle power are particularly relevant because power declines more rapidly than strength in old age.[6] Importantly, tests of strength and power correlate reasonably well with functional capacity in the elderly and interventions that improve strength are also effective at improving functional performance.[10] An example of this is ankle plantar-flexor power, which is primarily generated by the Triceps Surae muscles, and is critical for propelling the body forward, as well as for quickly recovering balance after a stumble or trip.[95–99] Muscle-driven simulations of human walking show that gait is most sensitive to weakness of the ankle plantar-flexors, hip abductors and hip flexors.[100] Therefore, it is important to utilize resistance training protocols to improve or maintain both concentric and eccentric strength and power of these muscles.

Gait

Any decline in an adult's ability to walk or a delay in a child's gait development can lead to disability, poor health and a heightened risk of falling.[101–103] Major gait changes typically occur during or after the seventh decade of life,[104] primarily through reductions in step length, cadence and walking speed, and an increase in step width.[105–109] These measures can now be assessed by instrumented walkways that are valid and reliable.[110]

Other gait changes involve reductions in trunk and lower-limb joint motion (e.g. hip extension), foot-ground/obstacle clearance and ankle plantar-flexor power.[106,109,111–116] Gait speed appears to be related to healthy ageing, with self-selected gait speeds faster than 1.0 m·s⁻¹ associated with healthier ageing and speeds slower than 0.6 m·s⁻¹ increasing the likelihood of poor health and function.[117,118] A single cut-off speed of 0.8 m·s⁻¹ has been proposed.[119] However, in a study involving 34,485 older adults (78.5 ± 5.9 years), a gait speed of 0.8 m·s⁻¹ was associated with median life expectancy, whereas a speed faster than 1.0 m·s⁻¹ suggested better-than-average life expectancy and above 1.2 m·s⁻¹ suggested exceptional life expectancy.[117] There are several databases that are integrated with instrumented walkways, which can be used to assess the gait patterns of children, adolescents and adults.[108,116,120–123] Ankle plantar-flexor power during walking is an important indicator of gait speed, and this can be measured by using 3D motion analysis techniques.[95] 3D motion analysis techniques are relatively reliable and exhibit high validity, but can be labour intensive and time consuming.[124]

Functional fitness

The stair climb test, which involves participants climbing and sometimes descending a flight of stairs, measures either the time taken to climb a set number of stairs or the number of stairs climbed in a set period of time.[125] Stair climb power can also be derived from the results of the stair climb test,[10] and is a useful measure due to its association with leg power, which is closely related to functional capacity in older adults.[126] This test might also be suitable for individuals diagnosed with respiratory diseases.[127]

The 6 minute walk test (6MWT) measures the distance walked by a participant within 6 minutes.[128] Performance in the 6MWT is correlated with a number of factors including age, weight, grip strength, symptoms of depression and decreased mental status.[129] The reliability and validity of this test have been demonstrated in a wide range of healthy and clinical populations.[130,131]

Functional fitness and mobility are closely related to muscle strength and power,[10] therefore exercise interventions designed to improve strength will result in improved functional fitness. This highlights the need to include resistance training and ballistic exercises in any exercise programme, regardless of age or functional capacity.

Balance and mobility

Common measures of balance are the functional reach test,[132] four-square step test,[133] Berg Balance Scale,[134] and parallel, semi-tandem and tandem stand.[135]

The functional reach test measures the distance that a participant can reach forward without moving the feet.[132] It can be used to measure the outer limit of stability[132] in a wide range of populations, such as children,[136] stroke patients[137] and older adults.[138] The test has been proven to be valid and reliable across a wide range of age groups,[132,136] and is easy and quick to administer as it requires minimal equipment and tester expertise. It should be noted, however, that researchers should carefully choose the method for measuring distance reached.[139] Also researchers should consider compensatory mechanisms, such as trunk rotation, when conducting the test.[140] There are also variations to this test, designed for testing different populations, and for testing limits of stability in the posterior and medial-lateral directions in addition to the forward direction.[141–144]

Other commonly used measures of balance are the parallel, semi-tandem and tandem stance tests with eyes open and closed.[135,145] Participants are timed for 10 seconds, and balance scored.[135] The Berg Balance Scale is also a widely used test of balance in the elderly.[134] However, these tests can have a ceiling effect when testing young adults. Therefore, these tests can be performed on a force plate to measure postural sway in the various stances, with the addition of single-leg stances and compliant surfaces.[146] Another reliable and valid test of balance for healthy and physically active individuals is the Star Excursion Balance Test.[147] Finally, the four-square step test is a valid and reliable tool for measuring dynamic balance in a wide range of clinical groups, such as stroke patients, lower-limb amputees, people with Parkinson disease and children with cerebral palsy or Down Syndrome.[133]

The timed-up-and-go test is a test of basic mobility that involves an individual standing up from a chair, walking 3 metres, turning around and sitting back down in the chair.[148] It is commonly used, mainly in research involving older adults.[145,148] However, its validity and reliability has been demonstrated in other populations such as people with Parkinson disease,[149] stroke patients,[150] lower-limb amputees [151] and in 3- to 9-year-old children.[152]

Exercise interventions that improve muscular strength and power will also improve mobility and balance.[6] Balance-specific training, such as using tilt boards, have been shown to improve balance ability.[153]

Flexibility

The sit-and-reach test is the most common test of lower-limb flexibility, used in many population groups, and aims to measure hamstring and lower-back flexibility.[154]

However, as research has indicated that it might not be a valid measure of lower-back flexibility,[155] modifications have been proposed that have higher validity.[156] The chair sit-and-reach is a modification of the sit-and-reach, and is a valid and reliable test of hamstring flexibility in older adults.[157]

The back scratch test, a test of upper-limb flexibility, involves an individual reaching over the shoulder with one hand with the other hand reaching up the middle of the back.[158] The distance between the extended middle fingers is measured.[158] Most research involving the use of the back scratch test has involved older adults,[158–161] and the validity and reliability of this measure has been demonstrated only in this population.[157] Static, dynamic, ballistic and proprioceptive neuromuscular facilitation stretching are all effective at improving flexibility for the specific body part/s, when performed on at least two days each week.[162]

Conclusion

Clinical and functional health and fitness can be accurately and repeatedly measured using an array of invasive and non-invasive measures, which can be conducted in laboratory or clinical environments. The outcomes of these measures should be used to guide exercise prescription, which has been demonstrated to have beneficial effects on all measures of clinical and functional health and fitness. Depending on the desired outcome, the practitioner needs to identify the optimal mode of exercise (i.e. aerobic or resistance), along with the frequency, intensity and time required to obtain the known positive benefits of physical activity and/or exercise participation. Muscle function appears to be a consistent contributor to both functional fitness and clinical health, and therefore measures of muscle strength and/or power should be strongly considered.

References

1 Eyler AA, Brownson RC, Bacak SJ, Housemann R. The epidemiology of walking for physical activity in the United States. *Med Sci Sports Exerc.* 2003; **35**(9):1529–36.
2 Penedo F, Dahn JR. Exercise and well-being: a review of mental and physical health benefits associated with physical activity. *Curr Opin Psychiatr.* 2005; **18**(2):189–93.
3 Janisse H, Nedd D, Escamilla S, Nies MA. Physical activity, social support, and family structure as determinants of mood among European-American and African-American women. *Women Health.* 2004; **39**(1):101–16.
4 Mang'eni Ojiambo R. Physical activity and well-being: a review of health benefits of physical activity on health outcomes. *J Appl Med Sci.* 2013; **2**(2):69–78.
5 Doherty TJ. Invited review: aging and sarcopenia. *J Appl Physiol.* 2003; **95**(4):1717–27.
6 Raj IS, Bird SR, Shield AJ. Aging and the force-velocity relationship of muscles. *Exp Gerontol.* 2010; **45**(2):81–90.
7 Bottaro M, Machado SN, Nogueira W, Scales R, Veloso J. Effect of high versus low-velocity resistance training on muscular fitness and functional performance in older men. *Eur J Appl Physiol.* 2007; **99**(3):257–64.
8 Henwood TR, Taaffe DR. Improved physical performance in older adults undertaking a short-term programme of high-velocity resistance training. *Gerontology.* 2005; **51**(2):108–15.
9 Kryger AI, Andersen JL. Resistance training in the oldest old: consequences for muscle strength, fiber types, fiber size, and MHC isoforms. *Scand J Med Sci Sports.* 2007; **17**(4):422–30.
10 Raj IS, Bird SR, Westfold BA, Shield AJ. Effects of eccentrically biased versus conventional weight training in older adults. *Med Sci Sports Exerc.* 2012; **44**(6):1167–76.

11 Whelton PK, Carey RM, Aronow WS, Casey DE, Collins KJ, Dennison Himmelfarb C, et al. 2017. ACC/AHA/AAPA/ABC/ACPM/AGS/APhA/ASH/ASPC/NMA/PCNA Guideline for the prevention, detection, evaluation, and management of high blood pressure in adults. *J Am Coll Cardiol.* 2017; pii: S0735–1097(17)41519–1. DOI: 10.1016/j.jacc.2017.11.006

12 Leung AA, Nerenberg K, Daskalopoulou SS, McBrien K, Zarnke KB, Dasgupta K, et al. Hypertension Canada's 2016 Canadian hypertension education program guidelines for blood pressure measurement, diagnosis, assessment of risk, prevention, and treatment of hypertension. *Can J Cardiol.* 2016; **32**(5):569–88.

13 Myers MG. Replacing manual sphygmomanometers with automated blood pressure measurement in routine clinical practice. *Clin Exp Pharmacol Physiol.* 2014; **41**(1):46–53.

14 Reino-Gonzalez S, Pita-Fernandez S, Cibiriain-Sola M, Seoane-Pillado T, Lopez-Calvino B, Pertega-Diaz S. Validity of clinic blood pressure compared to ambulatory monitoring in hypertensive patients in a primary care setting. *Blood Pressure.* 2015; **24**(2):111–8.

15 Campbell NR, Berbari AE, Cloutier L, Gelfer M, Kenerson JG, Khalsa TK, et al. Policy statement of the world hypertension league on noninvasive blood pressure measurement devices and blood pressure measurement in the clinical or community setting. *J Clin Hypertens (Greenwich, Conn).* 2014; **16**(5):320–2.

16 Pickering TG, Hall JE, Appel LJ, Falkner BE, Graves J, Hill MN, et al. Recommendations for blood pressure measurement in humans and experimental animals: part 1: blood pressure measurement in humans: a statement for professionals from the subcommittee of professional and public education of the American heart association council on high blood pressure research. *Circulation.* 2005; **111**(5):697–716.

17 Bonso E, Dorigatti F, Palatini P. Accuracy of the BP A100 blood pressure measuring device coupled with a single cuff with standard-size bladder over a wide range of arm circumferences. *Blood Pressure Monitor.* 2009; **14**(5):216–9.

18 MacRae HSH, Allen PJ. Automated blood pressure measurement at rest and during exercise: evaluation of the motion tolerant CardioDyne NBP 2000. *Med Sci Sports Exerc.* 1998; **30**(2):328–31.

19 Lightfoot JT, Tankersley C, Rowe SA, Freed AN, Fortney SM. Automated blood pressure measurement during exercise. *Med Sci Sports Exerc.* 1989; **21**(6):698–707.

20 Rasmussen PH, Driscoll DJ, Beck KC, Bonekat HW, Wilcox WD. Direct and indirect blood pressure during exercise. *Chest.* 1985 ;**87**(6):743–8.

21 Cameron JD, Stevenson I, Reed E, McGrath BP, Dart AM, Kingwell BA. Accuracy of automated auscultatory blood pressure measurement during supine exercise and treadmill stress electrocardiogram-testing. *Blood Pressure Monitor.* 2004; **9**(5):269–75.

22 Czarkowski M, Staszkow M, Kostyra K, Shebani Z, Niemczyk S, Matuszkiewicz-Rowinska J. Determining the accuracy of blood pressure measurement by the Omron HEM-907 before and after hemodialysis. *Blood Pressure Monitor.* 2009; **14**(5):232–8.

23 Dean E, Ross J, Bartz J, Purves S. Improving the validity of clinical exercise testing: the relationship between practice and performance. *Arch Phys Med Rehab.* 1989; **70**(8):599–604.

24 Carpio-Rivera E, Moncada-Jimenez J, Salazar-Rojas W, Solera-Herrera A. Acute effects of exercise on blood pressure: a meta-analytic investigation. *Arq Bras Cardiol.* 2016; **106**(5):422–33.

25 Cornelissen VA, Smart NA. Exercise training for blood pressure: a systematic review and meta-analysis. *J Am Heart Assoc.* 2013; **2**(1):e004473.

26 Guimaraes GV, Ciolac EG, Carvalho VO, D'Avila VM, Bortolotto LA, Bocchi EA. Effects of continuous vs. interval exercise training on blood pressure and arterial stiffness in treated hypertension. *Hypertens Res Off J Jap Soc Hypertens.* 2010; **33**(6):627–32.

27 Mota MR, de Oliveira RJ, Dutra MT, Pardono E, Terra DF, Lima RM, et al. Acute and chronic effects of resistive exercise on blood pressure in hypertensive elderly women. *J Strength Cond Res.* 2013; **27**(12):3475–80.

28 Tibana RA, Pereira GB, Navalta JW, Bottaro M, Prestes J. Acute effects of resistance exercise on 24-h blood pressure in middle aged overweight and obese women. *Int J Sports Med.* 2013; **34**(5):460–4.

29 Wyndham CH, Strydom NB, Maritz JS, Morrison JF, Peter J, Potgieter ZU. Maximum oxygen intake and maximum heart rate during strenuous work. *J Appl Physiol.* 1959; **14**:927–36.

30 Heart rate Variability: Standards of Measurement, Physiological Interpretation and Clinical Use. Task force of the european society of cardiology and the north american society of pacing and electrophysiology. *Circulation.* 1996; **93**(5):1043–65.

31 Gamelin FX, Berthoin S, Bosquet L. Validity of the polar S810 heart rate monitor to measure R-R intervals at rest. *Med Sci Sports Exerc.* 2006; **38**(5):887–93.

32 Kingsley M, Lewis MJ, Marson RE. Comparison of polar 810s and an ambulatory ECG system for RR interval measurement during progressive exercise. *Int J Sports Med.* 2005; **26**(1):39–44.

33 Hynynen E, Vesterinen V, Rusko H, Nummela A. Effects of moderate and heavy endurance exercise on nocturnal HRV. *Int J Sports Med.* 2010; **31**(6):428–32.

34 Kingsley JD, Figueroa A. Acute and training effects of resistance exercise on heart rate variability. *Clin Physiol Funct Imaging.* 2016; **36**(3):179–87.

35 Gkaliagkousi E, Gavriilaki E, Triantafyllou A, Douma S. Clinical significance of endothelial dysfunction in essential hypertension. *Curr Hypertens Rep.* 2015; **17**(11):85.

36 Sorensen KE, Celermajer DS, Spiegelhalter DJ, Georgakopoulos D, Robinson J, Thomas O, et al. Non-invasive measurement of human endothelium dependent arterial responses: accuracy and reproducibility. *Br Heart J.* 1995; **74**(3):247–53.

37 Rossman MJ, Groot HJ, Garten RS, Witman MAH, Richardson RS. Vascular function assessed by passive leg movement and flow-mediated dilation: initial evidence of construct validity. *Am J Physiol Heart Circ Physiol.* 2016; **311**(5):H1277.

38 Hwang MH, Yoo JK, Kim HK, Hwang CL, Mackay K, Hemstreet O, et al. Validity and reliability of aortic pulse wave velocity and augmentation index determined by the new cuff-based SphygmoCor Xcel. *J Hum Hypertens.* 2014; **28**(8):475–81.

39 Thiebaud RS, Fahs CA, Rossow LM, Loenneke JP, Kim D, Mouser JG, et al. Effects of age on arterial stiffness and central blood pressure after an acute bout of resistance exercise. *Eur J Appl Physiol.* 2016; **116**(1):39–48.

40 Morkedal B, Romundstad PR, Vatten LJ. Informativeness of indices of blood pressure, obesity and serum lipids in relation to ischaemic heart disease mortality: the HUNT-II study. *Eur J Epidemiol.* 2011; **26**(6):457–61.

41 Coqueiro Rda S, Santos MC, Neto Jde S, Queiroz BM, Brugger NA, Barbosa AR. Validity of a portable glucose, total cholesterol, and triglycerides multi-analyzer in adults. *Biol Res Nurs.* 2014; **16**(3):288–94.

42 Al-Humaidi MA, Abolfotouh MA, Sulaiman SA, Al-Kadoumi OF, Khattab MS, Al-Salmi HH, et al. The validity of the Reflotron as a screening tool for blood cholesterol. *J Egypt Public Health Assoc.* 1997; **72**(1–2):167–87.

43 Mann S, Beedie C, Jimenez A. Differential effects of aerobic exercise, resistance training and combined exercise modalities on cholesterol and the lipid profile: review, synthesis and recommendations. *Sports Med (Auckland, NZ).* 2014; **44**(2):211–21.

44 Wagganer JD, Robison CE, Ackerman TA, Davis PG. Effects of exercise accumulation on plasma lipids and lipoproteins. *Appl Physiol Nutr Metab.* 2015; **40**(5):441–7.

45 Kelley GA, Kelley KS, Roberts S, Haskell W. Comparison of aerobic exercise, diet or both on lipids and lipoproteins in adults: a meta-analysis of randomized controlled trials. *Clin Nutr (Edinburgh, Scotland).* 2012; **31**(2):156–67.

46 Kelley GA, Kelley KS. Impact of progressive resistance training on lipids and lipoproteins in adults: a meta-analysis of randomized controlled trials. *Prev Med.* 2009; **48**(1):9–19.

47 Yamashita S, Nakamura T, Shimomura I, Nishida M, Yoshida S, Kotani K, et al. Insulin resistance and body fat distribution. *Diabetes Care.* 1996; **19**(3):287–91.

48 Fujioka S, Matsuzawa Y, Tokunaga K, Tarui S. Contribution of intra-abdominal fat accumulation to the impairment of glucose and lipid metabolism in human obesity. *Metab Clin Exp.* 1987; **36**(1):54–9.

49   Despres JP, Lemieux I. Abdominal obesity and metabolic syndrome. *Nature.* 2006; **444**(7121):881–7.

50   Dutheil F, Gordon BA, Naughton G, Crendal E, Courteix D, Chaplais E, et al. Cardiovascular risk of adipokines: a review. *J Int Med Res.* 2018; **46**(6):2082–95.

51   Fosbol MO, Zerahn B. Contemporary methods of body composition measurement. *Clin Physiol Funct Imaging.* 2015; **35**(2):81–97.

52   Talma H, Chinapaw MJ, Bakker B, HiraSing RA, Terwee CB, Altenburg TM. Bioelectrical impedance analysis to estimate body composition in children and adolescents: a systematic review and evidence appraisal of validity, responsiveness, reliability and measurement error. *Obes Rev Off J Int Assoc Study Obes.* 2013; **14**(11):895–905.

53   Nana A, Slater GJ, Hopkins WG, Burke LM. Effects of daily activities on dual-energy X-ray absorptiometry measurements of body composition in active people. *Med Sci Sports Exerc.* 2012; **44**(1):180–9.

54   Melvin MN, Smith-Ryan AE, Wingfield HL, Fultz SN, Roelofs EJ. Evaluation of muscle quality reliability and racial differences in body composition of overweight individuals. *Ultrasound Med Biol.* 2014; **40**(9):1973–9.

55   Rona RJ, Sundin J, Wood P, Fear NT. Agreement between body mass index, waist circumference and skin-fold thickness in the United Kingdom Army. *Ann Hum Biol.* 2011; **38**(3):257–64.

56   Mooney SJ, Baecker A, Rundle AG. Comparison of anthropometric and body composition measures as predictors of components of the metabolic syndrome in a clinical setting. *Obes Res Clin Pract.* 2013; **7**(1):e55–66.

57   Gordon B, Chen S, Durstine JL. The effects of exercise training on the traditional lipid profile and beyond. *Curr Sports Med Rep.* 2014; **13**(4):253–9.

58   Tambalis K, Panagiotakos DB, Kavouras SA, Sidossis LS. Responses of blood lipids to aerobic, resistance, and combined aerobic with resistance exercise training: a systematic review of current evidence. *Angiology.* 2009; **60**(5):614–32.

59   Miller CT, Fraser SF, Levinger I, Straznicky NE, Dixon JB, Reynolds J, et al. The effects of exercise training in addition to energy restriction on functional capacities and body composition in obese adults during weight loss: a systematic review. *PloS One.* 2013; **8**(11):e81692.

60   Peake MJ, Bruns DE, Sacks DB, Horvath AR. It's time for a better blood collection tube to improve the reliability of glucose results. *Diabetes Care.* 2013; **36**(1):e2.

61   Inoue S, Egi M, Kotani J, Morita K. Accuracy of blood-glucose measurements using glucose meters and arterial blood gas analyzers in critically ill adult patients: systematic review. *Critical Care (London, England).* 2013; **17**(2):R48.

62   Terada T, Loehr S, Guigard E, McCargar LJ, Bell GJ, Senior P, et al. Test-retest reliability of a continuous glucose monitoring system in individuals with type 2 diabetes. *Diabetes Technol Ther.* 2014; **16**(8):491–8.

63   The accuracy of the CGMS in children with type 1 diabetes: results of the diabetes research in children network (DirecNet) accuracy study. *Diabetes Technol Ther.* 2003; **5**(5):781–9.

64   Bay C, Kristensen PL, Pedersen-Bjergaard U, Tarnow L, Thorsteinsson B. Nocturnal continuous glucose monitoring: accuracy and reliability of hypoglycemia detection in patients with type 1 diabetes at high risk of severe hypoglycemia. *Diabetes Technol Ther.* 2013; **15**(5):371–7.

65   Clarke WL, Anderson S, Farhy L, Breton M, Gonder-Frederick L, Cox D, et al. Evaluating the clinical accuracy of two continuous glucose sensors using continuous glucose-error grid analysis. *Diabetes Care.* 2005; **28**(10):2412–7.

66   World Health Organization. *Use of glycated haemoglobin (HbA1c) in the diagnosis of diabetes mellitus: abbreviated report of a WHO consultation.* Geneva, Switzerland: World Health Organization Press; 2011.

67   d'Emden MC, Shaw JE, Colman PG, Colagiuri S, Twigg SM, Jones GR, et al. The role of HbA1c in the diagnosis of diabetes mellitus in Australia. *Med J Aust.* 2012; **197**(4):220–1.

68 Venkataraman V, Anjana RM, Pradeepa R, Deepa M, Jayashri R, Anbalagan VP, et al. Stability and reliability of glycated haemoglobin measurements in blood samples stored at −20°C. *J Diabetes Comp.* 2016; **30**(1):121–5.

69 Arsie MP, Marchioro L, Lapolla A, Giacchetto GF, Bordin MR, Rizzotti P, et al. Evaluation of diagnostic reliability of DCA 2000 for rapid and simple monitoring of HbA1c. *Acta Diabetol.* 2000; **37**(1):1–7.

70 Bird SR, Hawley JA. Update on the effects of physical activity on insulin sensitivity in humans. *BMJ Open Sport Exerc Med.* 2017; **2**(1):e000143. DOI: 10.1136/bmjsem-2016-000143

71 Gutch M, Kumar S, Razi SM, Gupta KK, Gupta A. Assessment of insulin sensitivity/resistance. *Indian J Endocrinol Metab.* 2015; **19**(1):160–4.

72 Gordon BA, Fraser SF, Bird SR, Benson AC. Reproducibility of multiple repeated oral glucose tolerance tests. *Diabetes Res Clin Pract.* 2011; **94**(3):e78–82.

73 Ortega JF, Hamouti N, Fernandez-Elias VE, Mora-Rodriguez R. Comparison of glucose tolerance tests to detect the insulin sensitizing effects of a bout of continuous exercise. *Appl Phys Nutr Metab.* 2014; **39**(7):787–92.

74 Boule NG, Haddad E, Kenny GP, Wells GA, Sigal RJ. Effects of exercise on glycemic control and body mass in type 2 diabetes mellitus: a meta-analysis of controlled clinical trials. *JAMA.* 2001; **286**(10):1218–27.

75 Aune D, Norat T, Leitzmann M, Tonstad S, Vatten LJ. Physical activity and the risk of type 2 diabetes: a systematic review and dose-response meta-analysis. *Eur J Epidemiol.* 2015; **30**(7):529–42.

76 van Dijk JW, Manders RJ, Tummers K, Bonomi AG, Stehouwer CD, Hartgens F, et al. Both resistance- and endurance-type exercise reduce the prevalence of hyperglycaemia in individuals with impaired glucose tolerance and in insulin-treated and non-insulin-treated type 2 diabetic patients. *Diabetologia.* 2012; **55**(5):1273–82.

77 Gordon BA, Bird SR, MacIsaac RJ, Benson AC. Does a single bout of resistance or aerobic exercise after insulin dose reduction modulate glycaemic control in type 2 diabetes? A randomised cross-over trial. *J Sci Med Sport.* 2016; **19**(10):795–9.

78 Grace A, Chan E, Giallauria F, Graham PL, Smart NA. Clinical outcomes and glycaemic responses to different aerobic exercise training intensities in type II diabetes: a systematic review and meta-analysis. *Cardiovasc Diabetol.* 2017; **16**(1):37.

79 Snowling NJ, Hopkins WG. Effects of different modes of exercise training on glucose control and risk factors for complications in type 2 diabetic patients: a meta-analysis. *Diabetes Care.* 2006; **29**(11):2518–27.

80 Way KL, Hackett DA, Baker MK, Johnson NA. The effect of regular exercise on insulin sensitivity in type 2 diabetes mellitus: a systematic review and meta-analysis. *Diabetes Metab J.* 2016; **40**(4):253–71.

81 Gordon BA, Benson AC, Bird SR, Fraser SF. Resistance training improves metabolic health in type 2 diabetes: a systematic review. *Diabetes Res Clin Pract.* 2009; **83**(2):157–75.

82 Ishiguro H, Kodama S, Horikawa C, Fujihara K, Hirose AS, Hirasawa R, et al. In search of the ideal resistance training program to improve glycemic control and its indication for patients with type 2 diabetes mellitus: a systematic review and meta-analysis. *Sports Med (Auckland, NZ).* 2016; **46**(1):67–77.

83 Kim CH, Kim HK, Kim EH, Bae SJ, Park JY. Association between changes in body composition and risk of developing Type 2 diabetes in Koreans. *Diabetic Med J Br Diabetic Assoc.* 2014; **31**(11):1393–8.

84 Wewege M, van den Berg R, Ward RE, Keech A. The effects of high-intensity interval training vs. moderate-intensity continuous training on body composition in overweight and obese adults: a systematic review and meta-analysis. *Obes Rev Off J Int Assoc Study Obes.* 2017; **18**(6):635–46.

85 Peterson MD, Sen A, Gordon PM. Influence of resistance exercise on lean body mass in aging adults: a meta-analysis. *Med Sci Sports Exerc.* 2011; **43**(2):249–58.

206   *Brett Gordon et al.*

86 Hartmann A, Knols R, Murer K, de Bruin ED. Reproducibility of an isokinetic strength-testing protocol of the knee and ankle in older adults. *Gerontology.* 2009; **55**(3):259–68.

87 Webber SC, Porter MM. Reliability of ankle isometric, isotonic, and isokinetic strength and power testing in older women. *Phys Ther.* 2010; **90**(8):1165–75.

88 Mentiplay BF, Perraton LG, Bower KJ, Adair B, Pua YH, Williams GP, et al. Assessment of lower limb muscle strength and power using hand-held and fixed dynamometry: a reliability and validity study. *PLoS One.* 2015; **10**(10):e0140822.

89 Schroeder ET, Wang Y, Castaneda-Sceppa C, Cloutier G, Vallejo AF, Kawakubo M, et al. Reliability of maximal voluntary muscle strength and power testing in older men. *J Gerontol A Biol Sci Med Sci.* 2007; **62**(5):543–9.

90 Phillips WT, Batterham AM, Valenzuela JE, Burkett LN. Reliability of maximal strength testing in older adults. *Arch Phys Med Rehabil.* 2004; **85**(2):329–34.

91 Levinger I, Goodman C, Hare DL, Jerums G, Toia D, Selig S. The reliability of the 1RM strength test for untrained middle-aged individuals. *J Sci Med Sport.* 2009; **12**(2):310–6.

92 Reeves ND, Maganaris CN, Longo S, Narici MV. Differential adaptations to eccentric versus conventional resistance training in older humans. *Exp Physiol.* 2009; **94**(7):825–33.

93 Scaglioni G, Ferri A, Minetti AE, Martin A, Van Hoecke J, Capodaglio P, et al. Plantar flexor activation capacity and H reflex in older adults: adaptations to strength training. *J Appl Physiol.* 2002; **92**(6):2292–302.

94 Haykowsky M, Taylor D, Teo K, Quinney A, Humen D. Left ventricular wall stress during leg-press exercise performed with a brief Valsalva maneuver. *Chest.* 2001; **119**(1):150–4.

95 Cofre L, Lythgo N, Morgan D, Galea M. Aging modifies joint power and work when gait speeds are matched. *Gait Posture.* 2011; **33**(3):484–9.

96 Thelen D, Wojcik LA, Schultz AB, Ashton-Miller JA, Alexander NB. Age differences in using a rapid step to regain balance during a forward fall. *J Gerontol Biol Med Sci.* 1997; **52**(A):8–13.

97 Wojcik LA, Thelen D, Schultz AB, Ashton-Miller JA, Alexander NB. Age and gender differences in single-step recovery from a forward fall. *J Gerontol Biol Med Sci.* 1999; **54**(A):44–50.

98 Wojcik LA, Thelen D, Schultz AB, Ashton-Miller JA, Alexander NB. Age and gender differences in peak lower extremity joint torques and ranges of motion used during single-step balance recovery from a forward fall. *J Biomech.* 2001; **34**:67–73.

99 Thelen D, Schultz AB, Alexander NB, Ashton-Miller JA. Effects of age on rapid ankle torque development. *J Gerontol Biol Med Sci.* 1996; **51**:226–32.

100 van der Krogt M, Delp S, Schwartz MH. How robust is human gait to muscle weakness? *Gait Posture.* 2012; **36**:113–9.

101 Gallahue DL, Ozmun JC. *Understanding motor development: infants, children, adolescents, adults.* 5th ed. New York: McGraw-Hill Higher Education; 2002.

102 Hausdorf JM, Rios DA, Edelberg HK. Gait variability and fall risk in community-living older adults: a 1 year prospective study. *Arch Phys Med Rehab.* 2001; **82**:1050–6.

103 Hill K, Schwarz J, Flicker L, Carroll S. Falls among healthy, community-dwelling, older women: a prospective study of frequency, circumstances, consequences and prediction accuracy. *Aust N Z J Public Health.* 1999; **23**:41–8.

104 Prince F, Corriveau H, Hebert R, Winter DA. Gait in the elderly. *Gait Posture.* 1997; **5**:128–35.

105 Blanke DJ, Hageman PA. Comparison of gait of young men and elderly men. *Phys Ther.* 1989; **69**:144–8.

106 McGibbon CA. Toward a better understanding of gait changes with age and disablement neuromuscular adaptation. *Exerc Sport Sci Rev.* 2006; **31**(2):102–8.

107 Carmeli E, Coleman R, Llaguna O, Brown-Cross D. Do we allow elderly pedestrians sufficient time to cross the street in safety? *J Aging Phys Act.* 2000; **8**:51–8.

108 Oberg T, Karsznia A, Oberg K. Basic gait parameters: reference data for normal subjects, 10–79 years of age. *J Rehab Res Dev.* 1993; **30**(2):210–23.

109 Hageman PA, Blanke DJ. Comparison of young women and elderly women. *Phys Ther.* 1986; **66**:1382–7.

110 Menz HB, Latt MD, Tiedemann A, Mun San Kwan M, Lord SR. Reliability of the GAITRite walkway system for the quantification of temporo-spatial parameters of gait in young and older people. *Gait Posture.* 2004; **20**(1):20–5.

111 Chao EY, Laughman RK, Schneider E, Stauffer RN. Normative data of knee motion and ground reaction forces in adult level walking. *J Biomech.* 1983; **16**:219–33.

112 Crosbie J, Roongtiwa V, Smith R. Patterns of spinal motion during walking. *Gait Posture.* 1997; **5**:6–12.

113 Judge JO, Davis RB, Ounpuu S. Step length reductions in advanced age: the role of ankle and hip kinetics. *J Gerontol.* 1996; **51A**(6):303–12.

114 McGibbon CA, Krebs DE. Age-related changes in lower trunk coordinationand energy trnasfer during gait. *J Neurophys.* 2001; **85**:1923–31.

115 Lythgo N, Begg R. Age and speed effects on gait kinematics to negotiate surface height changes *J Aging Phys Act.* 2004; **12**(3):306–7.

116 Oberg T, Karsznia A, Oberg K. Joint angle parameters on gait: reference data for normal subjects, 10–79 years of age. *J Rehab Res Dev.* 1994; **31**(3):199–213.

117 Studenski S, Perera S, Patel K, Rosano C, Faulkner K, Inzitari M, et al. Gait speed and survival in older adults. *J Am Med Assoc.* 2011; **305**(1):51–8.

118 Cesari M, Kritchevsky SB, Penninx BW, Niklas BJ, Simonsick EM, Newman AB, et al. Prognostic value of usual gait speed in well-functioning older people-results from the health, aging and body composition. *J Am Geriatr Soc.* 2005; **53**(10):1675–80.

119 Abellan van Kan G, Rolland Y, Andrieu S, Bauer J, Beauchet O, Bonnefoy M, et al. Gait speed at usual pace as a predictor of adverse outcomes in community-dwelling older people. *J Nutr Health Aging.* 2009; **13**(10):881–9.

120 Dusing SC, Thorpe DE. A normative sample of temporal and spatial gait parameters in children using the GAITRite1 electronic walkway. *Gait Posture.* 2007; **25**:135–9.

121 Lythgo N, Wilson C, Galea M. Basic gait and symmetry measures for primary school aged children and young adults whilst walking barefoot and with shoes. *Gait Posture.* 2009; **30**(4):502–6.

122 Lythgo N, Wilson C, Galea M. Basic gait and symmetry measures for primary school-aged children and young adults II: walking at slow, free and fast speed. *Gait Posture.* 2011; **33**(1):29–35.

123 Schwartz M, Rozumalski A, Trost J. The effect of speed on the gait of typically developing children. *J Biomech.* 2008; **41**:1639–50.

124 McGinley JL, Baker R, Wolfe R, Morris ME. The reliability of three-dimensional kinematic gait measurements: a systematic review. *Gait Posture.* 2009; **29**(3):360–9.

125 Bennell K, Dobson F, Hinman R. Measures of physical performance assessments: Self-Paced Walk Test (SPWT), Stair Climb Test (SCT), Six-Minute Walk Test (6MWT), Chair Stand Test (CST), Timed Up & Go (TUG), Sock Test, Lift and Carry Test (LCT), and car task. *Arthritis Care Res.* 2011; **63**(S11):S350–70.

126 Suzuki T, Bean JF, Fielding RA. Muscle power of the ankle flexors predicts functional performance in community-dwelling older women. *J Am Geriatr Soc.* 2001; **49**(9):1161–7.

127 Roig M, Eng JJ, MacIntyre DL, Road JD, Reid WD. Associations of the stair climb power test with muscle strength and functional performance in people with chronic obstructive pulmonary disease: a cross-sectional study. *Phys Ther.* 2010; **90**(12):1774–82.

128 Gibbons WJ, Fruchter N, Sloan S, Levy RD. Reference values for a multiple repetition 6-minute walk test in healthy adults older than 20 years. *J Cardiopulm Rehabil Prev.* 2001; **21**(2):87–93.

129 Enright PL, McBurnie MA, Bittner V, Tracy RP, McNamara R, Arnold A, et al. The 6-min walk test: a quick measure of functional status in elderly adults. *Chest.* 2003; **123**(2):387–98.

130 Harada ND, Harada ND, Chiu V, Stewart AL. Mobility-related function in older adults: assessment with a 6-minute walk test. *Arch Phys Med Rehab.* 1999; **80**(7):837.

131 Sadaria K, Bohannon R. The 6-minute walk test: a brief review of literature. *Clin Exerc Physiol.* 2001; **3**:127–32.

132 Duncan PW, Weiner DK, Chandler J, Studenski S. Functional reach: a new clinical measure of balance. *J Gerontol.* 1990; **45**(6):M192–7.

133 Whitney SL, Marchetti GF, Morris LO, Sparto PJ. The reliability and validity of the four square step test for people with balance deficits secondary to a vestibular disorder. *Arch Phys Med Rehab.* 2007; **88**(1):99–104.

134 Berg K, Wood-Dauphine S, Williams JI, Gayton D. Measuring balance in the elderly: preliminary development of an instrument. *Physiother Can.* 1989; **41**(6):304–11.

135 Buchner DM, Hornbrook MC, Kutner NG, Tinetti ME, Ory MG, Mulrow CD, et al. Development of the common data base for the FICSIT trials. *J Am Geriatr Soc.* 1993; **41**(3):297–308.

136 Norris RA, Wilder E, Norton J. The functional reach test in 3-to 5-year-old children without disabilities. *Pediatr Phys Ther.* 2008; **20**(1):47–52.

137 Smith PS, Hembree JA, Thompson ME. Berg balance scale and functional reach: determining the best clinical tool for individuals post acute stroke. *Clin Rehab.* 2004; **18**(7):811–8.

138 Duncan PW, Studenski S, Chandler J, Prescott B. Functional reach: predictive validity in a sample of elderly male veterans. *J Gerontol.* 1992; **47**(3):M93–M8.

139 Volkman KG, Stergiou N, Stuberg W, Blanke D, Stoner J. Methods to improve the reliability of the functional reach test in children and adolescents with typical development. *Pediatr Phys Ther.* 2007; **19**(1):20–7.

140 Jonsson E, Henriksson M, Hirschfeld H. Does the functional reach test reflect stability limits in elderly people? *J Rehab Med.* 2003; **35**(1):26–30.

141 Lynch SM, Leahy P, Barker SP. Reliability of measurements obtained with a modified functional reach test in subjects with spinal cord injury. *Phys Ther.* 1998; **78**(2):128–33.

142 Katz-Leurer M, Fisher I, Neeb M, Schwartz I, Carmeli E. Reliability and validity of the modified functional reach test at the sub-acute stage post-stroke. *Disabil Rehab.* 2009; **31**(3):243–8.

143 Takahashi T, Ishida K, Yamamoto H, Takata J, Nishinaga M, Doi Y, et al. Modification of the functional reach test: analysis of lateral and anterior functional reach in community-dwelling older people. *Arch Gerontol Geriatr.* 2006; **42**(2):167–73.

144 Newton RA. Validity of the multi-directional reach test: a practical measure for limits of stability in older adults. *J Gerontol Ser A Biol Sci Med Sci.* 2001; **56**(4):M248–M52.

145 VanSwearingen JM, Brach JS. Making geriatric assessment work: selecting useful measures. *Phys Ther.* 2001; **81**(6):1233.

146 Bressel E, Yonker JC, Kras J, Heath EM. Comparison of static and dynamic balance in female collegiate soccer, basketball, and gymnastics athletes. *J Athl Train.* 2007; **42**(1):42–6.

147 Hertel J, Miller SJ, Denegar CR. Intratester and intertester reliability during the star excursion balance tests. *J Sport Rehab.* 2000; **9**(2):104–16.

148 Podsiadlo D, Richardson S. The timed "Up & Go": a test of basic functional mobility for frail elderly persons. *J Am Geriatr Soc.* 1991; **39**(2):142–8.

149 Morris S, Morris ME, Iansek R. Reliability of measurements obtained with the timed "Up & Go" test in people with Parkinson disease. *Phys Ther.* 2001; **81**(2):810–8.

150 Ng SS, Hui-Chan CW. The timed up & go test: its reliability and association with lower-limb impairments and locomotor capacities in people with chronic stroke. *Arch Phys Med Rehab.* 2005; **86**(8):1641–7.

151 Schoppen T, Boonstra A, Groothoff JW, de Vries J, Göeken LN, Eisma WH. The timed "up and go" test: reliability and validity in persons with unilateral lower limb amputation. *Arch Phys Med Rehab.* 1999; **80**(7):825–8.

152 Williams EN, Carroll SG, Reddihough DS, Phillips BA, Galea MP. Investigation of the timed 'up & go'test in children. *Dev Med Child Neurol.* 2005; **47**(8):518–24.

153 DiStefano LJ, Clark MA, Padua DA. Evidence supporting balance training in healthy individuals: a systemic review. *J Strength Cond Res.* 2009; **23**(9):2718–31.

154 Wells KF, Dillon EK. The sit and reach – a test of back and leg flexibility. *Res Quar Am Assoc Health Phys Educ Recreation.* 1952; **23**(1):115–8.

155 Jackson AW, Baker AA. The relationship of the sit and reach test to criterion measures of hamstring and back flexibility in young females. *Res Quar Exerc Sport.* 1986; **57**(3):183–6.

156 Hui SSC, Yuen PY. Validity of the modified back-saver sit-and-reach test: a comparison with other protocols. *Med Sci Sports Exerc.* 2000; **32**(9):1655–9.

157 Jones CJ, Rikli RE, Max J, Noffal G. The reliability and validity of a chair sit-and-reach test as a measure of hamstring flexibility in older adults. *Res Quar Exerc Sport.* 1998; **69**(4):338–43.

158 Rikli RE, Jones CJ. Functional fitness normative scores for community-residing older adults, ages 60–94. *J Aging Phys Act.* 1999; **7**(2):162–81.

159 Bautmans I, Van Hees E, Lemper JC, Mets T. The feasibility of whole body vibration in institutionalised elderly persons and its influence on muscle performance, balance and mobility: a randomised controlled trial [ISRCTN62535013]. *BMC Geriatr.* 2005; **5**(1):17.

160 Toraman A, Yıldırım NÜ. The falling risk and physical fitness in older people. *Arch Gerontol Geriatr.* 2010; **51**(2):222–6.

161 Bautmans I, Njemini R, Vasseur S, Chabert H, Moens L, Demanet C, et al. Biochemical changes in response to intensive resistance exercise training in the elderly. *Gerontology.* 2005; **51**(4):253–65.

162 Garber CE, Blissmer B, Deschenes MR, Franklin BA, Lamonte MJ, Lee IM, et al. Quantity and quality of exercise for developing and maintaining cardiorespiratory, musculoskeletal, and neuromotor fitness in apparently healthy adults: guidance for prescribing exercise. *Med Sci Sports Exerc.* 2011; **43**(7):1334–59.

20 Physical activity and the 'feel-good' effect

Challenges in researching the pleasure and displeasure people feel when they exercise

Panteleimon Ekkekakis, Matthew A. Ladwig and Mark E. Hartman

Chapter aims

This chapter provides methodological guidance for researchers interested in investigating the pleasures and displeasures that participants feel in response to exercise (termed 'affective responses'). A conclusion often found in textbooks is that exercise makes people 'feel better' but this statement seems to contrast with the low rates of regular participation in exercise and physical activity. This chapter explains how early methodological decisions that originally seemed reasonable inadvertently biased research results in favour of the 'feel-better' effect. Sections within this chapter address the implications deriving from several aspects of the research process including the sampling of participants, the choice of constructs (affect, mood, emotion), the timing of the assessment protocols, the methods of standardizing exercise intensity across participants and the approach used to examine change over time. In each case, the authors explain how the original methods may have led to bias and propose preferable alternatives.

Introduction

The study of the pleasure and displeasure responses to physical activity and exercise (hereafter referred to as 'affective responses') has been one of the most prolific research areas within the exercise sciences over the past half century. The interest in this topic is due to at least two reasons. First, if physical activity can help people regulate their mood (e.g. by reducing sadness or raising the level of perceived energy), it may benefit their overall mental health. Unlike commonly employed mental health interventions (i.e. pharmacotherapy), physical activity entails minimal or no financial cost and is accompanied by salubrious, rather than adverse, side-effects. Therefore, if physical activity is shown to be effective in reducing symptoms of prevalent mental health disorders (e.g. depression, anxiety, substance abuse), such a finding could have considerable implications for global mental health.[1] Second, if physical activity is consistently experienced as pleasant, this may strengthen the motivation of participants to remain physically active. While the health benefits of a physically active lifestyle are undeniable, public participation rates remain low and, of the people who initiate regular activity, most discontinue soon thereafter. Since it is generally presumed that people are more likely to pursue activities that make them feel better and avoid those that make them feel worse, improving the current understanding of the relationship between physical activity and pleasure-displeasure could help address the pandemic of physical inactivity.[2]

The research dilemma

A researcher entering this area for the first time would probably be surprised by a striking contrast. Textbooks and academic journals in exercise science are replete with confident assertions that physical activity makes people 'feel good'.[3] On the other hand, popular self-help books and the mass media are replete with advertisements for a seemingly endless array of substances or contraptions that promise to deliver many of the health benefits of regular physical activity (e.g. reduced body weight, higher cardiovascular and muscular fitness, better sleep) without doing any physical activity. These two phenomena seem contradictory; either the researchers are correct in stating that physical activity consistently makes people feel better or the marketers are correct in describing physical activity as something that most people would like to avoid (i.e. as painful, exhausting, or boring) and promising alternatives.

This contrast is, in fact, a demonstration of the importance of methodological rigour in research. In this chapter, we will illustrate how methodological choices can alter the conclusions that are drawn. For each of the issues we identify, we will highlight the important role of three factors. First, there should be open recognition of the fact that often, perhaps too often, research findings are false.[4] This is because of numerous forms of bias that are introduced in the process of research by fallible human agents,[5] either intentionally (e.g. due to financial or non-financial conflicts of interest) or unintentionally (e.g. due to carelessness or ignorance). It has been suggested that the likelihood of false findings may be highest in the social sciences, such as psychology, perhaps due to the fact that the theories do not allow for precise predictions, methods tend to not be fully standardized and researchers generally have more 'degrees of freedom' to influence the process toward a particular outcome.[6,7] Of particular interest here is the type of bias that is motivated by a form of 'prejudice' that may be overlooked or excused as 'well-intentioned' but constitutes serious bias nonetheless. This type of bias is the (usually, unabashed) pro-exercise agenda of exercise researchers. It is uncontroversial to suggest that most exercise researchers are also exercise proponents, if not exercise fanatics. This often places them emotionally closer to the subject of their research than other researchers and may blur the line between advocacy and scientific impartiality. For example, it may be tempting for an exercise researcher to highlight results showing that exercise makes people 'feel better' or to downplay results indicating that exercise has the opposite effects.

Second, our review underscores the importance of critical thinking and the willingness to 'swim against the current'. Entrenched methodological practices can be extremely difficult to change, even if they are convincingly shown to be problematic. The reason is that, if a certain methodological element has been part of the research platform used for the investigation of a certain phenomenon for many years, questioning its validity would challenge the credibility of that entire line of research and could thus place previous results in doubt. Questioning previous results also threatens the professional reputations of the researchers who produced those results, with potentially grave implications for their careers and their prospects of attracting further research funding. Thus, although, as researchers, we like to believe that science is ultimately self-correcting, such corrections may take a long time and a great deal of effort because there are often strong incentives to perpetuate erroneous approaches.[8] According to Ioannidis,[4] "Prestigious investigators may suppress via the peer-review process the appearance and dissemination of findings that refute their findings, thus condemning their field to perpetuate false dogma" (p. 698).

Third, we highlight the problem of 'secondary ignorance'. According to Eisner (1998):[9] "Primary ignorance . . . is when you do not know something but you know that you do not know it. In this situation, you can do something about it. Secondary ignorance is when you do not know something but you do not know you do not know it. In this case, you can do nothing about the problem" (p. 161). Investigating the relationship between physical activity and affect is hard because it requires expertise in two, quite diverse, scientific disciplines, namely the domain of psychology that focuses on the study of affective phenomena and the domain of physiology that investigates proper ways of quantifying and standardizing the dose of physical activity across individuals. Both of these disciplines have histories that extend for over a century and deal with complicated subject matters. Consequently, mastering even one of the two domains, let alone mastering both, requires extraordinary commitment and patience. As a result, researchers may be tempted to 'cut corners' by employing methodological approaches that are prevalent in the literature or approaches that simply 'seem' reasonable. The alternative, namely delving into the arcane primary literatures to perform a thorough critical analysis and form an independent, educated opinion on each issue, seems extremely onerous by comparison. Consequently, this option is likely to be regarded as unrealistic within an academic culture that rewards high productivity above all else.

A bit of history: the road to methodological artefacts is often paved with good intentions

To understand how honest methodological mistakes can initially be made, and can subsequently persist over a period of decades, it is instructive to revisit the early days of research on the exercise-affect relation. In December 1967, psychiatrists Pitts and McClure published an article in the prestigious *New England Journal of Medicine*,[10] claiming to have demonstrated a causal link between lactate and the likelihood of anxiety attacks among patients with anxiety. From this, they concluded that they had uncovered an important part of the biochemical basis of anxiety disorders. Moreover, they speculated that, since vigorous exercise leads to elevations in blood lactate, vigorous exercise could precipitate anxiety attacks and, therefore, patients, especially those at risk for anxiety disorders, should avoid it.

It turned out that both the experimental approach and the mechanistic conjectures of Pitts and McClure were flawed and, as such, they were widely rebuked in the psychiatric literature. Before the dust settled, however, the Pitts-McClure hypothesis captured the attention of the press and generated considerable – and understandable – public interest. Consequently, exercise scientists perceived the message 'exercise can cause anxiety attacks' as a potential threat to nascent efforts at that time to introduce exercise in clinical practice (e.g. for primary prevention and cardiac rehabilitation).

In the late 1960s, the evidence on the beneficial effects of exercise on the psyche consisted primarily of small-scale cross-sectional studies showing that those who are more aerobically fit or report larger amounts of physical activity or sport involvement also tended to give higher scores on measures of positive psychological traits (e.g. self-esteem) and lower scores on measures of negative traits (e.g. anxiousness, neuroticism). Experimental investigations, however, were non-existent. The Pitts-McClure hypothesis provided the motivation to initiate the line of research on the exercise-affect relation, which later developed into the field known today as exercise psychology.

In the first experimental study inspired by the Pitts-McClure hypothesis, Morgan, Roberts and Feinerman set out to demonstrate that exercise participation improves how people feel and should, therefore, reduce the likelihood of anxiety attacks.[11] This first attempt, however, failed to find any significant differences in post-treatment levels of anxiety and depression between participants assigned to groups that completed exercise sessions or equal periods of rest. Despite this finding, Morgan et al.[11] wrote that "even though significant psychologic changes were not observed, the majority of the subjects tested in these studies reported that the exercise bouts were exhilarating and they 'felt better' following the exercise" (p. 425). The researchers attributed the failure to formally document these beneficial effects to the questionnaires they used: "It is possible that the psychometric instruments were not sensitive enough to measure psychologic changes in normal subjects" (p. 425).

At approximately the same time, two new questionnaires were published that appeared to be good candidates for capturing the postulated 'feel-better' effect of exercise. There were two reasons for this. First, these new questionnaires could be used to assess transient psychological changes (such as those that may occur during and after a session of exercise). In contrast, questionnaires that existed up to that point were designed to assess chronic conditions (i.e. tap usual or frequently occurring symptoms of mental health disorders). Second, the two new questionnaires were appropriate for use with respondents from the general population. In contrast, earlier questionnaires had been mainly developed for clinical use (i.e. they were designed as screening or diagnostic instruments for mental health disorders).

One of these questionnaires was the State-Trait Anxiety Inventory (STAI).[12] It included 20 items designed to measure state anxiety (i.e. the negative emotional reaction that follows the perception of threat) and 20 items designed to measure trait anxiety (i.e. the predisposition to interpret situations as threatening and to respond to them with elevations in state anxiety that are disproportionate to the degree of objective danger). The second questionnaire was the Profile of Mood States (POMS).[13] It included 65 items divided into six scales, five of which were aimed to tap unpleasant mood states (tension, depression, anger, fatigue, confusion) and one that was aimed to tap a pleasant mood state (vigour). A composite 'mood disturbance' score can also be calculated by summing the scores of the five unpleasant scales and subtracting the score of the vigour scale.

Using these questionnaires, Morgan found that exercise bouts significantly reduced scores of state anxiety and mood disturbance.[14] These findings provided the evidence to substantiate anecdotal accounts that exercise makes participants 'feel better'. Thus, since exercise was found to result in reduced state anxiety and enhanced mood, Morgan claimed that this evidence amounted to a formal refutation of the Pitts-McClure hypothesis.[14]

The message 'exercise makes people feel better' proved very appealing to exercise researchers, who proceeded to replicate the initial findings by Morgan with numerous types of samples, exercise modes, intensities, durations and comparator conditions. Over the next 25 years, the number of studies that echoed the finding of an exercise-induced 'feel-better' effect numbered in the hundreds, causing Morgan to plead with the field to move on: "there is no need for further research or reviews dealing with the question of whether or not physical activity results in improved mood" (p. 230).[15]

While designing studies to replicate the exercise-induced 'feel-better' effect, researchers repeated the methodological approach that had been used by Morgan. They assessed how participants felt using the STAI, the POMS or both. They administered these questionnaires a few minutes before the start of exercise and again a few minutes after the end. They set exercise intensity to a certain level for all participants (usually, a percentage of measured or estimated maximal heart rate or oxygen uptake). And they analysed the data by standard statistical methods (e.g. a group by time analysis of variance, comparing the changes over time in the dependent variables between the exercise and the comparator group). All these choices seemed reasonable and were not questioned or altered for decades. Over time, researchers did not even feel the need to explain or defend the components of this methodological platform. In published reports, the sections describing the methods simply laid out what was done without articulating why things were done this way. The answer to this question was implied: the methodological approach that was followed was essentially the same as in the hundreds of similar previous studies.

What appears to have happened in this line of research is that the repetition of the same methodological approach over hundreds of studies suspended critical thinking. The 'popularity' of the approach was evidently interpreted as a proxy indicator of internal validity or methodological rigour and, as a result, the approach was accepted by investigators de facto. In other words, it can be said that, in the absence of any criticism or debate, repetition built a methodological 'paradigm'. Epistemologists have studied the processes leading to such phenomena. Perhaps unsurprisingly, the main culprit has been shown to be a criticism-averse and, therefore, innovation-averse culture in scientific gatekeeping, including the processes of blind peer-reviewing and editorial decision making.[16,17]

In research areas that operate under an established paradigm (i.e. a common, mostly unquestioned, way of thinking and doing research), a requisite condition for progress is what Kuhn (1962/1996) has called a 'crisis'.[18] A Kuhnian crisis occurs when there is a reliable demonstration of an inconsistency between the predictions of the paradigm and undeniable observations from nature. In the case of research on the exercise-affect relation, the crisis was arguably the inability to detect a dose-response pattern between different levels of exercise intensity and how people feel. Until the late 1990s, researchers concluded that the feel-better effect was not affected by exercise intensity. For example, according to Dunn and Blair,[19] "studies of both acute and chronic exercise indicate that intensity may not be an important factor for psychological benefits" (p. 58). This conclusion appeared to contrast with common sense and seemed hard to defend. Anyone with even the slightest experience with exercise would probably attest that, even if exercise can make someone feel better under certain circumstances, raising the intensity would eventually cause that individual to start feeling worse. Therefore, it became clear that a chasm had developed between what was considered 'textbook knowledge' within the exercise sciences (i.e. that exercise makes people 'feel better' – even regardless of intensity) and universally shared experiences. If the research were correct, exercise would have been the only known case of a human activity that made people feel better but was nonetheless almost universally avoided, according to objective data.[20] Alas, the research conclusions were wrong; research had been led astray by methodological choices that seemed reasonable but were, in fact, yielding data that were biased.[21]

In recent years, the field of exercise has been witnessing a revival of the same rift between conclusions prevalent in the research literature and shared public experience. This time, the controversy centres around "high-intensity interval training" (HIIT), a type of exercise that involves alternating between short periods of exercise performed at very high intensity and periods of recovery or rest. Reviewers have suggested that, despite the high intensity, HIIT represents a 'viable alternative' to the traditional format (i.e. moderate intensity continuous exercise) since several studies have shown no significant differences in affective and enjoyment responses between the two types of exercise.[22,23] Once again, it appears that the appeal of the message (i.e. that participants feel 'good' even with high-intensity exercise) may be suspending the critical consideration of the methods and opportunities for bias. In the following sections, we review several methodological elements, explain how they can lead to bias and summarize preferable alternatives.

Who should you study?

Research on the exercise-affect relation has a long history of using so-called analogue samples.[24] An example of this would be studying the effects of exercise on anxiety or depression in samples of participants who do not have a diagnosis or even elevated levels of anxiety or depression. Analogue research has a place in situations in which there is a need to test either a novel theoretical idea or a novel methodological approach without jeopardizing or inconveniencing vulnerable individuals or without the added expense of recruiting patients with a rare disease. After this preliminary, 'proof of concept' stage, however, continuing to study individuals who are not representative of the actual target population can compromise both external and internal validity.

A highly disconcerting phenomenon is the continued use of samples recruited from college campuses and consisting mainly of students. For example, according to a meta-analysis summarizing results based on 158 studies totalling 13,103 participants,[25] the average age of the participants was under 25 years. Moreover, approximately 75% represented highly select groups (62.4% were college students, 4.7% were a mix of students, faculty and college staff and 7.8% were athletes). In contrast, only 19.0% were individuals recruited from local communities and 3.9% were recruited from clinical settings. Besides characteristics that greatly restrict generalizability (i.e. young age, good health, average or above-average socioeconomic status and level of educational attainment, and generally satisfactory level of habitual physical activity), relying on college-student samples may introduce additional confounds that threaten internal validity: because most students are likely recruited from departments of exercise science or kinesiology, they probably have histories of athletic participation, presumably have a positive predisposition toward exercise and may have attended courses taught by the researchers themselves, thereby developing a good sense of what the researchers believe or expect to find. Imagine, for example, being taught by a professor who routinely appears on university promotional materials as an expert whose research has demonstrated that 'exercise makes people feel better', having to take exams that included questions on the results of studies conducted by the professor, and then volunteering for a study conducted by the same professor (or, worse, participating for course credit), in which, during and after an exercise session, you are asked 'how do you feel now?'

At this point, the continued use of college-student samples represents a significant challenge to the credibility of this line of research. This practice is problematic inasmuch as research has clearly progressed beyond the point at which 'analogue' samples could be justified by labelling the studies as novel, preliminary, exploratory or high risk. The interpretational leaps from data obtained from highly select samples to the adult population at large are too great and can be misleading. For example, one study found significantly higher enjoyment ratings after a bout of high-intensity interval exercise than after a bout of moderate intensity continuous exercise.[26] The authors interpreted this result as potentially "relevant for improving exercise adherence" (p. 547). Since non-adherence remains a great unresolved problem for exercise interventions, this finding has been cited hundreds of times as being, in fact, relevant to exercise adherence in the general adult population. Inspection of the methodological details, however, shows that this finding was based on a sample of eight male participants with a mean age of 25 years, who, despite being characterized as merely 'recreationally active' by the authors, had a mean aerobic capacity in the top 20% for their age.

To further intensify such interpretational challenges, authors often omit crucial information that would enable readers to assess the probability of selection bias. For example, the results could be different if a study was advertised generically as an 'exercise' study versus a study of 'high-intensity exercise' versus a study on 'how exercise makes people feel'. Similarly, the results could be different if participation for a study was solicited via an advertisement in the local community newspaper versus a flyer distributed to individuals entering the campus gymnasium versus a slide presentation to the campus triathlon club.

How many should you study

One of the most consequential methodological considerations related to the sample is deciding on the appropriate number of participants. This number should not be decided by how many volunteers were conveniently available or how many could be persuaded to sign up for the study within a given timeframe. The size of the sample has obvious implications for the width of the confidence intervals around estimates of population values (e.g. the means) and the generalizability of the conclusions. However, as most researchers recognize, one can also use the size of the sample to either increase or decrease the odds of detecting a difference as statistically significant by manipulating the statistical power of the analyses. In some cases, for example, researchers may have an 'equivalence' or 'non-inferiority hypothesis', namely that a novel exercise method would fare just as well as (or no worse than) an old method. One method of obtaining empirical support for such a hypothesis is by studying a small sample that affords a low level of statistical power. For example, suppose that the anticipated mean difference between two types of exercise is 'medium' (an effect size of one-half of a pooled standard deviation, $d = 0.50$). In order to attain 80% statistical power, which is considered (by convention) as the minimum acceptable level, a researcher would need to recruit 34 participants for a two-condition, within-subjects design. Therefore, when researchers compare affective and enjoyment responses to a bout of high-intensity interval exercise and a bout of moderate-intensity continuous exercise with a sample of 10 participants, the outcome is – statistically speaking – essentially known in advance: no significant differences for either ratings of affect or enjoyment.[27] This is because a sample size of 10 achieves only 29% statistical power to detect as 'significant' a medium-sized effect. In other words, there is a 71% chance that the analysis would produce a Type II error of statistical inference, i.e. a 'false negative', namely a failure to detect, in a small sample, an effect that actually exists in the population. For further details on statistical power and Type II errors see Chapter 17.

What should you measure?

As noted earlier, in the early days of research on the exercise-affect relation, Morgan was able to obtain evidence contradicting the Pitts-McClure hypothesis by using two questionnaires that became available at that time, namely the STAI and the POMS.[14] As the Pitts-McClure hypothesis was attracting the interest of physicians, it was essential to generate, in a timely manner, empirical evidence that the hypothesis was, in fact, false. The publication of the STAI and the POMS was, therefore, a well-timed, fortuitous or serendipitous occurrence.

Once Morgan demonstrated that bouts of exercise result in positive changes in state anxiety (STAI) and mood states (POMS),[14] these two questionnaires became the de facto measures of choice for all the subsequent investigators who wanted to replicate the initial results with other samples and types of exercise. In the numerous studies that followed, the STAI,[28] the POMS [29] or both were used based on the argument that these measures 'have been used before' and, therefore, would allow new findings to be compared to older ones.

Morgan himself was keenly aware that this was an unconvincing and insufficient rationale.[30] Even when combined, the STAI and the POMS measure seven distinct states, only one of which is positive: state anxiety, tension, depression, anger, fatigue, confusion and vigour. Nothing in the developmental histories of these measures implies that they can be interpreted as capturing a broader domain of content, such as 'mood' or 'emotion'. They were designed to capture only these seven distinct states. Therefore, it is clear that, when using the STAI and the POMS, researchers should discuss their findings only in relation to these seven specific states, without attempting to extrapolate to how exercise made the participants feel, in general. Morgan (1984) cautioned researchers on this point:

> Much, perhaps most, of the literature dealing with the psychologic effects of exercise has relied on the use of objective self-report inventories designed to measure constructs such as anxiety and depression . . . The extent to which these inventories can tap the psychometric domain of significance to the exerciser has not been evaluated. In other words, an investigator may employ an objective, reliable, valid test of anxiety or depression to quantify the psychologic effects of exercise only to find that no 'effects' have taken place when, in fact, there may have been numerous effects.
>
> (p. 134)[30]

A critical analysis should reveal that both the STAI and the POMS suffer from considerable limitations when used to investigate exercise effects. The STAI was developed on the basis of a cognitive theory,[12] according to which state anxiety is the emotional response that follows the cognitive appraisal of threat, with the 'threat' being mainly symbolic in nature (i.e. against one's ego, goals or self-identity) and originating mainly from the social environment. The questionnaire taps a range of symptoms that includes cognitive, experiential, behavioural and perceived autonomic manifestations of anxiety. These are assumed to emerge in unison when an individual experiences a state anxiety episode. Indeed, in most state-anxiety reactions that occur in social situations, this is what happens. However, acute exercise represents a unique case, in which autonomic symptoms that would otherwise reflect a state-anxiety response exhibit dramatic increases due to the physiological demands of the exercise stimulus. In such cases, respondents may report feeling less 'calm', less 'relaxed', less 'steady', not because they feel more anxious but because they are exercising. However, because this scenario was never considered in the development of the questionnaire, such changes are scored and interpreted as increases in state anxiety. Therefore, the validity of the STAI in the context of acute exercise should be considered dubious.[31]

The POMS[13] has a history that most of its users mysteriously ignore. The initials POMS initially stood for Psychiatric Outpatient Mood Scale. The questionnaire was developed as a screening tool for evaluating the reactions of psychiatric outpatients (primarily, war veterans) to various psychotropic drugs. This explains not only the emphasis on negative affective states (i.e. tension, depression, anger) but also the inclusion of somatic symptoms (i.e. fatigue, vigour) and the addition of a scale to measure confusion (i.e. a common side-effect of psychotropic medications), even though confusion is a cognitive symptom rather than a mood state. Given this history, it should be clear that the six-factor structure of the POMS was not theory-driven and was not meant to offer comprehensive coverage of the vastly broader content domain of 'mood'. As Morgan warned,[30] it is possible that a researcher using the POMS to investigate the effects of a certain exercise intervention on the broad domain of 'mood' may not detect changes on any of the six POMS factors even though changes may have occurred in other aspects of mood not tapped by this instrument.

So, what self-report measures should researchers interested in how exercise makes participants feel use in their studies? This is a difficult question, a complete answer to which is beyond the scope of this text. Therefore, interested readers must refer to specialized sources for more detailed guidance.[32,33] Here, we offer only the outline of the three-step decision-making process we recommend (also see Ekkekakis & Zenko, 2016).[34]

The **first step** should consist of choosing the most relevant affective phenomenon for the purpose of a given study. Three terms have been used interchangeably in this line of research but, in fact, represent substantively different phenomena: 'core affect', 'mood' and 'emotion'. Core affect is an elementary valenced (i.e. pleasant or unpleasant) feeling that is considered an inherent ingredient of the stream of consciousness. In other words, human beings have a constant readout of core affect, regardless of whether they find themselves in an affectively charged situation or not. Therefore, core affect is found in 'free-floating' form or it can be a component of broader and more complex phenomena, such as moods and emotions, to which it bestows the element of affective valence (the feeling of pleasure or displeasure). Core affect is assumed to have deep evolutionary roots but it has been preserved because it serves a crucial adaptational function: it compels an approach toward useful stimuli and avoidance of dangerous ones.

Emotions include the element of core affect but are much broader and more complex phenomena. Besides core affect, they include characteristic patterns of cognition (i.e. thoughts), a physiological 'signature' that may be more or less unique to each emotion, a pattern of behavioural expression and related coping efforts. Emotions are always in response to a stimulus and are always about something. Their instigator is the process of cognitive appraisal, by which individuals evaluate the relevance and potential implications of environmental stimuli for their goals and wellbeing. A particular appraisal theme is presumed to underlie each emotion. For example, for the emotion of state anxiety, the individual must appraise a situation as posing a threat, typically by comparing two subjective quantities: how much is expected in a situation and how prepared one is to meet the expectations. For the emotion of pride, the underlying appraisal theme is one of surpassing a subjectively defined standard of success. Because the variables being appraised are often symbolic rather than objectively quantifiable, emotions exhibit an extraordinary degree of malleability depending on individual developmental histories and the cultural context.

Moods also include core affect along with other ingredients, such as cognitions and characteristic behavioural expressions. They are often distinguished from emotions by being less intense but longer lasting (hours, days or even weeks). However, while emotions are clearly linked to a specific stimulus, the most important distinguishing feature of moods is their loose connection to the instigating stimulus (e.g. being in an irritable mood after a quarrel the previous day) and the diffuse nature of their underlying appraisals (e.g. 'the future', 'life as a whole').

Given these definitions, the appropriate construct for a given study depends on the purpose of that study. If the purpose is to describe how exercisers feel under different experimental conditions (e.g. levels of intensity or levels of ambient heat and humidity), especially when their responses cannot be predicted in advance on the basis of prior theory or empirical data, arguably the most appropriate target construct should be core affect. If the purpose is to assess the response to an experimental manipulation specifically designed to elicit a pattern of cognitive appraisal, then the appropriate target construct would be the emotion theorized to follow from the given appraisal (e.g. adding mirrors and critical observers to a gymnasium would be predicted to elicit a cognitive appraisal leading to the emotion of self-presentational anxiety). Finally, if the purpose is to examine the effects of exercise on a mood, such as the depression associated with a chronic disease diagnosis or the irritability associated with nicotine withdrawal, then the target construct should be that particular mood.

The **second step** should be deciding on the most appropriate conceptual model for the chosen construct. Unlike other psychological constructs that may be approached from a singular theoretical perspective or conceptual model, affective constructs are characterized by an overwhelming multiplicity of conceptualizations. Choosing among them can be a highly consequential decision and, therefore, this step requires careful contemplation.

The primary consideration should be to ensure that the conceptual model can offer comprehensive (or at least adequate) coverage of the targeted domain of content. For example, if the researcher wishes to study the global domain of 'mood', as was explained earlier, it would be nonsensical to attempt to study this domain through the prism of a conceptual model that only includes a few, distinct parts of it (as in the case of the POMS). In another example, many researchers have used the Positive and Negative Affect Schedule (PANAS),[35] which includes two 10-item scales that measure 'Positive Affect' and 'Negative Affect'. Researchers usually cite the popularity of the PANAS as the main justification that led them to the decision to select it. However, closer study of the conceptual basis of the PANAS reveals that its developers have intentionally excluded both pleasant low-activation states (such as calmness) and unpleasant low-activation states (such as fatigue) from the scope of this measure. It should be apparent, however, that both calmness and fatigue would be highly relevant to a study that involves exercise. Therefore, having a good understanding of the conceptual basis of a measure is of paramount importance.

If large content domains, such as 'mood', cannot be assessed in a comprehensive manner by sampling a few distinct parts, what is the alternative? Theoretical proposals and empirical studies attempting to address this challenge have been appearing in the psychological literature for over a century. These efforts have led to the formulation of so-called dimensional models that seek to identify a small set of elemental dimensions that can account for most of the similarities and differences among words that describe affective states. For example, a widely used dimensional model of the content domain of core affect, called the circumplex,[36] postulates that the affective domain can be adequately defined by two orthogonal and bipolar dimensions, namely affective valence (pleasant versus unpleasant states) and activation ('high' versus 'low' states). When considered in combination, these two dimensions can be thought of as the horizontal and vertical axes of a two-dimensional map of core affect, which is divided into four quadrants: (a) high-activation pleasant affect (e.g. excitement, enthusiasm, energy), (b) high-activation unpleasant affect (e.g. tension, distress, nervousness), (c) low-activation unpleasant affect (e.g. boredom, fatigue, exhaustion) and (d) low-activation pleasant affect (calmness, relaxation, serenity). For example, by asking exercise participants to rate themselves repeatedly on scales that tap the valence (e.g. with the Feeling Scale)[37] and activation dimensions (e.g. with the Felt Arousal Scale),[38] researchers can track their trajectory of change within the domain of core affect (see Figure 20.1).[39]

The **third step** consists of choosing the measure of the targeted construct, which was developed on the basis of the selected conceptual model, and has the strongest psychometric evidence to support it. Although providing information on internal consistency, test-retest reliability and construct validity is often the only justification that is offered for choosing a measure, we propose that this step only makes sense after the two preceding steps. In other words, it is insufficient to claim that a measure is 'valid'. This information is useful only after researchers have offered compelling evidence that the conceptual model of which the measure is a 'valid' representation is appropriate for the purpose of their study.

When should you measure?

As described earlier, in the early studies in this line of research, the questionnaires used to measure the outcome variables (i.e. state anxiety, mood states) were typically administered once before the start of an exercise session and again a few minutes after the end of the session. Presumably, this decision was driven by practical considerations; because the STAI and the POMS were multi-item questionnaires, it was deemed impractical or overly intrusive to ask participants to complete them while they were exercising.

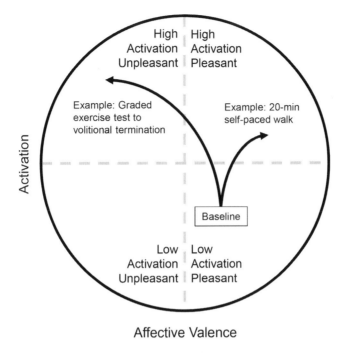

Figure 20.1 The circumplex model of core affect, defined by the orthogonal and bipolar dimensions of valence and activation. By repeatedly assessing valence and activation during and following exercise bouts, researchers can plot the trajectory of affective responses in this broad two-dimensional map. Typical responses to a self-paced walk and a graded exercise test to volitional termination are shown for illustration.

It has now become apparent that this decision led to a systematic misrepresentation of the shape of the affective response and, thus, to false conclusions. As it turns out, when exercise intensity exceeds a certain level (the ventilatory threshold),[40] most people report feeling worse. Thus, there may be substantial deterioration in how people feel over the course of a vigorous exercise bout. Upon cessation of the bout, however, most people experience a robust and nearly instantaneous positive 'rebound' in how they feel, which typically leads to reports that are better than those at baseline (see Figure 20.2).

Therefore, since two points can only define a straight line, obtaining only one measure before and another after the exercise bout may give the false impression that the participants went from the pre-exercise value to the (higher, better) post-exercise value via a straight, continuously improving path. However, it is possible that they arrived at the post-exercise value following a precipitous deterioration during the bout itself, followed by a positive rebound once the exercise was terminated (see Figure 20.2). It should be clear that, while the former scenario would support the conclusion that "exercise makes people feel better", the latter scenario would suggest that the exercise itself made people feel worse and it was only the cessation of exercise that made people feel better (i.e. a 'relief' effect). These two conclusions are obviously quite different. Therefore, detecting the during-exercise deterioration in how the participants feel is crucial. This is especially so since the available evidence

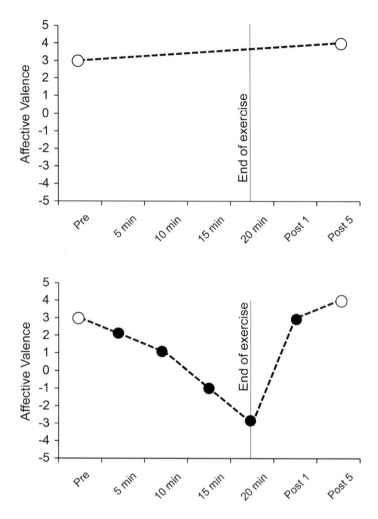

Figure 20.2 Assessing affective constructs only once before and once after the exercise bout
may lead to the impression that participants moved from the pre-exercise to a more
positive post-exercise rating via a path of continuous improvement over time (top
panel). Instead, assessing affect repeatedly during and after the exercise bout may
reveal a continuous decline during exercise, followed by a rapid and robust post-
exercise positive rebound (bottom panel). Therefore, the two assessment protocols
may lead to different conclusions.

suggests that affective responses during exercise are predictive of subsequent physical
activity behaviour, whereas the responses recorded post-exercise are not.[41]

Researchers should think about the timing of measurements as signal sampling:
if the 'signal' (i.e. the affective response) is expected to change at a certain rate, it
should be sampled with enough frequency to allow the faithful representation of
the shape of the response.[42] Sampling at a lower frequency (such as only before and
after exercise) can lead to what engineers call 'aliasing': the sampling can misrepre-
sent or distort the true shape of the signal. An apt example is investigating affective
responses to high-intensity interval exercise. In this case, the 'signal' oscillates. People
typically feel increasingly worse during the high-intensity intervals and better during

the intermittent periods of rest or active recovery. To faithfully represent the true shape of their affective response, affect should be sampled (at least) at each positive and each negative affective peak (i.e. at the very end of each high-intensity interval, when people presumably feel worst, and at the end of each recovery period, when people presumably feel best). When affect is assessed only after the end of each high-intensity interval, the sampling captures the positive 'rebound', misses the preceding precipitous decline and thus misrepresents the shape of the actual response.[43]

How should you measure?

Most psychological research deals with small (i.e. $d = \sim0.20$) to medium (i.e. $d = \sim0.50$) effect sizes. Given the challenges in obtaining large samples of participants to achieve adequate levels of statistical power for effects in this range, it is essential to take all necessary steps to reduce 'noise' variance. Such precautions include maintaining consistency in all experimental procedures, standardizing instructions and researcher-participant communications, eliminating confounds from the testing environment (e.g. ambient noise, temperature and humidity, visual distractors) and keeping the number of researchers present to a minimum. Any inconsistencies in the conditions under which different participants are tested will likely translate to variability that will negatively impact statistical power.

Besides these standard 'good practices', researchers should familiarize themselves with some of the less-known biases that may be inadvertently introduced in psychological research. In particular, we wish to emphasize so-called common method biases, namely distortions that may be introduced by measuring supposedly distinct constructs via similar measurement formats (such as rating scales) at the same time.[44] Consider, for example, what might happen when researchers place two rating scales side by side (see Figure 20.3), asking respondents to use one (ranging from 1: 'not at all' to 7: 'extremely') to rate their enjoyment and another (ranging from –5: 'I feel very bad' to +5: 'I feel very good') to rate their level of pleasure-displeasure.[45] Notice that, while the 'enjoyment' scale is unipolar (i.e. only encompasses gradations of enjoyment but not gradations of aversion), the scale of pleasure-displeasure is bipolar (i.e. it includes both gradations of pleasures and gradations of displeasure). In situations like this, a likely occurrence is 'variance transfer'. In other words, because of the similarities in the format of the scales, respondents may give similar numerical responses to the two scales, thereby obfuscating the substantive differences between the two measured constructs. For example, in one such example, respondents averaged ratings between 3.0 and 4.0 on both scales, even though these ratings were below the midpoint of the enjoyment scale (indicating only 'slight' to 'moderate' enjoyment) but near the top of the 'pleasure' scale.[45] To avoid such problems, it is recommended to vary the features of the scales (e.g. present one in vertical and the other in horizontal orientation), avoid presenting them side by side or on the same page and randomizing the order of presentation.

How should you standardize exercise intensity?

For meaningful conclusions to be drawn about the effects of exercise on affect, it is necessary to ensure that all participants receive the same exercise in terms of duration and intensity. While fixing duration is easy, standardizing intensity is exceedingly difficult. In early studies, researchers attempted to fix the intensity by having individuals

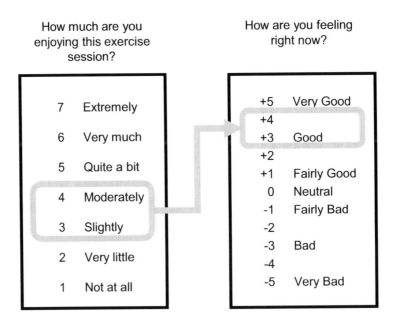

Figure 20.3 Juxtaposing two self-report instruments that are similarly oriented and use fully or partially overlapping numerical rating scales may lead to artificial 'variance transfer' from one to the other. This type of common method bias can obfuscate substantive differences between the constructs being assessed by the two measurement instruments.

exercise at the same absolute heart rate, such as 150 beats per min.[10] It soon became apparent, however, that this was inadequate, especially for samples that were heterogeneous with respect to age, since 150 beats per min may be near-maximal heart rate for an older person but relatively low for a younger person. Therefore, researchers started setting the intensity as a percentage of estimated or measured maximal exercise capacity, defined as maximal heart rate or maximal oxygen uptake. It was believed that this method, by taking cardiorespiratory fitness into account, offered adequate standardization of intensity across individuals.

It has now become apparent that the situation is even more complex. At a certain percentage of maximal capacity, some individuals may be above and others below important metabolic landmarks, such as the gas-exchange ventilatory threshold and the respiratory compensation point. Exceeding these landmarks can dramatically change the metabolic environment of the working muscles and can have widespread physiological effects.[46] To complicate matters, exercise prescription guidelines, such as those issued by the American College of Sports Medicine, continue to define exercise intensity in terms of percentages of maximal capacity. For example, the 'moderate' range of exercise intensity is defined as ranging from 64% to 76% of maximal heart rate and from 46% to 63% of maximal oxygen uptake.[47] Researchers who set the intensity in their studies by utilizing these conventional categorizations unwittingly introduce a major confound because, in most non-athletic adults, the ventilatory threshold typically occurs at approximately 60–70% of maximal heart rate or 50–60% of maximal oxygen uptake. Therefore, by setting the intensity within the range commonly labelled as 'moderate', researchers likely place some of their participants above and others below the ventilatory threshold, thus causing heterogeneous physiological responses and, consequently, heterogeneous affective responses.

A more effective method of standardizing exercise intensity consists of taking into account individually determined metabolic landmarks.[46] By doing so, one can divide the range of exercise intensity into three domains (see Figure 20.4). The first domain, termed the domain of 'moderate' exercise, includes the intensities up to the ventilatory threshold. Within the moderate domain, individuals can maintain a physiological steady-state over time (i.e. physiological parameters, such as oxygen uptake, heart rate, and blood lactate, remain stable). The second domain, termed the domain of 'heavy' exercise, extends from the ventilatory threshold to an intensity characterized as the 'maximal lactate steady-state' (i.e. the highest level of intensity at which the rate of lactate clearance can 'catch up' with the rate of production from the working muscles) or the respiratory compensation point (i.e. a second, abrupt breakpoint in the relation between oxygen uptake and carbon dioxide production). Within the heavy domain, reaching a physiological steady-state may be delayed compared to the moderate range but it is still feasible. The third domain, termed the domain of 'severe' exercise, extends from the maximal lactate steady-state or the respiratory compensation point to the point of maximal oxygen uptake. Within the severe domain, the maintenance of a physiological steady-state is no longer possible. Physiological parameters, such as oxygen uptake and blood lactate, rise continuously towards their maximal values and exercise is terminated within a few minutes. While the determination of the ventilatory threshold, the maximal lactate steady-state, and the respiratory compensation point require expensive equipment and technical expertise, implementing this three-domain typology is, at present, the most effective method of standardizing exercise intensity across individuals.

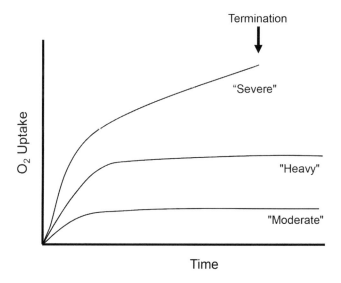

Figure 20.4 A three-domain typology of exercise intensity that takes into account important metabolic landmarks, such as the ventilatory threshold and the maximal lactate steady-state, can standardize exercise intensity across individuals more effectively than percentages of maximal exercise capacity. Each domain is associated with a different pattern of physiological responses over time.

How should you analyse the data?

Like most research areas, the standard approach of analysing data in this line of research has been to focus on the group means. Once again, this common approach, despite seeming reasonable and uncontroversial, has been shown to be problematic. Although it is widely accepted that individuals will differ in the magnitude of their response to any given stimulus, in the case of affective responses to exercise, individuals also differ in the direction of their response. In other words, in response to the same exercise stimulus (especially at intensities proximal to the ventilatory threshold) some individuals may report increases and others decreases in pleasure.[48]

This phenomenon raises the possibility of misinterpretations because, when some individuals change in one direction over time whereas others change in the opposite direction, the group mean appears stable, becoming a statistical abstraction that is no longer representative of the response of the actual participants (see Figure 20.5). It is, therefore, recommended to supplement any standard analyses at the level of group means with an examination of changes at the level of individuals and subgroups (i.e. specify how many participants felt progressively better over time, how many felt progressively worse and how many provided stable ratings).

Conclusion

As demonstrated in the previous sections, the study of the exercise-affect relation has come a long way over the past half century, critically revising its methodological platform and producing reliable data that have led to a radical revision of its original conclusions.[34] It has now become clear that the long-advertised 'feel-better' effect, while possible, is not universal and automatic but rather conditional. Most adults in

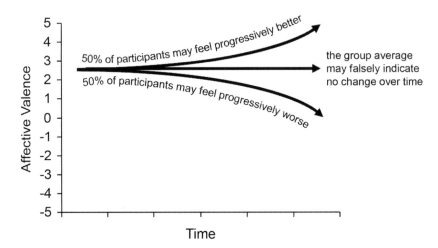

Figure 20.5 Affective responses to the same exercise stimulus may vary between individuals not only in terms of magnitude but also in terms of direction. This creates a significant analytic and interpretational challenge. In the hypothetical case in which half of the participants change in one direction and the other half in the opposite direction, an analysis of change focusing on the group mean would falsely suggest that there was no change over time.

industrialized countries, who are chronically sedentary and burdened by excess body mass, likely feel worse in response to exercise rather than better. This effect may contribute to physical inactivity.

Progress in clarifying the exercise-affect relation has been far from easy. As noted in the introduction, changing entrenched methodological practices is extraordinarily challenging. Demonstrating that a certain methodological approach is flawed is rarely a sufficient stimulus for changing research practices. Moreover, overcoming 'secondary ignorance' in an area of research that is inherently interdisciplinary is an additional barrier. As demonstrated in this chapter, the overhaul of the methodological platform would have been impossible without taking advantage of the knowledge bases of affective psychology and exercise physiology. Nevertheless, investigators now entering this line of research should not assume that the evolution and refinement of the methodological platform are now complete. Instead, they should continue to strive for enhancements and should always subject every detail to meticulous critical appraisal.

References

1   Ekkekakis P, Belvederi Murri M. Exercise as antidepressant treatment: time for the transition from trials to clinic? *Gen Hosp Psychiat.* 2017; **49**: A1–A5.
2   Ladwig MA, Hartman ME, Ekkekakis P. Affect-based exercise prescription: an idea whose time has come? *ACSM's Health Fit J.* 2017; **21**(5):10–15.
3   Faulkner H, Hefferon K, Mutrie N. Putting positive psychology into motion through physical activity. In: Joseph S, editor. *Positive psychology in practice: promoting human flourishing in work, health, education, and everyday life.* 2nd ed. Hoboken, NJ: John Wiley & Sons, Inc.; 2015. pp. 207–22.
4   Ioannidis JPA. Why most published research findings are false. *PLoS Med.* 2005; **2**(8):e124.
5   Podsakoff PM, MacKenzie SB, Podsakoff NP. Sources of method bias in social science research and recommendations on how to control it. *Ann Rev Psychol.* 2012; **63**: 539–69.
6   Fanelli D. "Positive" results increase down the hierarchy of the sciences. *PLoS One.* 2010; **5**(4):e10068.
7   Fanelli D, Ioannidis JP. US studies may overestimate effect sizes in softer research. *Proc Natl Acad Sci U S A.* 2013; **110**(37):15031–6.
8   Ioannidis JP. Why science is not necessarily self-correcting. *Perspect Psychol Sci.* 2012; **7**(6):645–54.
9   Eisner EW. *The kind of schools we need: personal essays.* Portsmouth, NH: William Heinemann; 1998.
10 Pitts FN Jr, McClure JN Jr. Lactate metabolism in anxiety neurosis. *N E J Med.* 1967; **277**(25):1329–36.
11 Morgan WP, Roberts JA, Feinerman AD. Psychologic effect of acute physical activity. *Arch Phys Med Rehab.* 1971; **52**(9):422–5.
12 Spielberger CD, Gorsuch RL, Lushene RE. *Manual for the state-trait anxiety inventory.* Palo Alto, CA: Consulting Psychologists Press; 1970.
13 McNair DM, Lorr M, Droppleman LF. *Profile of Mood States (POMS) manual.* San Diego, CA: Educational and Industrial Testing Service; 1971.
14 Morgan WP. Influence of acute physical activity on state anxiety. In: Mueller CE, editor. *Proceedings of the annual meeting of the national college physical education association for men.* Pittsburgh, PA: National College Physical Education Association for Men; 1973. pp. 113–21.
15 Morgan WP. Conclusion: State of the field and future research. In: Morgan WP, editor. *Physical activity and mental health.* Washington, DC: Taylor & Francis; 1997. pp. 227–32.

16   Park IU, Peacey MW, Munafò MR. Modelling the effects of subjective and objective decision making in scientific peer review. *Nature.* 2014; **506**(7486):93–6.

17   Siler K, Lee K, Bero L. Measuring the effectiveness of scientific gatekeeping. *Proc Natl Acad Sci U S A.* 2014; **112**(2):360–5.

18   Kuhn TS. *The structure of scientific revolutions.* Chicago: University of Chicago Press; 1962/1996.

19   Dunn AL, Blair SN. Exercise prescription. In: Morgan WP, editor. *Physical activity and mental health.* Washington, DC: Taylor & Francis; 1997; pp. 49–62.

20   Troiano RP, Berrigan D, Dodd KW, Mâsse LC, Tilert T, McDowell M. Physical activity in the United States measured by accelerometers. *Med Sci Sports Exerc.* 2008; **40**(1):181–8.

21   Backhouse SH, Ekkekakis P, Biddle SJH, Foskett A, Williams C. Exercise makes people feel better but people are inactive: paradox or artifact? *J Sport Exerc Psychol.* 2007; **29**(4):498–517.

22   Oliveira BRR, Santos TM, Kilpatrick M, Pires FO, Deslandes AC. Affective and enjoyment responses in high intensity interval training and continuous training: a systematic review and meta-analysis. *PLoS One.* 2018; **13**(6):e0197124.

23   Stork MJ, Banfield LE, Gibala MJ, Martin Ginis KA. A scoping review of the psychological responses to interval exercise: is interval exercise a viable alternative to traditional exercise? *Health Psychol Rev.* 2017; **11**(4):324–44.

24   Martinsen EW, Morgan WP. Antidepressant effects of physical activity. In: Morgan WP, editor. *Physical activity and mental health.* Washington, DC: Taylor & Francis; 1997. pp. 93–106.

25   Reed J, Ones DS. The effect of acute aerobic exercise on positive activated affect: a meta-analysis. *Psychol Sport Exerc.* 2006; **7**(5):477–514.

26   Bartlett JD, Close GL, MacLaren DP, Gregson W, Drust B, Morton JP. High-intensity interval running is perceived to be more enjoyable than moderate-intensity continuous exercise: implications for exercise adherence. *J Sports Sci.* 2011; **29**(6):547–53.

27   Little JP, Jung ME, Wright AE, Wright W, Manders RJF. Effects of high-intensity interval exercise versus continuous-moderate intensity exercise on postprandial glycemic control assessed by continuous glucose monitoring in obese adults. *Appl Physiol Nutr Metab.* 2014; **39**(7):835–41.

28   Ensari I, Greenlee TA, Motl RW, Petruzzello SJ. Meta-analysis of acute exercise effects on state anxiety: an update of randomized controlled trials over the past 25 years. *Anxiety Depress.* 2015; **32**(8):624–34.

29   Berger BG, Motl RW. Exercise and mood: a selective review and synthesis of research employing the profile of mood states. *J Appl Sport Psychol.* 2000; **12**(1):69–92.

30   Morgan WP. Physical activity and mental health. In: Eckert HM, Montoye HJ, editors. *Exercise and health.* Champaign, IL: Human Kinetics Publishers; 1984. pp. 132–45.

31   Ekkekakis P, Hall EE, Petruzzello SJ. Measuring state anxiety in the context of acute exercise using the State Anxiety Inventory: an attempt to resolve the brouhaha. *J Sport Exerc Psychol.* 1999; **21**(3):205–29.

32   Ekkekakis P. Affect, mood, and emotion. In: Tenenbaum G, Eklund RC, Kamata A, editors. *Measurement in sport and exercise psychology.* Champaign, IL: Human Kinetics Publishers; 2012. pp. 321–32.

33   Ekkekakis P. *The measurement of affect, mood, and emotion: a guide for health-behavioral research.* New York: Cambridge University Press; 2013.

34   Ekkekakis P, Zenko Z. Measurement of affective responses to exercise: from "affectless arousal" to "the most well-characterized" relationship between the body and affect. In: Meiselman HL, editor. *Emotion measurement.* Duxford, UK: Woodhead; 2016. pp. 299–321.

35   Watson D, Clark LA, Tellegen A. Development and validation of brief measures of positive and negative affect: the PANAS scales. *J Pers Soc Psychol.* 1988; **54**(6):1063–70.

36   Feldman Barrett L, Russell JA. The structure of current affect: controversies and emerging consensus. *Curr Dir Psychol Sci.* 1999; **8**(1):10–14.

37   Hardy CJ, Rejeski WJ. Not what, but how one feels: the measurement of affect during exercise. *J Sport Exerc Psychol.* 1989; **11**(3):304–17.

38 Svebak S, Murgatroyd S. Metamotivational dominance: a multimethod validation of reversal theory constructs. *J Pers Soc Psychol.* 1985; **48**(1):107–16.

39 Ekkekakis P, Hall EE, Petruzzello SJ. The relationship between exercise intensity and affective responses demystified: to crack the forty-year-old nut, replace the forty-year-old nutcracker! *Ann Behav Med.* 2008; **35**(2):136–49.

40 Ekkekakis P, Parfitt G, Petruzzello SJ. The pleasure and displeasure people feel when they exercise at different intensities: decennial update and progress towards a tripartite rationale for exercise intensity prescription. *Sports Med.* 2011; **41**(8):641–71.

41 Williams DM, Dunsiger S, Jennings EG, Marcus BH. Does affective valence during and immediately following a 10-min walk predict concurrent and future physical activity? *Ann Behav Med.* 2012; **44**(1):43–51.

42 Bixby WR, Spalding TW, Hatfield BD. Temporal dynamics and dimensional specificity of the affective response to exercise of varying intensity: differing pathways to a common outcome. *J Sport Exerc Psychol.* 2001; **23**(3):171–90.

43 Stork MJ, Kwan M, Gibala MJ, Martin Ginis KA. Music enhances performance and perceived enjoyment of sprint interval exercise. *Med Sci Sports Exerc.* 2015; **47**(5):1052–60.

44 Podsakoff PM, MacKenzie SB, Lee JY, Podsakoff NP. Common method biases in behavioral research: a critical review of the literature and recommended remedies. *J Appl Psychol.* 2003; **88**(5):879–903.

45 Martinez N, Kilpatrick MW, Salomon K, Jung ME, Little JP. Affective and enjoyment responses to high-intensity interval training in overweight-to-obese and insufficiently active adults. *J Sport Exerc Psychol.* 2015; **37**(2):138–49.

46 Gaesser GA, Poole DC. The slow component of oxygen uptake kinetics in humans. *Exerc Sport Sci Rev.* 1996; **24**:35–70.

47 American College of Sports Medicine (ACSM). Available from: www.acsm.org/

48 Van Landuyt LM, Ekkekakis P, Hall E, Petruzzello SJ. Throwing the mountains into the lakes: on the perils of nomothetic conceptions of the exercise-affect relationship. *J Sport Exerc Psychol.* 2000; **22**(2):208–34.

21 Studying the risks of exercise and its negative impacts

Andy Smith and Nathalie Noret

Aims of the chapter

The purpose of this chapter is to provide researchers studying the negative impact of exercise with a resource to help guide the development of their methodology. The chapter: (i) explains why it is important to study the negative impacts of exercise; (ii) suggests issues to be considered when researching the negative impact of exercise, signposting readers to examples of research in this area; (iii) presents a scenario on ethical and legal issues and (iv) suggests five research questions on the negative impact of exercise. This chapter also provides a worked example, based on bullying in sport, as an illustration of the methodologies that can be used to study the bad things in sport and exercise.

Why is it important to study the negative impacts of exercise?

The negative impacts of exercise should be studied to inform evidence-based practice, to retain our objectivity, to enable us to be value-led and because it might lead to a paradigm change.

Exercise is not a panacea for all ills. It is contradicted for some conditions and more research is needed in other areas before evidence-based practice can be developed. However, on occasions celebrity endorsements and media hype can create the impression that exercise is a miracle cure or the elixir of youth. Evidence-based practice should be based on a corpus of peer-reviewed papers that investigate both the good and the bad things about exercise. To base our professional practice on the evidence we need to know when exercise is contradicted, when it can do harm and when other (non-exercise-based) interventions are more effective.

If research in exercise science is to have credibility, particularly when it is intended to inform clinical practice or public health interventions, it has to be demonstrably objective. Clearly individual studies need to be objective but here we refer to the objectivity of the literature as a whole. Care needs to be taken to ensure that the canon of work includes studies which specifically go looking 'for the bad news'. It is only by challenging, contesting and problematizing everything that we can be confident that we are providing evidence that the public, policy makers and health professionals can rely upon. By studying the potential harm that exercise can do we demonstrate our objectivity and lack of bias. The evidence that exercise normally improves physical and mental health is so strong that the consensus of its beneficial effects will not be threatened by a concerted attempt to identify the boundaries of its positive impact.

A number of authors and initiatives have argued persuasively that values matter in both research and sport.[1-3] With colleagues at York St John University the first author has founded a new School of Sport based on *"social justice, the right to play, putting the performer before the performance, a focus on the healthy athlete, stressing participation over consumerism and holding to account those who seek elitism rather than sporting excellence"*. If one conducts research within such an ethos it is important to understand where the boundary is that separates the large areas where exercise is good for people from what appears to be the small areas, where it is not. It is only by conducting such work that we can 'put the performer before the performance' and know what is healthy both for the athlete and the public.

Research which challenges conventional wisdom by starting from the counter-intuitive perspective, that exercise is bad for people, might lead to new insights and even a paradigm shift. As the evidence strongly demonstrates that for most people, most of the time, exercise is health-enhancing: finding those cases and conditions when it is not may reveal new insights. In addition, the challenge of finding such cases and conditions may challenge researchers to develop new methodologies and/or improve existing modes of enquiries.

Issues to be considered when researching the negative impact of exercise and examples of research in this area

Good research design is good research design irrespective of whether the investigation is into the possible benefits of exercise (e.g. cardiac rehabilitation) or possible risks (e.g. sudden cardiac death in marathons). Nonetheless, those designing research methods to investigate the negative impact of exercise might benefit from considering the following angles.

Go looking for trouble

Asking the right question is the essential starting point in the design of any good methodology. Formulating the right question, in the experience of the authors, begins either with a moment of inspiration or is the informed outcome of review of literature. As all good research methods books should, we strongly recommend that it is best if the questions we ask emerge from reading the literature. If one goes 'looking for trouble' and reads the literature with an open and sceptical mind it may be possible to establish research questions that look at the negative impact of exercise. Nonetheless, we should not forget that researchers are first and foremost people who no matter how hard they train to be objective have their own passions, enthusiasms and loves and are prone, thankfully, to moments of wonder and inspiration. Indeed a strong case can be made that without the power of inspiration scientific enquiry would stagnate. If one is persuaded by this argument, might it be that those of us who conduct research on exercise are more likely to have inspirations concerning the positive impact of exercise rather than on the possible negative impact? Might it be that the optimism inherent in the human condition predisposes us to ask 'how can exercise help people?' rather than 'how can exercise harm people?' If this is the case, and even if it isn't, in our endeavour to be objective scientists and to serve the public we must, from time to time, go looking for trouble and spend some of our research careers investigating the negative impact of exercise.

An example from the authors' own work of when we have gone 'looking for trouble' is our research on bullying in school sport. Through our work on bullying we have identified an unintended consequence of school sport i.e. bullying and the negative impact it can have in terms of turning children and adolescents away from health-enhancing physical activity. We have begun to examine this phenomenon from a number of perspectives. Firstly, we interrogated pre-existing data collected as part of a school survey, conducted with primary and secondary schools in one school district in England. Although the data were not collected with the intention of testing any hypotheses related to bullying in sport, a piece of exploratory research identified trends related to: (i) the prevalence of bullying in sport facilities, and (ii) bullying related to sporting ability. Results of the analysis also found a relationship between being bullied in sport and doing less physical activity. Adopting a secondary data analysis approach was an important first step in identifying the scale and nature of the bullying phenomenon in school sport.[4] When 'looking for trouble' it can be difficult to access participants as gatekeepers (such as school head teachers or coaches) may be unwilling to participate for fear of any negative impact on their organization's reputation. Identifying initial prevalence rates can be an important first step to start the conversation with organizations and gain access to additional participants. As a result of this initial analysis we have developed this programme of work to look at: (i) retrospective reports of bullying in sport, (ii) experiences of bullying in university sport and (iii) focused surveys with children and adolescents of bullying in school and community sport.

Ethical and legal issues

Not surprisingly ethics committees find submissions that want to see if an intervention will cause harm to the participants challenging. Applicants, therefore, need to locate their work within the 'big picture' that we have articulated in this chapter. This may mean attempting to justify clearly defined and limited harm to a small group of participants in terms of the benefits that may accrue to a larger population. Such applications clearly challenge both the applicants and the members of ethical committees. Both parties in such application 'earn their money' when dealing with such issues and there are clearly no right or wrong answers, simply the judgement of individuals doing their best with the information they have available at the time and their value systems.

Given the importance of ethical and legal issues to conducting research on the negative impact of exercise this subsection is followed by a scenario designed to promote thought and reflection.

Outliers

The evidence-based consensus is that exercise is, for most people, a safe and effective way to enhance and maintain the individual's health and wellbeing. As a result, conducting research into the negative impacts of exercise may often involve studying outliers. Hypothetical outliers who may be of importance in advancing the sum of human knowledge include:

- Individuals who have an adverse response to an exercise programme which is normally beneficial.
- Individuals who do not respond in terms of health and fitness gain to a normal 'dose' of exercise.

- Individuals who are fit and healthy, but who don't exercise.
- Individuals who suffer catastrophic medical emergencies during exercise and sports events.
- Individuals who 'over-dose' on exercise.

Studying outliers can be achieved in a number of ways including the use of case studies. Single-subject case studies can adopt a quantitative or qualitative approach. In 2011 Barker et al.[5] broke new ground when they wrote a book whose "*primary purpose [. . .] is to provide a resource of single-case designs, procedures and analysis strategies*" (p. xvi). We strongly recommend this book to readers considering such a methodology. Qualitative case studies are a well-developed methodology in the social sciences. For example, they have proved useful in illustrating social problems in sport.[6]

Manage the media

Those who go 'looking for trouble' and find it have a responsibility to make sure they manage the media fall-out from their work responsibly. For example, the work of one of our teams on sudden cardiac death in marathons demonstrates that the phenomenon exists and whilst worthy of further study the chances of dying in a marathon are very low.[7] Nonetheless, sadly deaths in marathons are 'newsworthy'. It is their rarity and the huge impact on all those concerned that make them of interest to the media.

Scenarios

As with all research, addressing and managing the ethical issues should be at the forefront of the research design. Alongside issues relating to consent, debrief and the protection from harm (physical and psychological) researchers need to be mindful of two key interrelated issues related to researching risk: (1) protection of participants, the researcher and the discipline, and (2) ethical issues related to dissemination. Regarding protection, and aligned with managing the potential harm to participants, researchers need to define 'participants' inclusively. Using bullying in sport as an example, when managing the risk of harm, we ensured that participants had sources of support available to them should they become upset regarding reports of their bullying experiences. But alongside protecting participants, we also had the ethical requirement to protect participating schools. Bullying is an emotive subject, and any suggestion of bullying occurring can have negative consequences, and therefore the assurance of confidentiality and anonymity are key to ensure an effective working relationship with schools.

Often the most troubling issues of interest to researchers involve the study of illegal behaviour(s), such as sexual abuse in exercise settings and doping. Such topics pose some challenging ethical and methodological issues. If you are investigating illegal behaviour you will need to address the following issues:

- How can you ensure participants will tell the truth?
- If participants report engaging in illegal behaviour, are you legally obliged to share this information with law enforcement agencies?
- Is there a serious risk of distress to the participants? If so how will this be managed?

- Is there a risk to the researcher, can their safety be guaranteed?
- Is there a risk that the results may damage the reputation of sport and exercise?

With these questions in mind, consider the following two scenarios:

Scenario 1

A researcher is interested in studying the social experiences of swimmers. The researcher conducts a series of one-to-one interviews with swimmers where they are asked questions on any negative social experiences they may have experienced. One participant describes a situation when as a young swimmer she felt pressured to take illegal drugs. She explains the situation in harrowing detail.

Scenario 2

A researcher is interested in studying the prevalence of doping using illegal drugs in swimming. The researcher plans to send a questionnaire to professional swimmers asking about all aspects of doping in swimming.

Whilst both scenarios are related to the use of illegal drugs, there are important differences between the two.

Scenario 1 highlights a situation where illegal behaviour is reported, but is not the focus of the research project. Participants are not directly asked about illegal behaviour; instead experiences of substance use were raised by the participant. Under current UK law, there is no legal requirement for such information to be reported and such reports are likened to witnessing a crime. While there may be ethical or moral reasons for reporting the crime, there is no legal obligation to do so. When planning a research study, you need to think carefully about whether there is a risk that illegal behaviour may be reported. If such a risk exists we would encourage you to consider:

- Supporting participants – It may be helpful to provide sources of support for participants, such as contact details for organizations that can provide guidance or counselling.
- Providing the 'right to withdraw' – After completing a study, participants may change their mind about their data being used. Ensure you provide a clear outline of how participants can withdraw their data, and any time limits associated with this.
- Checking with your local ethics committee/institutional review board – This chapter is based on our experience of conducting research in the UK. Therefore, we strongly advise that you seek support and guidance from your local ethics committee/institutional review board. Ensure you get up-to-date advice and guidance (laws change and differ under different jurisdictions).

Scenario 2 sets out to investigate illegal substance use and asks directly about the issue. As such participants would be reporting on, and possibly admitting to, engaging in illegal activities. Some ethical guidelines provide guidance on such research. For example, Harriss and Atkinson state:[8] "*Athletes as participants in studies on doping agents. In principle, recreational and elite athletes should not be recruited to participate in research that exposes them to violations of the World Anti-Doping Code*". That said, the authors also acknowledge, that while such research should be avoided, it may be of value in certain circumstances. If you are to undertake such research you need to consider:

- Speaking to the relevant authorities about your research, to help protect your participants and yourself as the researcher. This could include your local ethics committee, sports organizations and anti-doping organizations, and local legal authorities.[8]
- How will you access participants and what is the likelihood of people wanting to take part in your study? Any contact with gatekeepers and participants should wait until you have acquired ethical approval for your study.
- Do you have the required experience and skill to undertake such research? Some ethics guidelines and ethics review committees will factor this into their decision on any ethics application pertaining to research on illegal behaviour.[9]
- What method of data collection will you use? How best can you reduce socially desirable responses?[10]

Doing research into illegal activity in exercise and sport raises many ethical and legal issues. However, what is sometimes overlooked is avoiding such challenging research questions and 'playing it safe' and not 'going looking for trouble' raises equally challenging ethical issues. Ignoring potential problems in exercise and sport because to conduct such research is difficult is moral cowardice and an affront to the scientific ideal.

Suggested research questions on the negative impact of exercise

In a spirit of intellectual generosity, we conclude this chapter by sharing with readers 5 five research questions that we wonder what the answers to will be.

- *What is the impact on an individual's confidence and self-esteem of not adhering to an exercise intervention?* A reasonably foreseeable outcome for many participants in a community or research-based exercise intervention is that they will 'drop out'. Non-adherence to exercise interventions has been widely reported in the literature since Dishman's seminal work in the area.[11,12] Whilst drop-out rates are often reported in research studies or in the evaluation of community interventions, little is known about the consequences of dropping out for the individuals concerned. Based on what we know at present all we can say is that they do not receive any benefit that may have resulted from the intervention. However, might it be possible that 'dropping out' has a negative psychological impact? Might it reduce perceived behavioural control over future attempts to be active or other health-enhancing behaviours like diet?
- *What is the prevalence of the body's acute and/or chronic response to exercise leading to errors in medical diagnostics?* The authors know, anecdotally, of a number of cases where the extreme fitness of individuals appear to have caused problems in medical diagnosis or the misreporting of symptoms.

- *Does a culture of alcohol, abuse and bullying in some sport outweigh the health benefit of the exercise?* In some countries might this be of particular concern in relation to student sport at universities?
- *What is the opportunity cost of funding exercise and sport-based health interventions?* If a financial investment is made to set up an exercise intervention to the improve health of a community, that money can only be spent once. The opportunity cost being what else the money could have been invested in. One can imagine a situation where $1,000 spent on an exercise-based intervention resulted in a hypothesized health benefit of $2,000 being evaluated positively. However, unless the opportunity cost was factored into the evaluation it might be that an investment of $1,000 into a smoking cessation programme may have yielded a benefit of $5,000.
- *What is the health and financial cost of exercise-related injury?* Arguably our colleagues in sports science are far ahead of exercise science in knowing the cost of sports injury and its impact on the individual.[13] We need to know more about the toll of muscular skeletal injury on those who exercise.

Conclusion

Exercise is a complex phenomenon and set of behaviours. Exercisers are even more complex and bring to the park, gym or sport a wide variety of body shapes, workload capacities and sometimes disease states. Added to this mix is the changing nature of exercise and those who participate. Given these factors it is logical to assume that from time to time exercise can do more harm than good. So stop reading and go looking for trouble, and tell us what you found.

References

1   Cleret L, McNamee M, Page S. 'Sports integrity' needs sports ethics (and sports philosophers and sports ethicists too). *Sport Ethics Philos.* 2015; 9(1):1–15.
2   MINEPS. *Declaration of Berlin.* United Nations Education Scientific and Cultural Organisation. 2013. Available from: http://unesdoc.unesco.org/images/0022/002211/221114e.pdf
3   Treagus M, Cover R, Beasley C. *Integrity in sport.* The University of Adelaide. 2011. Available from: www.ausport.gov.au/__data/assets/pdf_file/0011/516782/Integrity_in_Sport_Literature_Review-.pdf
4   Noret N, Smith A, Birbeck N, Velija P, Mierzwinski M. *Bullying in school sport.* York, UK: St John University; 2015.
5   Barker JB, McCarthy PJ, Jones MV, Moran A. *Single-case research methods in sport and exercise psychology.* London: Routledge; 2011.
6   Anderson E, White A. *Sport, theory and social problems: a critical introduction.* Abingdon, UK: Routledge; 2017.
7   Waite O, Smith A, Madge L, Spring H, Noret N. Sudden cardiac death in marathons: a systematic review. *Physician Sportsmed.* 2016; 44(1):79–84.
8   Harriss DJ, Atkinson G. Ethical standards in sport and exercise science research: 2016 update. *Int J Sports Med.* 2015; 36(14):1121–4.
9   Health & Care Professions Council (HCPC). *Standards of conduct, performance and ethics.* London: HCPC; 2016.
10 Tourangeau R, Yan T. Sensitive questions in surveys. *Psychol Bull.* 2007; 133(5):859.

11 Dishman RK. *Advances in exercise adherence.* Champaign, IL: Human Kinetics Publishers; 1994.

12 Dishman RK. Compliance/adherence in health-related exercise. *Health Psychol.* 1982; **1**(3):237.

13 Forsdyke D, Smith A, Jones M, Gledhill A. Psychosocial factors associated with outcomes of sports injury rehabilitation in competitive athletes: a mixed studies systematic review. *Br J Sports Med.* 2016; **50**:537–44.

22 Research studies with children

Michael J. Duncan and Keith Tolfrey

Aims of the chapter

This chapter aims to provide insight into the issues associated with researching with children and to provide guidelines for researchers intending to work with this group.

Introduction

Research has demonstrated the importance of physical activity and exercise participation on multiple and varied outcomes relating to physical, psychological, social and emotional health and wellbeing.[1] With children and adolescents (young people; typically less than 18 years old) in particular, physical activity and exercise have significant and long-lasting effects, which has led to increasing practical and research activity focused on this population. It is imperative to acknowledge, however, that children are not simply smaller adults; thus, working with young people requires consideration of numerous different factors compared with adult-based research and practice. It is essential for researchers planning to work with this population to understand these issues in addition to some of the practical issues and implications that arise when working with young people. This chapter aims to provide insight into the key issues associated with conducting research with young people and to provide guidelines and a checklist for researchers intending to work with this group. Examples illustrating good practice will also be provided. The chapter will, in the first instance, consider the ethics of research with young people and then explore other research issues when working with this special population.

Ethics

From the outset, it is important to assert that there can be strong ethical grounds to conduct non-therapeutic research with children or adolescents; research with this population can be valuable and legitimate.[2] While many of the key tenets of good research ethics with adults hold when working with children and adolescents, there are other considerations that arise when working with a paediatric population. The British Association of Sport and Exercise Sciences (BASES) expert statement on ethics and participation of research with young people[3] provides a key resource for researchers and scientists intending to work with children and adolescents in a research setting and offers a robust framework when read in conjunction with other related authoritative guidance.[2]

Irrespective of research focus or topic, the key overarching pillar of any research activity with young people is that their welfare as participants in the research study or project is upheld at all times.[2] In the context of good research ethics and from a moral viewpoint of wanting to treat research participants in an appropriate manner, Williams et al.[3] identified two fundamental issues that underpin any decisions related to upholding the welfare of child research participants: (1) that the child is likely to gain personal benefit from the procedure or intervention; (2) the level of risk of the research (i.e. is there potential for physical or psychological harm to the participant and what is the extent of this potential harm?). In some cases there are personal benefits to participating in a research study; however, it has been suggested that the majority of exercise and sport-related research may result in no direct benefit to the participant, but the work exposes the participants to 'minimal risk'. For the latter, the key criterion to consider is that research studies involving young people may be deemed ethical if procedures do not pose a risk of harm that is greater than those the child would encounter in daily life. For example, maximal exercise testing with healthy young people, in the absence of pre-defined contraindications, is normally considered to be ethical, whereas a tissue biopsy is not. Likewise, interventions examining manipulations in breakfast composition on cognitive or exercise performance are ethical, but the influence of creatine monohydrate consumption on the same outcome variables would not be because young people do not normally consume this supplement in isolation and the long-term side-effects have not been established in this population.

All research that involves children or adolescents as research participants should have formal ethics approval that outlines the relevance, merits, risks and benefits of the research study being undertaken as well as clearly identifying the extent to which the participants (and their primary carers) have been properly informed. It is also key that any research project with young people adheres to current good practice for safeguarding and is conducted by researchers/individuals who have the requisite safeguarding and police conviction disclosure or governmental check (e.g. Disclosure and Barring Service checks in the UK, Working with Children Check in Australia, Local Police Check in the United States or a Police Certificate in Spain) in place before any measurements commence.

Informed consent

The need for informed consent to participate in a scientific research study is well established, irrespective of participant age, but this is not as straightforward when working with children or adolescents. Consent is considered "the positive agreement of an individual" whereas providing assent is "to go along with".[4] Normally, informed consent for research studies involving children and adolescents is characterized by parental (or legal carer) consent and child assent, as participants are minors. Gaining valid consent from parents is recognized legally where the participant is under 18 years of age. Provision of assent to participate has no legal basis; however, it should be seen as good (best) practice, and as an essential facet of 'participation' in the research by the children or adolescents involved. Parental informed consent should be both given freely and informed.

Within research studies, and as part of the informed consent process, it is normal for participants to be provided with information sheets detailing the procedures, demands, requirements and risks of what is being asked of the participants. Importantly, researchers should always provide two versions of the participating information sheet when working with children or adolescents. The information contained within these versions should not differ particularly, but the expression is different. The language needs to be developmentally appropriate and specialized technical terms should be avoided to increase primary carer and participant understanding. The written information sheet might need to be supplemented with verbal and/or visual information for young people to maximize their understanding of their involvement in the research.

Safeguarding

It is essential that conduct and practice before, during and after a research study with children and adolescents are established from a safeguarding standpoint. The safeguarding, rights, dignity, welfare and safety of the participants should be protected at all times. These safeguarding issues are not restricted solely to protecting paediatric participants from abuse or impairment to health, but also relate to reducing any hazard (or situation) that may cause physical, social or psychological harm or distress. This can be as simple as young people thinking their scores/results/responses on a research protocol will be revealed to other people. Consequently, it is important that researchers consider safeguarding as a proactive framework to promote a safe and positive environment for research. Anyone working with young people should be clear about protocols for reporting child safety and welfare issues and appropriate actions where necessary – these are likely to be specific to organizations or research settings (e.g. sports clubs, schools, universities, etc).

The overall conduct of research staff is also a key aspect of the safeguarding process. Researchers need to remember that the interests of the young participant should be paramount. They should use jargon-free language that the young people and their carers can understand easily and avoid unnecessary physical contact with paediatric participants. This latter point sometimes causes concern with researchers examining physical activity and exercise-related questions with paediatric populations. Physical contact is unavoidable for numerous procedures, including: surface anthropometry, electrocardiogram electrode placement, hip-based accelerometer positioning and waist circumference measurement. Importantly, the emphasis is placed on avoiding *unnecessary* contact with participants. Where physical contact is required, experience has shown that if researchers describe the procedure clearly and explain it is standard practice, children and adolescents are normally happy to be involved. These procedures must always be conducted in the presence of another adult chaperone (i.e. researcher or carer) whilst retaining the participant's privacy. Moreover, standard ethics procedures that allow any participant to opt-out or decline specific measurements, without the need for an explanation, must always be enforced.

For the safeguarding of both the young person and researcher, arrangements should be made to ensure they are not isolated one-to-one – this includes transportation to/from the laboratory or field setting (appropriate ethics procedures must include chaperoning guidelines). The researchers themselves also need to be clear to the child and parent/carer (if present) of who is in charge during the research data collection, particularly if in a laboratory setting, and to outline what is acceptable conduct for the children. Relevant health and safety procedures/regulations should be communicated to participants and adhered to.

Recruitment and retention

Excellent research design that is highly standardized and controlled, and rigorously executed, can place a significant burden on young participants and their carers.[5] This may often lead to low initial uptake and/or poor compliance.[6] Recent qualitative research has provided novel insights to issues related to recruitment, retention and adherence of children and adolescents in physical activity and exercise-related research,[5,7] which is useful for researchers to consider when planning their work.

In their study, Massie et al.[5] conducted focus group interviews with 26, 12- to 15-year-old girls using a purposive sampling strategy, which identified individuals who expressed an interest in being more physically active or increasing their cardiorespiratory fitness. The focus groups discussed issues relating specifically to recruitment and retention in exercise settings that included a chronic exercise training programme with physiological outcome variables (e.g. body composition, cardiorespiratory fitness and resting metabolic rate). Using a six-phase thematic analysis procedure,[8] eight main themes were identified inductively; these led to seven evidence-based practical recommendations (see recommendations column in Table 22.1) to improve recruitment and retention for future exercise training studies.[5] Although this work was conducted with adolescent girls, the key themes that emerged from their analyses are more widely relevant and could be applied to boys or girls spanning childhood and adolescence. The key themes, subthemes and recommendations from this research are presented in Table 22.1.

Table 22.1 Recommendations to improve recruitment and retention for exercise training studies in adolescents, taken from Massie et al. (2015)[5]

Process	Theme	Subtheme	Recommendations
Recruitment	1. Dynamics of Communication	1.1 Presenter 1.2 Peers	1. Define key terms
	2. Presentation of Content	2.1 Images 2.2 Choice of words and phrases	1. Define key terms 2. Representative images
	3. Motives to Participate	–	2. Images capture motives 4. Understand and monitor the motivations
Retention	4. Barriers	4.1 Logistical Barriers 4.2 Comparative Barriers	5. Address the barriers 6. Participant grouping – size/composition
	5. Exercise Training Programme	5.1 Activity Characteristics 5.2 Group Composition 5.3 Session Details	6. Participant grouping – size/composition 7. Activity variety
	6. Benefits of Participation	6.1 Fun and enjoyment 6.2 Body image 6.3 Physical/ psychological self	3. Maximize enjoyment 4. Understand and monitor the motivations 7. Activity variety
Retention	7. Participant Characteristics and Peer Relationships	–	3. Maximize enjoyment 6. Participant grouping – size/composition
	8. Instructor Characteristics	–	3. Maximize enjoyment

According to Massie et al.,[5] successful recruitment requires:

- Clear definitions of exercise-related terms;
- Appropriate choice of recruitment material;
- An understanding of participant motivations to engage in the research study.

Once recruited, participant retention can then be enhanced by:

- Regular monitoring of participant motives;
- Small group exercise sessions to foster peer and researcher support;
- Structuring sessions using friendship and/or ability groups;
- Employing a variety of activities to promote exercise adherence.

A consistent finding from this qualitative research was that imagery in the recruitment process was important. Using images that are an accurate representation of the planned research and also, where possible, reflect the potential motives of the targeted participants may maximize recruitment and subsequent retention. This is because the young people have been provided with a more informed and realistic overview of the research project from the outset.

Another key issue reflected in the suggestions made by Massie et al.,[5] and others for researchers working with young people is that enjoyment needs to be prioritized throughout.[9] Enjoyment may be an underplayed factor in many research studies, but is cited consistently as critical in the decision to participate and adhere to exercise.[9–11] Thus, it must be considered in the planning phase of all studies. This is likely to vary depending on the paediatric population of interest; the type and choice of activities, exercise and/or training, the training environment and the composition of the exercise group (if applicable): all require careful consideration. Where possible, arrangements for young people to complete most or all of the study measurements in friendship groups appears to be the most preferable approach.[12]

Study logistics

Study logistics can be an under-considered aspect of research with children and adolescents. School or community settings for research pose fewer logistical challenges for parents or carers, particularly if the measurements with the young participants are completed during regular school hours. Travel to laboratories or field settings will require more careful planning. A comprehensive overview of this aspect of research planning is beyond the scope of this chapter but, briefly, researchers need to consider key logistical barriers that have been cited in the literature,[5,13–15] namely:

- Time
- Location
- Transport
- Cost

Paediatric research requires careful consideration of parents/carers in addition to the participants. Participants in sport, exercise and physical activity research are often involved in numerous other activities (e.g. music, drama, competitive sport, extra-tuition, caring for siblings) outside of school, which are in addition to the research study demands. Therefore, scheduling study components needs to be as flexible as possible to accommodate participant, but also parental/carer commitments. Restricting children and adolescents to timetables best suited to researchers will result in poor recruitment and high attrition or low adherence. Thus, measurements are often required after school hours, at weekends, in half-term or holiday periods, or skilful negotiation with head teachers may be required for the young people to complete measurements during school time in off-site locations.

Simple as it may sound, the study location is a critical factor in planning and recruitment; measurements in a scientific laboratory or a novel sporting venue can be attractive features of the research for young participants, which aid recruitment. However, clear directions and parking arrangements must be conveyed to parents/carers and/or consideration of public transport, each of which have cost implications that need to be built into the study budget. Viewing research participation from a parent or carer's standpoint will help in ensuring access to the research is maximized. Patient and public involvement (PPI) in research planning has become an essential component of research grant funding (e.g. National Institute for Health Research INVOLVE, see www.invo.org.uk/ for more information) – getting children and adolescents involved in the planning phase of research is likely to lead to greater initial buy-in from them and sustained involvement.[16] INVOLVE provides an excellent list of top tips for researchers, which are specific to this special population.[16] Giving financial incentives to children or adolescents to participate in research brings its own ethical issues;[17] however, participant engagement is unlikely to be maximized if the parents/carers are meaningfully out of pocket.

Physical activity monitoring issues: a special case

Over the last 20 years, there has also been a considerable increase in the volume of paediatric-based research studies using objective measures of physical activity (e.g. accelerometry). Aside from the well-documented decisions that need to be made when using methods such as accelerometry with children and adolescents (e.g. position of accelerometer placement, wear time),[18] other more practical issues have arisen which are relevant for researchers considering work on the topic of physical activity assessment using accelerometers in young people. McCann et al.[7] have provided qualitative insight recently to issues surrounding physical activity monitoring in children and adolescents. Of practical use for researchers, McCann et al.[7] also provide a protocol for future studies to improve adherence to physical activity monitoring protocols.

Using deductive content analysis and an interpretivist methodology with a series of semi-structured interviews with children and adolescents, McCann et al.[7] identified four general dimensions, which helped explain young people's adherence to physical activity monitor wear time protocols. The four dimensions were: (1) participant-driven compliance strategies; (2) reasons for non-compliance; (3) strategies to improve accelerometer care and (4) reasons for non-compliance to study conditions. These were then translated into practical strategies that could be used to increase compliance to physical activity study protocols. It is important to note that these strategies also differed between children and adolescents. For children, the

Study Design

Where possible encourage a comprehensive formative research phase that is based upon established theoretical models and acknowledges the developmental differences in determinants with age.

Compliance

Compliance strategies should accommodate the differing preferences of children and young people. In the absence of a formative research phase future accelerometry based research should consider these informed strategies to improve compliance to habitual physical activity monitoring:

Children (8–11 yrs.): 1) sticky note reminders; 2) mobile phone reminders; 3) social conformity.

Young people (12–15 yrs.): 1) social conformity; 2) mobile phone reminders; 3) monetary compensation.

Recruitment

Children and Young People:

Where possible target friendship groups to enhance social conformity. If not possible then inform class/forms/sets so that peers who are connected socially are involved in the study. It is suggested that friendship groups have the potential to contribute to behavioural reinforcement.

Parents and gatekeepers:

Invite parents, siblings and teachers of participants to a small group discussion. The social environment of children and young people primarily includes, parents, siblings, friends and teachers. All should be briefed on the study and in particular wear time criteria, asking for support in terms of reminding the participants to wear the accelerometer and enforcing the positive aspects of the study.

Small group familiarity sessions

Accelerometers: allow participants time to pick up and look at the accelerometer in detail, asking any questions they may have. Once fitted, let participants practice taking the accelerometer on and off, and sitting/standing/writing with the accelerometer so they are familiar with how it feels and are comfortable with adjusting the accelerometer for comfort.

Instructions and wear time diaries: Combine the two documents into a simple format to reduce participant burden, and emphasize the importance of completing this document each day. If funding allows create an electronic version so that participants can access this through mobile phone and computer technology.

Wear time

Participants should wear waterproof accelerometers at all times during waking hours and remove others only for water-based activities. Provide participants with supporting letters to hand to sports coaches to prevent removal. Only if the accelerometer is deemed unsafe by the coach should the accelerometer be removed.

Care of accelerometers

To instil a sense of trust inform participants that accelerometers remain the property of the institution. For each accelerometer that is broken or damaged that would cost the institution the equivalent of a PS3 or XBOX 360.

Figure 22.1 Proposed protocol to maximize provision of data in accelerometer-based physical activity research with children and adolescents, taken from McCann et al. (2016)[7]

The Study Protocol

This protocol was created from the suggestions of young people to maximize the provision of adequate data in future accelerometer-based research.

following strategies were considered popular as means to optimize physical activity monitor wear time:

- Sticky note reminders (attached to a prominent place in the home);
- Mobile phone reminders;
- Social conformity (adherence was more likely if peer groups engaged in the study together).

For adolescents the following were considered as popular means to optimize wear time:

- Social conformity;
- Mobile phone reminders;
- Monetary compensation (for achieving wear time thresholds).

This process then informed the development of a protocol to maximize data acquisition in studies employing objective monitoring of physical activity with children and adolescents (Figure 22.1). The informal protocol provided by McCann et al.[7] provides a solid framework for researchers intending to monitor free-living physical activity with children and adolescents. In lieu of any other available protocols, the McCann et al.[7] framework provides a useful focal point from which researchers can plan optimal physical activity data acquisition with confidence.

Conclusion

Working in physical activity and sport and exercise-related research with young people requires different considerations in terms of ethics, informed consent, safeguarding, recruitment and retention and study logistics that differ from research with adults. Understanding these differences, being proactive in following guidance published on behalf of the Royal College of Paediatrics and Child Health,[2] considering involving young people in the planning phase of research and using the top tips for researchers working with this population via INVOLVE will provide a solid foundation to ensure good practice when conducting research with children and adolescents.[16]

References

1 Janssen I, LeBlanc AG. Systematic review of the health benefits of physical activity and fitness in school-aged children and youth. *Int J Behav Nutr Phys Act.* 2010; **7**:40.
2 Modi N, Vohra J, Preston J, for a Working Party of the Royal College of Paediatrics and Child Health, et al. Guidance on clinical research involving infants, children and young people: an update for researchers and research ethics committees. *Arch Dis Child.* 2014; **99**:887–91.
3 Williams C, Cobb M, Rowland R, Winter E. The BASES expert statement on ethics and participation in research of young people. *Sport Exerc Sci.* 2011; **29**:12–13.
4 Royal College of Paediatrics and Child Health: Ethics Advisory Committee. Guidelines for the ethical conduct of medical research involving children. *Arch Dis Child.* 2000; **82**:177–82.
5 Massie R, Smith B, Tolfrey K. Recommendations for recruiting and retaining adolescent girls in chronic exercise (Training) research studies. *Sports.* 2015; **3**:219–35.
6 Steinbeck K, Baur, L, Cowell C, Pietrobelli A. Clinical research in adolescents: challenges and opportunities using obesity as a model. *Int J Obes.* 2009; **33**:2–7.

7   McCann DA, Knowles ZR, Fairclough SJ, Graves LEF. A protocol to encourage accelerometer wear in children and young people. *Qual Res Sport Exerc Health*. 2016; **8**:319–31.

8   Braun V, Clarke V. Using thematic analysis in psychology. *Qual Res Psychol*. 2006; **3**:77–101.

9   Jago R, Davis L, McNeill J, Sebire SJ, Haase A, Powell J, Cooper AR. Adolescent girls' and parents' views on recruiting and retaining girls into an after-school dance intervention: implications for extracurricular physical activity provisions. *Int J Behav Nutr Phys Act*. 2011; **8**:1–9.

10   Whitehead S, Biddle S. Adolescent girls' perceptions of physical activity: a focus group study. *Eur Phys Educ Rev*. 2008; **14**:243–62.

11   Phoenix C, Orr N. Please: a forgotten dimension of physical activity in older age. *Soc Sci Med*. 2014; **115**:94–102.

12   Jago R, Brockman R, Fox KR, Cartwright K, Page AS, Thompson JL. Friendship groups and physical activity: qualitative findings on how physical activity is initiated and maintained among 10-11 year old children. *Int J Behav Nutr Phys Act*. 2009; **6**:4.

13   Biddle SJH, Whitehead SH, O'Donovan TM, Nevill ME. Correlates of participation in physical activity for adolescent girls: a systematic review of recent literature. *J Phys Act Health*. 2005; **2**:423–34.

14   Coday M, Boutlin-Foster C, Goldman Sher T, Tennant J, Greaney ML, Saunders SD, Somes GW. Strategies for retaining study participants in behavioural intervention trials: retention experience of the NIH behaviour change consortium. *Ann Behav Med*. 2005; **29**:55–65.

15   Dwyer JJ, Allison KR, Goldenberg ER, Fein AJ, Yoshida KK, Boutilier MA. Adolescent girls' perceived barriers to participation in physical activity. *Adolescence*. 2006; **41**:75–89.

16   INVOLVE. *Involving children and young people in research: top tips and essential key issues for researchers*. Eastleigh, UK: INVOLVE; 2016.

17   Wendler D, Rackoff JE, Emanuel EJ, Grady C. The ethics of paying for children's participation in research. *J Pediatr*. 2002; **141**:166–71.

18   Ridgers N, Fairclough S. Assessing free-living physical activity using accelerometry: practical issues for researchers and practitioners. *Eur J Sport Sci*. 2011; **11**:205–13.

23 Research studies with older people

Jane Sims and Harriet Radermacher

Aims of the chapter

This chapter aims to provide insight into the issues associated with undertaking research with older people, and to provide guidance for researchers intending to work with this group. The prevalence of physical activity, and sedentary behaviour, among older people in Western countries is noted. Reference is made to the current physical activity recommendations for older people. A brief discussion of engagement strategies for older people is provided. The potential contextual influences of ageism, environment and cultural factors are considered. A critique of the subjective and objective measurement tools available for data collection in older people is presented. Evidence gaps and future research opportunities are highlighted to promote ongoing physical activity in older people and its effective evaluation.

Introduction

The benefits of physical activity have been discussed elsewhere in this book: they are well established and include a lower incidence of hypertension, heart disease, osteoporosis, arthritis, colonic cancer and diabetes mellitus, improved mood and memory function, and the greater likelihood of a maintained social network.[1] With ageing, the prevalence of chronic health problems increases; physical inactivity and sedentary behaviour compound the effects of chronological ageing and place older people at greater absolute risk of ill health. At a population level, the increasing proportion of older people in society means that there will be more people with chronic health problems and more people with conditions associated with ageing. Old age does not necessarily mean ill-health, but there are a number of health conditions, known as geriatric syndromes, that are more common in older people.[2] These conditions tend to be multicausal and multisystemic, e.g. dementia, sarcopaenia, frailty, immobility, gait disturbances and falls. Physical activity can also assist with many of these health and functional impairments. For example, there is level 1 evidence for the role of physical activity in falls prevention,[3,4] and growing evidence for physical activity's role in ameliorating the impact of Alzheimer's disease.[5,6] Whilst it is beyond the scope of this chapter to discuss the evidence base for specific health conditions, the key message is that physical activity can impact on the range of comorbidities an older person may live with.

Unfortunately inactivity remains common amongst older people and as a consequence, there is a great imperative for individual and public health interventions that promote physical activity in older people. As Evans stated "there is no segment of the population that can benefit more from exercise than the elderly" (p. 12).[7]

Who are older people?

Older people represent the largest age cohort in society, spanning several generations and an age range of many years. Older people are a heterogenous group of adults, with varying capacities. There are clearly potential differences between a 65-year-old and an 85-year-old, not simply in terms of chronological age, but also in life circumstances and behaviours. Gerontologists have classified older people into several categories: the young-old (65–74), the old (75–84) and the oldest-old (85+). Although there are difficulties in ascribing a particular chronological age to define 'older people', and while it is recognized that there is wide variability in health status, function and wellbeing at any age, in this chapter the term 'older people' primarily refers to those aged over 65 years. For Indigenous populations, a lower chronological age is usually used to define older people in acknowledgement of their reduced life expectancy; for example in Australia, for Aboriginal and Torres Strait Islanders, the age of 55 years and above is used.

The WHO Heidelberg guidelines identify three groups of older people along the health-fitness gradient:[8] the physically fit-healthy; the physically unfit-unhealthy but independent living; and the physically unfit-unhealthy and dependent individuals. Within each of these categories, people may display a variety of physical activity and sedentary behaviour profiles. The contemporary context for physical activity promotion centres on a wellness model of care, where physical activity is meant to complement other restorative and reablement activities, to optimize the health and wellbeing of older people across the spectrum. It is acknowledged that many of the factors associated with physical activity adoption in older people may have applicability for other age groups, for example, younger people with disability.

The terms 'physical activity', 'exercise' and 'sport' were defined in Chapter 3. It is worth noting that whilst here the term 'physical activity' encompasses exercise in the sporting as well as the therapeutic context, much of the literature focuses on the latter, whilst the former tends to deal with elite senior athletes, who are not representative of the general population.

Prevalence of physical activity

Prevalence rates for physical activity vary widely for older people. This is partly due to the heterogeneous nature of this group, but also because of the variety of data sources used to determine prevalence.[9] Potentially, the most reliable source is a population-based survey, such as a government census. National physical activity surveys to date have included older people, but the reported data is often aggregated. Even an age band such as '75 years and over' can contain more than one generation of older people. A detailed breakdown of the older population would allow us to see which subgroups may need further targeting. There is also scope to distinguish between community-dwelling older people and those living in residential care, but the latter are often excluded from national surveys. Further, whilst a population-based survey necessarily gathers data from adults of all ages, enabling intergenerational comparisons, there are potential limitations in interpreting older peoples' responses to the tools used. These methodological issues will be discussed further below.

Methodological limitations notwithstanding, statistics from many Western countries highlight the degree of inactivity amongst older people. In Australia, for example, fewer than half of older Australians are sufficiently active to achieve a health benefit;[10]

they are more sedentary than younger adult cohorts, and this rate has remained consistent over the last decade.

Given this background, the need for physical activity promotion and interventions, guided by recommendations, can clearly be seen. The next section provides a summary of the physical activity recommendations from a sample of English language resources.

Physical activity recommendations

Several countries have produced recommendations and evidence-based guidelines on physical activity for older people, including the USA,[11] UK,[12] Canada,[13,14] New Zealand[15] and Australia (Table 23.1).[16] With the exception of the latter, these have been directed at healthcare providers. The Australian recommendations were explicitly intended for older people themselves.

Table 23.1 Physical activity recommendations for older people: key examples[†]

Source	Recommendation
Australia[16]	1 Older people should do some form of physical activity, no matter what their age, weight, health problems or abilities.
	2 Older people should be active every day in as many ways as possible, doing a range of physical activities that incorporate fitness, strength, balance and flexibility.
	3 Older people should accumulate at least 30 minutes of moderate intensity physical activity on most, preferably all, days.
	4 Older people who have stopped physical activity, or who are starting a new physical activity, should start at a level that is easily manageable and gradually build up the amount, type and frequency of activity.
	5 Older people who have enjoyed a lifetime of vigorous physical activity should continue to participate at this level in a manner suited to their capability into later life, provided recommended safety procedures and guidelines are adhered to.
United Kingdom[12]	§1 Older adults who participate in any amount of physical activity gain some health benefits, including maintenance of good physical and cognitive function. Some physical activity is better than none, and more physical activity provides greater health benefits.
	2 Older adults should aim to be active daily. Over a week, activity should add up to at least 150 minutes (2½ hours) of moderate intensity activity in bouts of 10 minutes or more – one way to approach this is to do 30 minutes on at least 5 days a week.
	3 For those who are already regularly active at moderate intensity, comparable benefits can be achieved through 75 minutes of vigorous intensity activity spread across the week or a combination of moderate and vigorous activity.
	4 Older adults should also undertake physical activity to improve muscle strength on at least two days a week.
	5 Older adults at risk of falls should incorporate physical activity to improve balance and co-ordination on at least two days a week.
	6 Older adults should minimise the amount of time spent being sedentary (sitting) for extended periods.

(Continued)

Table 23.1 (Continued)

Source	Recommendation
New Zealand[15]	1 Be as physically active as possible and limit sedentary behaviour.

1 Be as physically active as possible and limit sedentary behaviour.

- View movement as an opportunity, not an inconvenience, as every bit helps. Older people should be encouraged to increase their physical activity levels (especially their ADLs) and reduce their sedentary behaviour. Incremental increases in physical activity and decreases in sedentary behaviour can both reduce mortality and morbidity risk.

2 Consult an appropriate health practitioner before starting or increasing physical activity.

- This recommendation applies particularly to insufficiently active and physically inactive older people, or those who have a health condition (or co-morbidities), to ensure they will be able to do it safely.

3 Start off slowly and build up to the recommended daily physical activity levels.

- As fitness tends to decrease with age, older people tend to have lower exercise capacity than younger people. Older people are advised to slowly build up to the recommended amount of physical activity to prevent injury.

4 Aim to do aerobic activity on five days per week for at least 30 minutes if the activity is of moderate intensity; or for 15 minutes if it is of vigorous intensity; or a mixture of moderate- and vigorous-intensity aerobic activity.

- No amount of physical activity can prevent ageing, but people can gain significant health benefits from doing at least 30 minutes of moderate-intensity aerobic activity on five days per week, in sessions of at least 10 minutes at a time.

5 Aim to do three sessions of flexibility and balance activities, and two sessions of muscle-strengthening activities per week.

- Flexibility and balance are essential for older people to do everyday activities such as climbing stairs, getting on and off the bus, and hanging out the washing. Strong muscles and bones are needed for everyday activities such as carrying shopping.

Older people who are **frail** should:

- be as physically active as possible and limit sedentary behaviour
- consult an appropriate health practitioner before starting or increasing physical activity
- start off slowly and build up to the recommended physical activity levels
- aim for a mixture of low impact aerobic, resistance, balance and flexibility activities

Source	Recommendation
	• Physical activity is beneficial for older people who are frail to maintain strength and improve muscular functions which are important for everyday activities
	○ discuss with their doctor about whether vitamin D tablets would benefit the older person.
	• Low levels of vitamin D can lead to muscle weakness and poor balance which can cause falls. Taking vitamin D tablets has been shown to significantly reduce falls in older people in residential care.
World Health Organisation[81]	For adults of this age group (65 years old and above) physical activity includes recreational or leisure-time physical activity, transportation (e.g walking or cycling), occupational (if the person is still engaged in work), household chores, play, games, sports or planned exercise, in the context of daily, family, and community activities. In order to improve cardiorespiratory and muscular fitness, bone and functional health, and reduce the risk of NCDs, depression and cognitive decline, the following are recommended:
	1 Adults aged 65 years and above should do at least 150 minutes of moderate-intensity aerobic physical activity throughout the week, or do at least 75 minutes of vigorous-intensity aerobic physical activity throughout the week, or an equivalent combination of moderate- and vigorous-intensity activity.
	2 Aerobic activity should be performed in bouts of at least 10 minutes duration.
	3 For additional health benefits, adults aged 65 years and above should increase their moderate intensity aerobic physical activity to 300 minutes per week, or engage in 150 minutes of vigorous intensity aerobic physical activity per week, or an equivalent combination of moderate- and vigorous intensity activity.
	4 Adults of this age group with poor mobility should perform physical activity to enhance balance and prevent falls on 3 or more days per week.
	5 Muscle-strengthening activities should be done involving major muscle groups, on 2 or more days a week.
	6 When adults of this age group cannot do the recommended amounts of physical activity due to health conditions, they should be as physically active as their abilities and conditions allow.

† The US[11] and Canadian[13,14] guidelines can be viewed online. § Crown copyright © ADLs activities of daily living; NCDs non-communicable diseases

The recommendations support the conduct of both aerobic and non-aerobic, e.g. strength training forms of activity. Their inclusion of balance and flexibility exercises highlights a distinction with those for younger adults and represents a focus on prevention of the conditions of ageing that are associated with frailty.

The extent to which guidelines have been disseminated has varied, leaving scope for research into their reach and impact on behaviour change and subsequent health and organizational changes. In addition to systematic assessment of the effect of a physical activity intervention programme, the impact of physical activity recommendations on older peoples' physical activity behaviour requires surveillance and monitoring.

Recommendations and programmes are necessary, but not sufficient, for physical activity adoption to occur amongst older people. There are contextual factors to consider: social, environmental and cultural. These will be discussed in the following sections.

Contextual influences on physical activity behaviour in older people

Engagement of older people in physical activity

The research literature about engagement of older people in physical activity programmes is dominated by studies to promote improvements in a particular health condition. In this context there is a specific incentive for the target population to join a study programme: the potential to ameliorate the negative effects of a particular disease. From a population health perspective, the potential benefits of engagement in physical activity are more generic. Health literacy plays a role in the likelihood of being physically active.[17] Overall, the evidence base confirms that older people are aware of the benefits of physical activity,[18] but as the prevalence rates indicate, this knowledge doesn't necessarily translate into behaviour change. Seminal research by King and colleagues provides a comprehensive overview of factors that enable older people to become physically active.[19,20] These include:

- Preceding and ongoing education
- Pre-screening
- Motivational techniques
- Activity choice
- Flexibility in meeting goals and targets
- Individualized schedules

Education is critical. Misconceptions about exercise need to be addressed, amongst both older people and the general public. For example, a systematic review of barriers and enablers for participating in resistance training found older people had misperceptions that hamper participation, ranging from 'looking muscular' to increased risk of heart attack, stroke or death.[21] The acknowledged health benefits, e.g. improved muscle strength and endurance, bone density and reduced risk of sarcopaenia, cannot be capitalized upon unless people have the correct information to remove unwarranted fears.

A common barrier to the uptake of physical activity is concerns about the risks of doing exercise, particularly in those with pre-existing health conditions.[18] Cohen-Mansfield and colleagues reported that 20% of their sample cited age as a barrier. Both of these concerns can be addressed by appropriate education from a trusted health professional. Other barriers, such as perceived lack of time, access, cost, weather, poor self-esteem, health and energy levels can be partially addressed by motivational techniques.[22] These have been discussed elsewhere in this book. Burbank and Riebe's monograph focusing on using the transtheoretical model to promote physical activity in older people is also a useful resource.[23]

The form the physical activity takes will depend on the older person's goals. Compared to younger adults, older people seek to become physically active not simply to remain healthy, but to maintain function and most importantly, independent living. Even for frail older people, physical activity can enable some autonomy. The value of tailored programmes has been noted elsewhere in this book: this is particularly pertinent for older people, given their diverse capacities. Several researchers have highlighted older people's preference for age-appropriate programmes, with an expert facilitator.[21]

Ageism

In Chapter 7 the ethical review process was discussed, with a focus on vulnerable populations and issues of power. With regard to older people, we provide an overview of ethical considerations through the ageism lens. Ageism influences many aspects of society's relationships with older people. A brief commentary is included here, with the aim of offsetting the potentially negative impact of an ageist approach to physical activity promotion.

Ageism is likely to impact the process and interpretation of research with older people on a number of levels. For older people themselves, community perceptions that older people are frail, shouldn't be active or only participate in certain activities can result in internalized ageist beliefs that consequently limit the nature and likelihood of physical activity.

Researchers are also subject to their own biases and make assumptions about older people, influenced by their own age and experience. For this reason, qualitative researchers in particular have embraced the notion of reflexivity which encourages researchers to be open and reflective about the impact of their own attitudes and background and how this might impact on the data they collect and their interpretations of the research findings.[24] Reflexivity is a useful tool with respect to other characteristics, such as socioeconomic background, education and ethnicity.

Important for the interpretation of any data about older people is that they come with a long history of physical activity as a younger person – whether this is inactive or active, sporadic or continuous, or injury riddled. Younger researchers, in particular, may tend to overlook that older people were once young.

In a methodological sense, older people are consistently excluded from clinical research trials (maximum age limits are often 65 years) which has big implications for the applicability and relevance of research findings.[25] This will be addressed in more detail in the measurement section below.

Environment

At a practical level, environmental factors are also important. A study conducted by the authors to assess determinants of physical activity uptake in people from culturally diverse communities identified factors such as the weather, clothing, location, community attitudes, family commitments and available time.[26] More broadly, there has been a growth in research about physical environment features that promote physical activity. This has been driven in part by the WHO's Age-Friendly Cities framework.[27] The work is now focusing on age-friendly communities also, to capture the needs of those living in rural, as well as urban, areas.

A recent review, on behalf of the Council for the Environment and Physical Activity, explored the environmental factors associated with active travel in older people.[28] As with other adults, accessibility, aesthetics and destinations relevant to their needs influenced older people's active transport patterns. Enabling factors included walkability, street connectivity, residential density/urbanization, land use mix, pedestrian-friendly features, overall access to destinations/services and access to several types of destination. Common barriers include vandalism and environmental decay, but for older people, fear of crime and perceived safety are more likely to be cited.[29]

Cultural diversity

Despite increasing levels of cultural and linguistic diversity worldwide, much research continues to exclude these diverse perspectives.[30] Proportions of people born overseas range from 12% in the UK, 13% in the US and 27% in Australia. In Australia, the proportion grows to 37% in people over age 65.[31] Given that insufficient levels of physical activity are more prevalent among culturally diverse people born overseas than among the Australian-born, and likely to be the case elsewhere, strategies to increase the cultural diversity of participants and to ensure samples are more reflective of the current population are paramount.[32]

In an Australian study exploring the impact of the environment on physical activity of older people from different ethnic backgrounds, the challenges of recruitment and retention of older people were specifically examined.[33] The impact of dominant white and Western ideologies on research approaches and methodologies, as well as power relations between researchers and participants, were identified as important considerations when conducting research with culturally diverse groups. These issues tend to perpetuate the marginalization and exclusion of culturally diverse people in research. Using key informants from the respective communities and bilingual researchers, building trusting relationships, using participatory research methods and critical reflexivity are all strategies that can enable more effective recruitment and retention, and therefore greater diversity of participant samples.

People have different conceptualizations and understandings about physical activity – its definition, purpose and importance – as well as there being different cultural norms about what is acceptable (e.g. quantity and type).[26] For example, some older people may not perceive themselves as doing any physical activity and self-report as such. However, this would be an inaccurate reflection of many older people from culturally diverse backgrounds who, depending on the definition used, may score highly if daily housework and caring for grandchildren are included.

Overall, people from culturally diverse backgrounds tend to have fewer years of formal education, limited English-language proficiency, lower health literacy and migrant histories which will significantly shape understanding, beliefs and attitudes about physical activity and research as well as physical activity histories. Greater levels of informal family and caring responsibilities will also impact on opportunities to be physically active. And barriers for being physically active may relate to stigmas about one's public appearance (e.g. not being acceptable to wear active clothing, exposing skin or being hot and sweaty).

All these factors have significant implications for measuring physical activity (e.g. selection of culturally appropriate tools), recruitment and retention, as well as for the appropriate design and targeting of interventions to promote more activity amongst older people from culturally and linguistically diverse backgrounds.

Measurement: addressing validity and reliability

To determine whether – and how – physical activity interventions are impacting on older people's behaviour and ultimately their health, we need suitable measurement tools. Physical activity behaviour in older people has been examined using both direct and indirect data collection methodologies. Broadly speaking, the approaches used for older people mirror those outlined in Chapter 18 of this book. As do the methodological issues common to physical activity research in general (Chapters 5–21). These include: small samples, lack of detail regarding the intervention, variable means of recording physical activity behaviour, absence of intention to treat analyses and limited follow-up periods.

However, there are particular challenges in ensuring the internal and external validity of measurement tools for older people. A summary of the key issues follows. Whilst a statistical or clinical benefit may be reported, there is often little reference to whether national guideline criteria have been met, i.e. whether the physical activity behaviour level is sufficient to produce health benefits. Indeed, several studies with older people may have reported statistically significant differences between intervention and control groups, but the additional amount of physical activity achieved may be relatively modest. Chase and colleagues highlight the importance of assessing clinically meaningful changes, such as improvements in physical function.[34]

Secondly, there are concerns about generalizing findings from studies of the adult population to older people. Hillsdon and colleagues' review of physical activity interventions contained only four studies that focused on older people.[35] Whilst 10 studies included people 60 or above, aggregated findings were presented, preventing any discrimination of differences amongst different subgroups of older participants. Stewart et al.[36] in the Community Healthy Activities Model Program for Seniors (CHAMPS) study did compare outcomes between those above and below 75 years old and found no difference in outcomes between these two age groups, but greater attention to assessing potential subgroup variation within the older population is vital.

Thirdly, there has been relatively limited use of data collection instruments specifically designed for older people. Many studies use instruments designed for the general adult population. For example, the International Physical Activity Questionnaire (IPAQ) has been widely used, both in surveillance and intervention studies.[37] The strength of the IPAQ is that findings can be compared against recommendations and across age groups. It also benefits from the inclusion of specific questions on walking, probably the most common form of activity amongst older people.[38] Whilst questions refer to vigorous household activities, such as gardening or yard work, there is specific exclusion of other household activities. This means that a key activity source amongst older people may not be systematically captured. Such questionnaires may also fail to capture lower-intensity physical activity, the type often seen in older adults.[39] For specific monitoring of the older population, it is important to use instruments shown to be valid and reliable for use with this population group.

Indirect measurement

To date, relatively few instruments have been developed for use with older people.[40] These include the Physical Activity Scale for the Elderly (PASE),[41] the Yale Physical Activity Survey,[42] the Zutphen Physical Activity Questionnaire,[43] the Modified Baecke Questionnaire for Older Adults[44] and the Community Health Activities Model

Program for Seniors (CHAMPS) Questionnaire.[45] These instruments have been psychometrically tested and are reasonably robust, but have limitations with regard to their validity, reliability and responsivity. A review of physical activity tools suitable for fall prevention trials found that none of the available tools was wholly suitable.[46] The authors recommended that new tools be developed, or the more robust ones, such as the CHAMPS questionnaire, be further developed. Two recent systematic reviews provide extensive discussion of the limitations of currently available self-report instruments for older people.[47,48]

The heterogeneous nature of the older population makes measurement challenging even when age-relevant tools are used. Disability and impairments associated with chronic disease can influence the conduct of physical activity and the reporting of its duration and intensity. For example, the absolute intensity of activity measured on a scale may not reflect the relative underlying capacity of the person to exercise. It can take longer for a mobility-impaired person to walk a set distance and it can involve more effort. This means that their reporting of such activity can be skewed to make it appear to be longer and of greater intensity than in a healthy person. Thus it is preferable to focus on the frequency of physical activity rather than duration or intensity. Alternatively, data could be adjusted according to the person's functional status.

There is the potential that routine, incidental activity may not be captured. People find it more difficult to recall such activity, whereas less regular bouts of more intense activity are more likely to be remembered. Researchers recently developed an incidental and planned exercise tool (IPEQ), particularly for older people, to address this concern.[49] The tool has reasonable criterion validity and has the potential to be particularly useful in studies that are aiming to move people from sedentary behaviour to some physical activity.[50]

To date, only the CHAMPS and the IPEQ have been assessed for responsivity, that is, the degree of responsiveness to change when an intervention is undertaken. Using data from a controlled trial of a fall prevention physical activity intervention, Merom and colleagues tested the responsiveness of the IPEQ.[50] The responsiveness index was calculated using baseline and 12-month follow-up data (the mean IPEQ change in the intervention group divided by the SD of the mean change in the control group). The responsiveness index was 0.45 for planned walking and 0.34 for combined moderate and vigorous physical activity (planned exercise, walking for exercise, walking for errands and outdoor chores).

Self-report measures, even those that have been validated, are impeded by recall and over-reporting bias. Further, the instruments have often been designed for males living in Western cultures, so their appropriateness for not only older people, but women and those from culturally and linguistically diverse backgrounds, is unclear.[51] Evaluation of the impact of future programmes clearly requires accurate measurement of physical activity behaviour, using measures appropriate for a multicultural older population.

Direct measurement tools

Given the limitations of self-report tools, there has been a move towards alternative, more direct measurement of physical activity. Whilst measures such as calorimetry and doubly labelled water techniques are usually infeasible in community implementation trials, using activity monitors may enable researchers to measure physical activity more directly. The past decade has seen technological advances in the production of 'wearable' devices and there are many products available, not only for research purposes, but also in the public domain. These so-called objective measurement tools may remove self-reporting bias, but are not without their own technical and logistical challenges. This section will focus on factors related to using activity tracking tools in older people.

Accelerometry (or actigraphy) can be used to quantify physical activity in daily life.[52] As with self-report measures, the key issue is whether the instrument is suitably calibrated for use in older people. Research is gathering about how to produce appropriate algorithms for older people, where to place the device and the timeframe required for data collection to enable accurate recording of different types of activity. Most commonly the hip or lower back is used for single-site monitoring. The lower-back position may be more accurate than other positions to detect falls, bodily orientation, gait characteristics, low intensity and transitional activity.[53] Trunk accelerometry, using a lower-back-positioned instrument, can identify different forms of activity.[54] It can also quantify spatiotemporal gait characteristics.[55]

Day-to-day variation in the quantity of physical activity is well acknowledged.[56] To obtain reliable estimates of the amount and type of activity, repeated measurement across different days is required. Researchers have been exploring measurement regimes to achieve reliable estimates of the frequency, duration and intensity of a range of activities.[56] To date, few studies have included older people and those that did limited data collection to daytime.[57] For older people night-time activities could provide additional information, given the potential for increased falls risk.[58] Recently, van Schooten et al.,[59] measured total duration of locomotion, lying, sitting, standing and shuffling, movement intensity, the number of locomotion bouts per day, the median and maximum locomotion bout duration within a day and the number of transitions to standing. They determined that a trunk accelerometer should be worn for at least 2 days to accurately measure activity (ICC $\geq$ 0.7), with lying and median duration locomotion bouts requiring up to 5 days' measurement. Such an approach is recommended for studies of older people with a range of mobility capacities, to capture the lower-intensity patterns that could be indicative of more than simply sedentary behaviour. The quantity and quality of gait and of sit-to-stand and stand-to-sit movements are associated with mortality and fall risk.[60]

There is general agreement that a cut-off point of 100 counts per minute can be used to define sedentary behaviour, but for different intensity physical activities, no consensus has been reached.[61] Few studies have calibrated activity in older people.[62] Copland and Dale conducted a calibration study where participants walked on a treadmill at 3.2 km/h (3.7 METs).[63] A good correlation was found with oxygen consumption for a medium intensity cut-point of 1,040 counts per minute. Matthews proposed a cut-point of 760 counts per minute,[61] based upon calibration studies across a range of moderate-intensity domestic and leisure activities in community-living adults.

Pedometry

Pedometry can also be used to quantify the volume of physical activity. Pedometers don't measure activity intensity but they capture both intentional and incidental activity. Pedometers cannot be worn during some activities, such as swimming, but data imputation is possible.

Although '10,000 steps' has been used in social marketing campaigns, there are no national guidelines on daily step counts for older people. Tudor-Locke and colleagues reported normative data for healthy older adults ranging from 2,000 to 9,000 steps, reflecting the heterogenous nature of this cohort.[64] Tudor-Locke and colleagues estimated, based on adult cadence data, that older people should do 3,000 steps at moderate intensity, in addition to 5,000 steps from incidental activity.[65] The latter value is likely to be lower in those who have a disability or chronic condition that impedes mobility.

The lack of guidelines hampers interpretation of data. However, the importance of clinical meaningfulness is reiterated. Luna de Melo and colleagues found that greater functional fitness was associated with high amounts of walking (> 6,500 steps/day) but not with smaller amounts,[66] so clinically relevant doses need to be considered.

Combining tools

Clearly both indirect and direct measures have strengths and weaknesses. The choice of tool(s) will be guided by the research question, study design considerations and pragmatism. For example, walking is a common activity in older people, but given varying functional capacities, it may be preferable to assess walking speed rather than simply ask about 'walking'.[67] This focus makes accelerometry preferable to pedometry or self-report. Studies show that accelerometers are good for measuring sedentary, walking, moderate and vigorous activity.[68] Capturing and distinguishing low-intensity activities with low ambulatory component and low frequency gait movement, such as Tai Chi, Pilates, balance activities, requires further consideration. Adding a 24-hour diary to the data collection suite may be useful here.[50]

Output: reporting met·minutes with older people

It is becoming more usual to measure physical activity as volume. Here, frequency and duration are multiplied then the sum multiplied by a measure of intensity, the MET, to give volume in MET·min/wk.[69] Moderate activity is equivalent to about 3 METs so that a MET·min·wk^{-1} value of between 500 and 1,000 relates to the physical activity recommendation of 150 plus minutes of moderate/vigorous intensity activity additional to incidental activity.

The authors of the American and the Canadian physical activity recommendations highlight the importance of using relative intensity with regard to older people.[14,70] In absolute terms, moderate-intensity activities are defined as 3.0 to 5.9 METs. The American guidelines note that intensities in this range may actually be vigorous or physiologically infeasible for older people with low levels of fitness, and recommend intensity be defined relative to fitness. That is, the intensity is expressed in terms of a proportion (%) of an individual person's maximal heart rate, heart rate reserve or aerobic capacity reserve ($\dot{V}O_2$). The American guidelines define relatively moderate-intensity activity as 40–59% – and relatively vigorous-intensity activity as 60–84% – of reserve.

The use of relative intensity allows comparison to other adults. Performance time measured using a relative intensity marker such as $\dot{V}O_2$ max produces similar results to younger adults.[71] Paterson and Warburton refer to moderate walking at 3 mph as being of 3.3 METs intensity, with vigorous walking at 4 mph being equivalent to 4.2 METs.[14] Paterson and Warburton refer to their dose-related recommendation for older people:[14]

> Physical activity (above baseline 'normal' daily activity levels) at an intensity of moderate to moderately vigorous aerobic (endurance) activity (3.3 to 4.2 METS;

3–4 mph walk; >50% $\dot{V}O_2$max), with a total weekly volume of 150–180 min/wk (3 hours at moderate pace or 2.5 hours of a more vigorous 'brisk' walking, or other types of aerobic activities, with each physical activity session of greater than 10 minutes) and, a gain of 0.5 MET (~2 ml·kg^{-1}·min^{-1}) in cardiorespiratory fitness.

(p. 18)

A caveat to the comparability of younger and older adults is that any multiplier between moderate- and vigorous-intensity activity is likely to be less for older adults, as generally speaking there is a much narrower range between what constitutes moderate and what constitutes vigorous activity for them.

The summary checklist below (Box 23.1) for researchers is in addition to the general principles that apply when working with any group, such as ethical issues, potential risks, discomfort, inconvenience to the participants and potential benefits to the individual participants.

Box 23.1 Checklist for researchers intending to work with older people

- Have the tools selected been validated for use with older people? Are they appropriate? Are they overly burdensome?
- What factors might influence how older people engage with my research? Who isn't represented?
- How might the research findings be explained?
- How can my research better include the voices, experiences and values of older people?
- What ageist assumptions am I making? Are all older people vulnerable and inactive?

Future directions

The 2010 Technical Review of Physical Activity Guidelines in the UK noted the following research gaps:[72]

- Effective promotion and targeting of physical activity for older adults;
- The benefits of a long-term exercise referral programme;
- Socio-environmental determinants of physical activity participation of older adults who live in institutions and those living in rural areas.

This chapter has highlighted some of the issues that researchers need to be aware of and provided some guidance on how to optimize engagement of older people. Further research to confirm the impact of engagement strategies in different contexts and settings is required.

Because research programmes have tended to be short-term, we have limited evidence about the longer-term benefits of physical activity programmes. There is also limited evidence for the sustainability of physical activity behaviour change and associated health outcomes over time. Recent reviews of physical activity programmes for older people have reported that the impact is often short term and relatively small.[73] Notable exceptions are the CHAMPS study,[36] which had a one-year follow-up and a New Zealand home-based falls prevention exercise programme that had a two-year follow-up period.[74] The LIFE-P study evaluated a 12-month programme and reported higher physical performance outcomes in the intervention group compared to controls at two-year follow-up, although the effect size (0.4) barely reached significance, possibly due to the small sample.[75] A two-year study with older, postmenopausal women (50–65 years old) participating in walking groups reported good levels of compliance with the three miles, three times per week schedule.[76] The relative impact of self-monitoring, phone prompts and incentives on compliance was not reported. We have known for some time that integration of physical activity into one's daily life is key to maintenance,[77] but we need more information about how to support such sustained behaviour change. There is scope for further research in this area.

There remains limited information about those living in institutions and rural areas. A recent review highlighted the paucity of evidence about physical activity interventions in rural communities:[78] more information is needed on contextual and programme characteristics in that setting. There is promising evidence emerging where physical activity has been trialled in aged care facilities,[6] with positive impacts on physical, mental and cognitive function (mobility, agitation, mood) reported. It may not always be practicable to conduct a randomized controlled trial to assess programme impact, but a robust evaluation of an intervention operated as part of a facility's lifestyle programme would be valuable. An illustrative example is given in Box 23.2.

This chapter highlights that these groups, given access to tailored programmes, are as likely to benefit as other older people. The challenges are likely to be organizational: discussion of this topic is beyond the scope of this chapter.

Given the prevalence of sedentary behaviour amongst older people, a focus on moving people to become more active is critical. The impact on functionality and associated independence has both individual and societal implications. Mobility can be maintained by regular activity such as walking,[79] yet there has been limited intervention to reduce the risk of frailty. In recent times there has been a move to care for people in their homes to extend independence and prevent admission to aged care facilities. However, there is little evidence that the home care setting has been used to introduce activity programmes that aim to promote functional health.[80]

Box 23.2 Case study of physical activity promotion in an aged care facility

A lifestyle and wellbeing programme was conducted at a residential aged care facility operated by a not-for-profit organization. The Life in Motion (LIM) programme used information and communication technologies (ICT) to improve the health and wellbeing of older people living in a New South Wales aged care facility. The study explored the physical, mental and social health benefits of a three-month pilot physical activity programme using Xbox Kinect™.

A range of appropriate games were identified and adapted where necessary to enable participants to play. Lifestyle and wellbeing staff facilitated the sessions and provided prompting, physical and social support to participants. Participating residents had a range of physical and cognitive limitations.

The staff reported some functional improvement in participating residents, notably in balance and upper-limb movement. Progression through the activities produced physical and cognitive benefits. The sessions also afforded great social interaction and engagement. Participants enjoyed the sessions and were happy to continue attending, engaging with fellow residents to have fun. There were cognitive gains in terms of concentration, stimulation and repetition during the sessions. Some reminiscence occurred about previous sporting and daily activities. Maintained engagement and participation was achieved.

These data, albeit limited, illustrate that the introduction of the LIM programme decreased sedentary behaviour amongst residents.

Conclusion

There is compelling evidence for the benefits of exercise across an array of biopsychosocial health outcomes in older people. The challenge for researchers is that a diverse collection of tools have been used for measuring activity types and health-related outcome variables, making cross-study comparison problematic when trying to determine what methods to use to conduct further research.

Such measurement limitations impact on our ability to accurately measure physical activity prevalence and assess the effectiveness of physical activity interventions across settings and among different cohorts of older people. Measurement tools have given us some understanding of physical activity patterns and barriers to physical activity. There is an ongoing need for methodologies that allow researchers to capture why people do maintain physical activity behaviours, so that this information can be used in motivating others whose health may be at risk from their sedentary lifestyles.

Future research will need to systematically employ well-validated, age- and culturally appropriate measurement instruments. In order to contextualize observed changes in an individual's behaviour, researchers and evaluators need to incorporate both individual-level data collection and ecological-level data to determine mediators and predictors operating across individual, societal and system levels of influence.

References

1 Pate R, Pratt, M, Blair SN, Haskell WL, Macera CA, Bouchard C, et al. Physical activity and public health: a recommendation from the centers for disease control and prevention and the American college of sports medicine. *J Am Med Assoc.* 1995; **273**:402–7.
2 Inouye S, Studenski S, Tinetti ME, Kuchel GA. Geriatric syndromes; clinical, research and policy implications of a core geriatric concept. *J Am Geriatr Soc.* 2007; **55**:780–91.
3 Cameron I, Gillespie LD, Robertson MC, Murray GR, Hill KD, Cumming RG, Kerse N. Interventions for preventing falls in older people in care facilities and hospitals. *Cochrane Database Syst Rev* [Internet] 2012; Issue 12. Art. No.: CD005465. DOI: 10.1002/14651858. CD005465.pub3.

4 Gillespie L, Robertson MC, Gillespie WJ, Sherrington C, Gates S, Clemson LM, Lamb SE. Interventions for preventing falls in older people living in the community. *Cochrane Database Syst Rev* [Internet] 2012; Issue 9. Art. No.: CD007146. DOI: 10.1002/14651858. CD007146.pub3.

5 Groot C, Hooghiemstra AM, Raijmakers PG, van Berckel BN, Scheltens P, Scherder EJ, et al. The effect of physical activity on cognitive function in patients with dementia: a meta-analysis of randomized control trials. *Ageing Res Rev.* 2016; **31**(25):13–23.

6 Brett L, Traynor V, Stapley P. Effects of physical exercise on health and well-being of individuals living with a dementia in nursing homes: a systematic review. *J Am Med Dir Assoc.* 2016; **17**(2):104–16.

7 Evans W. Exercise training guidelines for the elderly. *Med Sci Sports Exerc.* 1999; **31**(1):12–7.

8 World Health Organisation. Heidelberg guidelines for promoting physical activities among older person. *J Ageing Phys Act.* 1997; **5**:2–8.

9 Hill R, Brown WJ. Older Australians and physical activity guidelines: do we know how many are meeting guidelines? *Australas J Ageing.* 2012; **31**(4):208–17.

10 Australian Bureau of Statistics. *Australian health survey: physical activity, 2011–12.* Canberra: ABS, Australian Bureau of Statistics; 2013.

11 Nelson M, Rejeski W, Blair SN, et al. Physical activity and public health in older adults: recommendation from the American college of sports medicine and the American heart association. *Circulation.* 2007; **116**:1094–105.

12 Department of Health. UK physical activity guidelines. Fact sheet 5: older adults (65+ years) 2011. Available from: www.gov.uk/government/publications/uk-physical-activity-guidelines

13 Canadian Society of Exercise Physiology. Canadian physical activity guidelines for older adults: 65 years and older 2011. Available from: http://www.csep.ca/cmfiles/guidelines/ canadianphysicalactivityguidelinesstatements_e_2012.pdf

14 Paterson D, Warburton DER. Physical activity and functional limitations in older adults: a systematic review related to Canada's physical activity guidelines. *Int J Behav Nutr Phys Act.* 2010; **7**:38. Available from: www.ijbnpa.org/content/7/1/38

15 Ministry of Health. *Guidelines on physical activity for older people* (aged 65 years and over). Wellington: Ministry of Health; 2013, HP5612.

16 Sims J, Hill K, Hunt S, Haralambous B. Physical activity recommendations for older Australians. *Australas J Ageing.* 2010; **29**(2):81–7.

17 Al Sayah F, Johnson ST, Vallance J. Health literacy, pedometer, and self-reported walking among older adults. *Am J Public Health.* 2016; **106**(2):327–33.

18 Cohen-Mansfield J, Marx M, Guralnik J. Motivators and barriers to exercise in an older community-dwelling population. *J Aging Phys Act.* 2003; **11**:242–53.

19 King A, Rijeski W, Buchner D. Physical activity interventions targeting older adults: a critical review and recommendations. *Am J Prev Med.* 1998; **15**:316–33.

20 King A. Interventions to promote physical activity by older adults. *J Gerontol A Biol Sci Med Sci.* 2001; **56**:36–46.

21 Burton E, Farrier K, Lewin G, Pettigrew S, Hill AM, Airey P, et al. Motivators and barriers for older people participating in resistance training: a systematic review. *J Aging Phys Act.* 2017; **25**:311–24.

22 Baert V, Gorus E, Mets T, Geerts C, Bautmans I. Motivators and barriers for physical activity in the oldest old: a systematic review. *Ageing Res Rev.* 2011; **10**(4):464–74.

23 Burbank P, Riebe D. *Promoting exercise and behaviur change in older adults: interventions with the transtheoretical model.* New York: Springer; 2002.

24 Finlay L. 'Outing' the researcher: the provenance, process, and practice of reflexivity. *Qual Health Res.* 2002; **12**:531–45.

25 McMurdo M. Clinical research must include more older people. *Br Med J.* 2013; **346**:27.

26 Bird S, Radermacher H, Feldman S, Sims J, Kurowski W, Browning C, Thomas S. Factors influencing the physical activity levels of older people from culturally diverse communities: an Australian experience. *Ageing Soc.* 2009; **8**(Special Issue):1275–94.

27 World Health Organisation WHO. Checklist of essential features of age-friendly cities. Available from: www.who.int/ageing/age_friendly_cities_material/en/

28 Cerin E, Nathan A, van Cauwenberg J, Barnett DW, Barnett A, on behalf of the Council on Environment and Physical Activity (CEPA) – Older Adults working group. The neighbourhood physical environment and active travel in older adults: a systematic review and meta-analysis. *Int J Behav Nutr Phys Act.* 2017; **14**:15.

29 Van Dyck D, Cerin E, De Bourdeaudhuij I, Salvo D, Christiansen LB, Macfarlane D, et al. Moderating effects of age, gender and education on the associations of perceived neighborhood environment attributes with accelerometer-based physical activity: the IPEN adult study. *Health Place.* 2015; **36**:65–73.

30 Bhopal R, Sheikh A. Inclusion and exclusion of ethnic-minority populations in research on the effectiveness of interventions. *Divers Equal Health Care.* 2009; **6**:223–6.

31 Australian Institute of Health and Welfare. Ageing. *AIHW.* 2017 [cited 2017 May 16]; Available from: www.aihw.gov.au/ageing/

32 Holdenson Z, Catanzariti L, Phillips G, Waters AM. *A picture of diabetes in overseas-born Australians. AIHW Bulletin. Cat. no. AUS 38.* Canberra: Australian Institute of Health and Welfare; 2003.

33 Feldman S, Radermacher H, Bird S, Browning C, Thomas S. Challenges of recruitment and retention of older people from culturally diverse backgrounds in research. *Ageing Soc.* 2008; **28**(4):473–93.

34 Chase J, Phillips LJ, Brown M. Physical activity intervention effects on physical function among community-dwelling older adults: a systematic review and meta-analysis. *J Aging Phys Act.* 2017; **25**:149–70.

35 Hillsdon M, Foster C, Thorogood M. Interventions for promoting physical activity. *Cochrane Database Syst Rev.* 2005; (1).

36 Stewart A, Mills K, King A, et al. CHAMPS physical activity questionnaire for older adults outcomes for interventions. *Med Sci Sports Exerc.* 2001; **33**:1126–41.

37 Craig C, Marshall AL, Sjostrom M, Bauman AE, Booth ML, Ainsworth BE, et al. International physical activity questionnaire: 12-country reliability and validity. *Med Sci Sports Exerc.* 2003; **35**(8):1381–95.

38 Lim K, Taylor L. Factors associated with physical activity among older people–a population-based study. *Prev Med.* 2005; **40**:33–40.

39 Tudor-Locke C, Myers AM. Challenges and opportunities for measuring physical activity in sedentary adults. *Sports Med.* 2001; **31**(2):91–100.

40 Washburn R. Assessment of physical activity in older adults. *Res Quar Exerc Sports.* 2000; **71**:S79–S88.

41 Washburn R, Smith KW, Jette AM, Janney CA. The physical activity scale for the elderly (PASE): development and evaluation. *J Clin Epidemiol.* 1993; **46**:153–62.

42 DiPietro L, Caspersen CJ, Ostfeld AM, Nadel ER. A survey for assessing physical activity among older adults. *Med Sci Sports Exerc.* 1993; **25**:628–42.

43 Caspersen CJ, Bloemberg BPM, Saris WHM, Merritt RK, Kromhout D. The prevalence of selected physical activities and their relation with coronary heart disease risk factors in elderly men: the Zutphen study. *Am J Epidemiol.* 1991; **5**:116–9.

44 Baecke JAH, Burema J, Britjers JER. A short questionnaire of the measurement of habitual physical activity in epidemiological studies. *Am J Clin Nutr.* 1982; **36**:936–42.

45 Stewart A, Mills A, King AC, Haskell WL, Gills D, Ritter PL. CHAMPS Physical activity questionnaire for older adults: outcome for interventions. *Med Sci Sports Exerc.* 2001; **33**:1126–41.

46 Jorstad-Stein EC, Hauer K, Becker C, Bonnefoy M, Nakash RA, Skelton DA, et al. Suitability of physical activity questionnaires for older adults in fall-prevention trials: a systematic review. *J Aging Phys Act.* 2005; **13**:461–81.

47 Forsen L, Loland MW, Vuillemin A, et al. Self-administered physical activity questionnaires for elderly. *Sports Med.* 2010; **40**(7):601–23.

48 Krol-Zielinska M, Ciekot M. Assessing physical activity in the elderly: a comparative study of most popular questionnaires. *Trends Sport Sci.* 2015; **3**(22):133–44.

49 Dalbaere K, Hauer, K, Lord, S. Evaluation of the Incidental and Planned Activity Questionnaire (IPAQ) for older people. *Br J Sports Med.* 2010; **44**:1029–34.

50 Merom D, Delbaere K, Cumming R, Voukelatos A, Rissel C, van der Ploeg HP, Lord SR. Incidental and planned exercise questionnaire for seniors: validity and responsiveness. *Med Sci Sports Exerc.* 2014; **46**(5):947–54.

51 Seefeldt V, Malina RM, Clark MA. Factors affecting levels of physical activity in adults. *Sports Med.* 2002; **32**(3):143–68.

52 Taraldsen K, Chastin SFM, Riphagen II, Vereijken B, Helbostad JL. Physical activity monitoring by use of accelerometerbased body-worn sensors in older adults: a systematic literature review of current knowledge and applications. *Maturitas.* 2012; **71**(1):13–9.

53 Sumukadas D, Laidlaw S, Witham MD. Using the RT3 accelerometer to measure everyday activity in functionally impaired older people. *Aging Clin Exp Res.* 2008; **20**(1):15–8.

54 de Groot S, Nieuwenhuizen MG. Validity and reliability of measuring activities, movement intensity and energy expenditure with the DynaPort MoveMonitor. *Med Eng Phys.* 2013; **35**(10):1499–505.

55 Houdijk H, Appelman M, Van Velzen JM, Van der Woude LH, Van Bennekom CA. Validity of dynaPort gaitMonitor for assessment of spatiotemporal parameters in amputee gait. *J Rehab Res Dev.* 2008; **45**(9):1335–42.

56 Hart TL, Swartz A, Cashin S, Strath S. How many days of monitoring predict physical activity and sedentary behaviour in older adults? *Int J Behav Nutr Phys Act.* 2011; **8**(1):62.

57 Nicolai S, Benzinger P, Skelton DA, Aminian K, Becker C, Lindemann U. Day-to-day variability of physical activity of older adults living in the community. *J Aging Phys Act.* 2010; **18**(1):75–86.

58 Lehtola S, Koistinen P, Luukinen H. Falls and injurious falls late in home-dwelling life. *Arch Gerontol Geriatr.* 2006; **42**(2):217–24.

59 van Schooten K, Rispens SM, Elders PJM, Lips P, van Dieën JH, Pijnappels M. Assessing physical activity in older adults: required days of trunk accelerometer measurements for reliable estimation *J Ageing Phys Act.* 2015; **23**(1):9–17.

60 Studenski S, Perera S, Patel K, Rosano C, Faulkner K, Inzitari M. Gait speed and survival in older adults. *J Am Med Assoc.* 2011; **305**(1):50–8.

61 Matthews C. Calibration of accelerometer output for adults. *Med Sci Sports Exerc.* 2005; **37**(Suppl 11):S512–S22.

62 Strath S, Pfeiffer KA, Whitt-Glover MC. Accelerometer use with children, older adults, and adults with functional limitations. *Med Sci Sports Exerc.* 2012; **44**:S77–85.

63 Copland J, Dale EW. Accelerometer assessment of physical activity in active healthy older adults. *J Ageing Phys Act.* 2009; **17**:17–30.

64 Tudor-Locke C, Bassett DR Jr. How many steps/day are enough? Preliminary pedometer indices for public health. *Sports Med.* 2004; **34**(1):1–8.

65 Tudor-Locke C, Craig CL, Aoyage Y, Bell RC, Croteau KA, de Bourdeauduij I, et al. How many steps/day are enough? For older adults and special populations. *Int J Behav Nutr Phys Act* [Internet]. 2011; **8**. Available from: www.ijbnpa.org/content/8/1/80

66 Luna de Melo L, Menec, VH, Ready, AE. Relationship of functional fitness with daily steps in community-dwelling older adults. *Geriatr Phys Ther.* 2014; **37**:116–20.

67 van Holle V, De Bourdeaudhuij I, Deforche B, van Cauwenberg J, van Dyck D. Assessment of physical activity in older Belgian adults: validity and reliability of an adapted interview version of the long International Physical Activity Questionnaire (IPAQ-L). *BMC Public Health* [Internet]. 2015; **15**:433.

68 Klenk J, Bichele G, Lindemann U, Kaufmann S, Peter R, Laszlo R, et al. Concurrent validity of activPAL and activPAL3 accelerometers in older adults. *J Aging Phys Act.* 2016; **24**:444–50.

69 Ainsworth B, Haskell WL, Herrmann SD, et al. Compendium of physical activities: a second update of codes and MET values. *Med Sci Sports Exerc.* 2011; **43**:1575–81.

70 Office of Disease Prevention and Health Promotion. Appendix 1. Translating scientific evidence about total amount and intensity of physical activity into guidelines. 2008. Available from: https://health.gov/paguidelines/guidelines/Appendix1.aspx

71 Poulin M, Paterson D, Cunningham D, Govindasamy D. Endurance training of elderly men: responses to submaximal exercise. *J Appl Phys.* 1992; **73**:453–7.

72 Bull F. *Expert working groups. Physical activity guidelines in the U.K.: review and recommendations.* Loughborough: School of Sport, Exercise and Health Sciences, Loughborough University; 2010.

73 van der Bij A, Laurent M, et al. Effectiveness of physical activity interventions for older adults. *Am J Prev Med.* 2002; **22**(2):120–33.

74 Campbell AJ, Robertson MC, Gardner MM, Norton RN, Buchner DM. Falls prevention over 2 years: a randomised controlled trial in women 80 years and older. *Age Ageing.* 1999; **28**:513–8.

75 Rejeski W, Marsh A, Chmelo E, Prescott A, Dobrosielski M, Walkup MP, et al. The Lifestyle Interventions and Independence for Elders Pilot (LIFE-P): 2-year follow-up. *J Gerontol Ser A.* 2009; **64**:462–7.

76 Kriska A, Bayles C, et al. A randomized exercise trial in older women: increased activity over two years and the factors associated with compliance. *Med Sci Sports Exerc.* 1986; **18**(5):557–62.

77 King A. Community intervention for promotion of physical activity and fitness. *Exerc Sports Sci Rev.* 1991; **19**:211–60.

78 Moore M, Warburton J, O'Halloran PD, Shields N, Kingsley M. Effective community-based physical activity interventions for older adults living in rural and regional areas: a systematic review. *J Ageing Phys Act.* 2016; **24**:158–67.

79 Field B, Cochrane T, Davey R, Kinfu Y. Walking up to one hour per week maintains mobility as older women age: findings from an Australian longitudinal study. *J Ageing Phys Act.* 2017; **25**:269–76.

80 Burton E, Lewin G, Boldy D. A systematic review of physical activity programs for older people receiving home care services. *J Aging Phys Act.* 2015; **23**:460–70.

81 World Health Organisation. *Global recommendations on physical activity for health.* Geneva, Switzerland: World Health Organization Press; 2010.

24 Working with Indigenous and other cultural groups

Aunty Kerrie Doyle and Elizabeth Pressick

Aims of the chapter

Given the diversity of human societies and cultures, researchers need to be cognizant of cultural issues and practises of the groups with whom they wish to research. Being aware of such matters can facilitate the development of good working relationships, whilst a failure to do so may present barriers. In this chapter we use the example of working with Indigenous Australians and Indigenous Australian communities to illustrate some of the issues to which researchers should be aware. Whilst each culture will have different specific practices, being aware of such cultural matters, such as those presented here, will enable the researcher to be better informed of the type of cultural issues and practices that they should themselves become familiar with as they prepare to work with other cultural groups.

The following chapter outlines the considerations that need to be made by researchers when working with one specific cultural group, Indigenous Australians, and is therefore presented as an example and awareness raiser. The issues raised within this chapter should thereby sensitize researchers to the considerations that need to be made when working with any cultural group. Moreover the principles raised in this chapter should be vigorously applied to any research that involves working with cultural groups, regardless of the culture.

The chapter closes with the inclusion of guidance provided by the World Health Authority for working in such contexts.

Researching in Indigenous communities

Aboriginal and Torres Strait Islanders are the Indigenous peoples of Australia (hereafter called 'Indigenous Australians'). As a population group, Indigenous Australians suffer a substantial gap in life expectancy compared to non-Indigenous-Australians.[1,2] The urgency to close the gap has led to the ongoing growth in multi-disciplinary research in Indigenous communities, making Indigenous people some of the most researched of all people.[3] In order to assert sovereignty in the research process, Indigenous communities now require research to have an *Indigenist* focus that resists any ongoing colonizing influences, and facilitates self-determination and healing.[4] This support will allow Indigenous communities to create and control research processes that self-define their relationships with others and the environment.[5] For researchers to be successful in their projects requires an understanding of how to apply the processes of Indigenist research, and engage with Indigenist knowledges.

Indigenous knowledges in Indigenist research

Indigenous knowledges are generally accepted as the distinct ideas, information and skills held by Indigenous people, and are usually contrasted or compared with Western scientific knowledge,[6] although definitions are highly contested.[4] Castree et al.[7] explain three characteristics that differentiate Indigenist knowledges from mainstream, or Western, knowledge (Table 24.1).

Indigenous knowledges are often presented and perceived as opposite to Western knowledge, although the utility of this stance has been questioned.[8-10] Dei et al.[11] conceptualize Indigenous knowledge as:

> a body of knowledge associated with the long-term occupancy of a certain place. This knowledge refers to traditional norms and social values, as well as to mental constructs that guide, organize, and regulate the people's ways of living and making sense of their world. It is the sum of the experience and knowledge of a given social group, and forms the basis of decision making in the face of challenges both familiar and unfamiliar. It is accumulated by the social group through both historical and current experience. This body of knowledge is diverse and complex given the histories, cultures, and lived realities of people.
>
> (p. 6)

In Australia, the range of definitions of Indigenous knowledge reinforces the diversity across and within Indigenous people and knowledges.[11-13] The diversity amongst Indigenous communities reinforces the complexity involved in cross-cultural research, where outcomes usually need to be expressed in Western terms. For this reason, both Indigenous and non-Indigenous researchers need to privilege Indigenous knowledge by making use of Indigenous methodologies in ethical research.

Principles of ethical research in Indigenous communities

There are 14 principles of ethical research with which all researchers need to comply, as described by the Australian Institute of Aboriginal and Torres Strait Islander Studies (AIATSIS) that are widely accepted as the gold standard for directing research

Table 24.1 Characteristics of Indigenist knowledge

	Characteristic	*Example*
1	Context-dependent to locale; adaptable circumstances:	Knowing what animal to hunt, when and where in a changeable environment may not be readily transferred to another geographical area.
2	Shared by individuals and communities:	Oral transmission by stories, songs, dances, or through learning by observing and copying others.
3	Holistic, or embedded in lived experience:	Not readily translated into analytical categories such as economy, ecology, and society.

Note: Adapted from Castree, Kitchin and Rogers (2013),[7] Copyright (2013) Oxford University Press; and Hill et al. (2012),[40] Copyright (2012) Resilience Alliance.

in Indigenous communities. For examples see: Dunbar and Scrimgeour,[14] Lawrance et al.,[15] Ritchie and Janke,[16] Smith,[17] Thomson, Breen, & Chalmers.[18] Even though there is considerable difference in protocols between communities, the AIATSIS principles are based on the United Nations (UN) Declaration of the Rights of Indigenous Peoples (see Coulter[19]), and are considered suitable as the basis for all Indigenist research.

It is inadvisable to attempt to create an Indigenist methodology that fits all 200 distinct nations and knowledges in Indigenous communities in Australia.[20] A point that extends to the wider context, whereby a researcher from a different culture may not be aware of diversity in a group that they may erroneously assume to be a single culture. Even so, there is a need to develop approaches to Indigenist research that challenge the ongoing colonization of Indigenous peoples, communities and knowledges; and are culturally appropriate. The most effective way of ensuring cultural proficiency is to ensure the congruence between core values of the researcher with the researched.

Core values of Indigenist research

According to Denzin and Lincoln,[21] ethical research rests upon the principles of respect, reciprocity and feedback, regardless of the group that is being researched or the method(s) employed. Creating an individualized model for context and place of research for Indigenous researchers is considered de rigour. Smith (1999) considers this to be part of the decolonizing process. This permissions Indigenous researchers such as Bessarab and Ng'andu,[22] Walter and Anderson,[23] West et al.[24] and Doyle et al.[25] to tailor research methodologies to meet the needs of the research project, the community, the research and the host organization, and still meet the requirement to adopt critical theory to local participants to avoid the risk of having the Indigenous person as an outsider "unable to speak for him or herself".[26] These Indigenist methodologies are considered briefly below.

Indigenist research methodologies

Yarning

Bessarab takes the Aboriginal concept of 'yarning', where '(y)arning is an informal conversation that is culturally friendly and recognised by Aboriginal people as meaning to talk about something, someone or provide and receive information' and uses it as a tool for engaging Aboriginal people in conversation.[27] Using yarning builds on oral traditions of 'handing down' information and comfortably sits with Indigenous pedagogy as it is 'relaxed and informal', with diverse types of yarning (collaborative, research topic, social and therapeutic) used in research in various Indigenous issues.[22,27]

Dadirri

Dadirri is the "search for meaning and understanding at a profound level by 'listening with the heart'".[28] West et al.[24] use *Dadirri*, the language of the Daly River mob, the Ngangikurungkurr people of the Northern Territory, to create an Indigenist research model. The *Dadirri* model is a collection of values to inform research practice, and is based on political and critical methodologies such as Freire's transformative education process,[29] and Habermas's theory of communicative action,[30] mixed with critical theory. West et al.,[24] claim this methodology provides a significant framework for Indigenous researchers undertaking liberatory studies that promote change.

nayri kata

The *palawa* people are the Aboriginal people of Tasmania and the words '*nayri kata*' mean 'good numbers' in that language.[23] The *palawa* prefer not to capitalize their words, so lowercase is used in these examples. The *palawa* is Maggie Walter's language group, and she created her model to align with her Indigenist standpoint for research.[23] According to Walter, the *nayri kata* model is a quantitative Indigenous methodology that consists of two key methodological purposes.[23]

The first purpose of *nayri kata* is to generate statistical data through 'an Indigenous lens', to: "privilege Indigenous voices, knowledges, and understandings . . . refuse to take Euro-Australians or their accompanying value systems as the unacknowledged norm . . . and to refute the presumption of Indigenous deficit as a starting point".[23] The second purpose is to "challenge the hegemony of Indigenous statistical practice by exposing the standpoint from which it operates".[23]

Yerin dilly bag model

Doyle et al.,[3] created a model based on the Doyle's language and values. It is a values-based model that offers researchers guidance to cultural proficiency. The word for

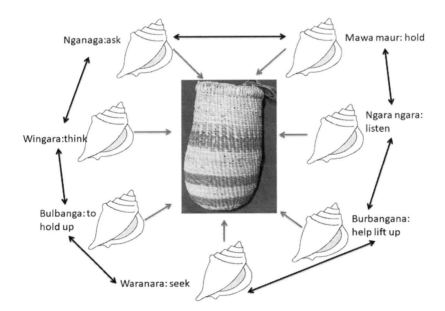

Figure 24.1 Cyclic nature of the Dilly Bag Model, describing the links to the values of this research. Note: the dilly bag in this figure was gifted to the author by Aunty Evonne Munuyunu from Miwatj mob at Yirrkala, NT, and used with permission to demonstrate respect for elders.

Table 24.2 Yerin Dilly Bag Values in practice

Mawa maur: hold	Waranara: seek	Ngara ngara: listen	Nganaga: ask
'Holding' means that the information shared between people is regarded and kept as sacred. Researchers only 'hold' the knowledge; they cannot keep it, or own it. An example of *holding* in the dilly bag model is when an Aboriginal person shares their story. That story, either positive or negative, is held, and is not used to stigmatize or sensationalize an issue in community. It demonstrates respect and engenders trust in the researcher, as to 'hold' a community, person or issue is to communicate to the participants the importance of the individual or group to the researcher.	To 'seek' means to actively look for an item of interest, or path. In a research setting, it means to look in order to learn. Aboriginal people often learn by observation, and 'too many worry' questions will cause a researcher to be avoided. Seeking makes sure the behaviours of the research are in harmony with the Indigenous community.	'Listening' is important – not just for what a researcher might hear, but also for that which is not heard. Silence is not always uncomfortable for Indigenous people, and a researcher needs to know when to hold, when to seek, and when to listen. Respect is the core value informing listening.	Oftimes, non-Indigenous people 'walk on eggshells' around Indigenous people. Even Indigenous people on other groups' country will be reticent about 'big-noting' themselves. Putting 'ask' in your research dilly bag means that researchers have enough humility to recognize they are not the keepers of all knowledge, that researching in Indigenous communities is a privileged position. One way to make sure a researcher does not breech cultural and a community protocol is to ask for cultural assistance. To ask someone for clarity regarding an issue in a respectful manner is to demonstrate respect for that culture. Asking the Indigenous people in the research programme to clarify and contribute to the research will be emancipatory for some communities. No Indigenous people like a 'big noter', so cultural humility is the core value that informs 'ask'.

Wingara: think	Burbangana: help lift up	Bulbanga: to hold up
When entering an Indigenous community, it is necessary to be ever-mindful, until the researcher is culturally proficient and safe. A researcher with cultural humility will have an observable understanding of power relationships, and a respectful demeanour towards Aboriginal participants. This researcher will think of the effect his or her actions will have on the community pre, during and post the research event. Thinking requires time to reflect. Indigenous people might prefer that researchers take time to consider an Indigenous perspective, rather than imposing a Western parameter on the interactions. Researchers are expected to consider, reflect and think about the stories shared, and seek clarification in a respectful manner.	Indigenous people have always been a collectivist people. Even in relative poverty, Indigenous people will share resources. It is a core value of many Indigenous people to strengthen their community. Research and researchers can do this. This does not mean that researchers should give away their resources, but it does mean they have to leave the community, person or issue in a better condition, as defined in conjunction with community. Leaving the community in a stronger position will help lift up that community. Having burbangana in the researcher's dilly bag will remind that researcher of the long-term issues arising from a piece of research. It might be as simple as increasing the skills and knowledge in a community, or the self-esteem of an individual. Research in Indigenous communities should be conducted with a view to adding to that community.	This value is in every facet of any research project. After a research project or intervention is completed (or burbangana), there is still a responsibility to ensure that community is 'held up' – or supported. It is not appropriate for a community to participate in research, and not to benefit from that research. Researchers have an ongoing responsibility to the communities that have contributed to their research. Researchers need to consider what will happen to that community when the research is over. It is not acceptable to enter a community, perform an intervention and then leave with no thought of the effects on that community. For example, a researcher cannot enter a community and take measurements for psychological distress, then leave the community without organizing access to counselling or specialist follow-up. Knowledge transfer must include and consider the community, while keeping the reputation of the community should be considered of paramount importance.

the mixing of salt sea and creek fresh waters in Eora/Cadigal is '*yerin*', and means not only brackish water, but when two ideas or stories are intermingled, or two people are intermingled. It is a cultural site of enrichment, embodying unconditional positive regard for other. Aboriginal people in coastal New South Wales (NSW) used to, and in many places still do, weave 'dilly bags'.[31,32] These bags were woven from grasses and reeds, especially those found near the ocean,[33] and were used to transport food, sometimes weapons, and often small treasures of the owner. Dilly bags could have short or long 'handles' and generally went around the head and/or carried over a shoulder. Whilst predominantly used by women, men also used them at need.[34] Dilly bags keep cultural valuables,[35] either as food stuffs or artefacts.[36] In this research methodology, the core value is unconditional positive regard for other, and the dilly bag is the metaphorical holder of the core behaviours used to inform the practice of research as demonstrated in Figure 24.1 and explained in Table 24.2.

Applying Indigenist methodologies to research

Each community that is the target of any research will need to be considered individually. The building of trust between researcher and community is of paramount importance, and gaining trust requires an understanding of Indigenous protocols. Indigenous communities can be discreet (i.e. mostly comprised of people who identify as having an Indigenous heritage, such as remote communities, or mission/reserves in rural and urban settings) or non-discreet (such as professional communities, or work-related communities). Entering an Indigenous community requires a working understanding of the protocols in cross-cultural research.

Protocols of cross-cultural research

Non-Indigenous people can of course conduct Indigenist research, with an expectation that the research will add value to the community, and an understanding of the protocols in cross-cultural research. Cultural humility is important, where the researchers are coachable, and use reflection to determine the cultural appropriateness of their behaviours and values in the research relationships.[37] Approaching community negotiators to gain entry into the community, either elders, liaison officers or representatives of Indigenous organizations, needs a culturally humble approach. A researcher might need to negotiate with more than one community representative or organization from the same community to get full permission from most of the community. While this first step can seem time consuming, it is the only way to get a participatory approach to any research or project, especially if a researcher has no Indigenous person who can 'vouch for' that researcher.

The community will then need to approve the research, if it is something they see of benefit, and if the processes are collaborative and participatory. This will require multiple community meetings with the understanding that sometimes meetings might be cancelled suddenly due to sorry business or other community reasons. Some communities will have their own requirements, for example, a project might need to be actively mentoring Indigenous researchers,[38] or that research outcomes are workshopped with the whole community.[39] The diversity in Indigenous communities reinforces the need for an individuated model for researchers, however, there are some commonalities that can be addressed with a pre-research checklist.

Table 24.3 The North Australian Indigenous Land and Sea Management Alliance (NAILSMA) checklist for research

- Meets community and landowner goals and aspirations.
- Promotes Indigenous management and control and helps protect Indigenous rights under Aboriginal law.
- Promotes and supports Indigenous Natural and Cultural Resource Management (NCRM)-based enterprise and economic activity, especially when linked to customary practice.
- Increases respect, understanding and the use of traditional knowledge and skills.
- Assists getting Indigenous people 'on country'.
- Has an adequate funding base, particularly in relation to the costs incurred by Indigenous organisations that are partners.
- Has a realistic time frame that takes account of the dictates of Indigenous life patterns.
- Makes a contribution to the viability of Indigenous organisations.
- Supports and strengthens Indigenous leadership.
- Yields results that can be of direct and immediate benefit.
- Helps record, collate and store Indigenous knowledge for generational transmission, education and management.
- Provides robust physical, biophysical and ecological baseline data to inform management, leaving ownership of the data with Indigenous custodians.
- Presents and explains the research project in clear understandable terms.
- Involves Indigenous people at all stages of the research process, including early planning and formulation.
- Employs Indigenous people as researchers, informants, cultural advisors, translators, and technical support using levels of remuneration in line with mainstream scales.
- Has provision for continuous monitoring, reporting and evaluation of the research process.
- Provides training, particularly when formally accredited and available to young people.
- Promotes communication and understanding between the research community and Indigenous people, between NCRM agencies and Indigenous people and between Indigenous people and between Indigenous land and sea managers.
- Promotes cooperative approaches to NCRM involving government agencies, Indigenous land owners and managers and other land owners. Strengthens control and tenure over Indigenous estates.
- Helps reduce the limited and uncertain tenure Indigenous people have over marine estates.
- Promotes recognition of Indigenous rights in the water reform agenda including water allocation.
- Promotes recognition of Indigenous rights in the emerging carbon trading agenda.
- Increases Indigenous contribution and participation in the development of government NCRM policy and management.
- Increases capacity to regulate and manage recreational use and tourism of land and sea areas.
- Assists in the protection of sacred sites.
- Promotes understanding of the research process.
- Adopts a flexible and adaptable approach that provides the opportunity to modify project methodology once the project has commenced.
- Uses translators where necessary to improve communication.
- Is controlled and supervised by a relevant community organisation or a project management group drawn from and supported by community leadership.
- Effectively restricts and protects sensitive information.
- Involves non-Indigenous researchers who have demonstrable cross-cultural engagement expertise.

Adapted from *Guidelines and protocols for the conduct of research* (p. 9) NAILSMA, Copyright (2007) North Australian Indigenous Land and Sea Management Alliance.

Table 24.4 Components, self-questions and rationale for cross-cultural research

Component	Self-question	Rationale
Funding	Have you considered the expenses for community consultation, including issues of reciprocity?	Funds should be jointly sought by the Indigenous communities and the research institution. Funding arrangements need to be transparent, and declared at the beginning of the research process. Consider catering your community consultation and focus groups. Research proposals should be prepared in collaboration, after appropriate consultation.
Ethics and consent	Have you got community consent before you start?	Community consent is required in addition to the participant consent process. Have you gained consent to enter the community? By the appropriate people? (eg health liaison officer, school liaison officer, or land council representative?)
Partnership	Are your processes transparent, and consider Indigenous people as equal?	The researcher and researched must be considered as equals, with a privileging of Indigenous knowledge. There must be an agreement of goals, objectives, methods, and any reimbursement must be negotiated at the outset. Authorship on publications, intellectual or commercial property rights, should be clearly negotiated with all community organisations.
Mutual benefits	Have you considered all benefits – economic? Political?	Tangible and intangible benefits include knowledge gained. Community members, where possible, should be employed on the project. Research should benefit Indigenous communities, in terms of better living outcomes, but also research training for participants and organisations. If there are any economic benefits, an equitable distribution should be agreed on prior to the start of any research project.
Cultural respect and competence	Have you considered cultural humility in every step in the research process?	All research should be in the language best understood by the Indigenous people for knowledge to be transferred, and research results and outcomes to be utilised independently of the researchers. Researchers need an understanding of the diversity of protocols in and between communities.
Capacity building	Have you planned to build capacity in the Indigenous community?	Capacity is considered at both an individual and organisational level – can be increase of skills, education, information, experience, and social capital of all partners.
Transparency in all process	Are all your processes easily understood and agreed upon?	All resourcing and financial decisions must be declared openly to all partners, and frequent checking against a risk management matrix should occur.
Research competency	Are you able to manage and monitor the collaboration?	All research project managers must have adequate management and leadership skills and competency as required by the project. Evaluations should assess the project from all stakeholders' perspectives.

Adapted from: WHO (2007);[42] and AIATSIS (2012).[43]

Checklist for research considerations

Indigenist research has the same considerations as all other research in terms of ethics, beneficence, etc., but there are other considerations that will make the research process and translation of knowledge more acceptable. Some organizations, the North Australian Indigenous Land and Sea Management Alliance (NAILSMA), have created their own checklist (see Tables 24.3–24.4), while others have a more generic approach.[40,41]

Table 24.4 demonstrates considerations for researching in most Indigenous communities based on the World Health Authority's recommendations and the AIATSIS protocols and guidelines for cross-cultural research.

Conclusion

Research in Indigenous communities is vitally important to close the gap in all indices of health and education. Without culturally competent researchers, the gap will never close. The take-home message to working in Indigenous communities is to be culturally humble by asking for clarity, apologizing if an error is made and respect and privilege Indigenous voices. Working together is the only way forward for the future.

References

1 Rosenstock A, Mukandi B, Zw AB, Hill PS. Closing the gaps: competing estimates of indigenous Australian life expectancy in the scientific literature. *Aust N Z J Public Health.* 2013; **37**(4):356–64.

2 Taylor A, Barnes T. 'Closing the Gap' in indigenous life expectancies: what if we succeed? *J Popul Res.* 2013; **30**(2):117–32.

3 Doyle KE. Australian Aboriginal peoples and evidence-based policies: closing the gap in social interventions. *J Evid Inf Soc Work.* 2015; **12**(2):166–74.

4 Shahjahan RA. Decolonizing the evidence-based education and policy movement: revealing the colonial vestiges in educational policy, research, and neoliberal reform. *J Educ Policy.* 2011; **26**(2):181–206.

5 Carm E. Inclusion of Indigenous Knowledge System (IKS) – a precondition for sustainable development and an integral part of environmental studies. *J Educ Res.* 2014; **4**(1):58–76.

6 Bohensky EL, Maru Y. Indigenous knowledge, science, and resilience: what have we learned from a decade of international literature on "integration". *Ecol Soc.* 2011; **16**(4):6–15.

7 Castree N, Kitchin R, Rogers A. *A dictionary of human geography.* Abington: Oxford University Press; 2013. pp. 230–4.

8 Agrawal A. Dismantling the divide between indigenous and scientific knowledge. *Dev Change.* 1995; **26**(3):413–59.

9 Nakata M. *Disciplining the savages, savaging the disciplines.* Canberra, ACT: Aboriginal Studies Press; 2007.

10 Peat FD. Traditional knowledge and western science. In: Hendry J, Fitznor L, editors. *Anthropologists, indigenous scholars and the research endeavour: seeking bridges towards mutual respect.* New York: Routledge; 2012. pp.118–27.

11 Dei GJ, Hall B, Rosenberg DG. Introduction. In: Dei GJS, Hall B, Rosenberg DG, editors. *Indigenous knowledges in the global contexts: multiple readings of the world.* Toronto, Canada: University of Toronto Press; 2000. pp. 1–32.

12 Semali LM, Kincheloe JL. What is indigenous knowledge and why should we study it? In: Semali LM, Kincheloe JL, editors. *What is indigenous knowledge? Voices from the academy.* New York: Routledge; 1999. pp. 125–32. ISBN 1135578508

13 Kincheloe J, McLaren, P. Rethinking critical theory and qualitative research. In: Denzin NK, Lincoln YS, editors. *The landscape of qualitative research: theories and issues.* 2nd ed. Thousand Oaks, CA: Sage; 2005. pp. 433–88.

14 Dunbar T, Scrimgeour M. LSIC: procedural ethics through an indigenous ethical lens. In: Walter M, Martin KK, Bodkin-Andrews G, editors. *Indigenous children growing up strong.* London: Palgrave Macmillan; 2017. pp. 61–78. ISBN: 978-1-137-53434-7

15 Lawrance M, Sayers SM, Singh GR. Challenges and strategies for cohort retention and data collection in an indigenous population: Australian aboriginal birth cohort. *BMC Med Res Methodol.* 2014; **14**(1):31–45. Available from: https://bmcmedresmethodol.biomedcentral.com/articles/10.1186/1471-2288-14-31

16 Ritchie E, Janke T. Who owns copyright in native title connection reports? *Indigen Law Bull.* 2015; **8**(20):8–11.

17 Smith L. Ethics or social justice? Heritage and the politics of recognition. *Aust Aborig Stud.* 2010; **2**:60–8.

18 Thomson C, Breen KJ, Chalmers D. Human research ethics guidelines in Australia. In: Dodds S, Ankeny RA, editors. *Big picture bioethics: developing democratic policy in contested domains.* Switzerland: Springer. 2016. pp. 165–90.

19 Coulter RT. UN Declaration on the rights of indigenous peoples: a historic change in international law, the. *Idaho L Rev.* 2008; **45**:539.

20 Kingsley J, Townsend M, Henderson-Wilson C, Bolam B. Developing an exploratory framework linking Australian Aboriginal peoples' connection to country and concepts of wellbeing. *Int J Env Res Public Health.* 2013; **10**(2):678–98.

21 Denzin N, Lincoln Y. *The SAGE handbook of qualitative research.* Thousand Oaks, CA: Sage; 2011.

22 Bessarab D, Ng'andu B. Yarning about yarning as a legitimate method in indigenous research. *Int J Crit Indigen Stud.* 2010; **3**(1):37–50.

23 Walter M, Anderson C. *Indigenous statistics: a quantitative research methodology.* Abingdon, UK: Routledge; 2013. IBSN 978-1-61132-293-4

24 West R, Stewart L, Foster K, Usher K. Through a critical lens indigenist research and the dadirri method. *Qual Health Res.* 2012; **22**(11):1582–90.

25 Doyle K, Cleary M, Blanchard D, Hungerford C. The yerin dilly bag model of indigenist health research. *Qual Health Res.* 2017; **27**(9):1288–301.

26 Vicary D, Bishop B. Western psychotherapeutic practice: engaging aboriginal people in culturally appropriate and respectful ways. *Aust Psychol.* 2005; **40**(1):8–19.

27 Bessarab B. *Yarning- a culturally safe method of indigenous conversation.* Paper presented at Dementia Networking Seminar, Curtin Health Innovation Research Institute, Curtin University, Perth, Australia; 2012.

28 Atkinson J. *Trauma trails, recreating song lines: the transgenerational effects of trauma in Indigenous Australia.* Melbourne, VIC: Spinifex Press; 2002.

29 Freire P. *Cultural action for freedom.* Cambridge, PA: Harvard Educational Review; 1972.

30 Habermas, Jürgen. *Reason and the rationalization of society, volume 1 of the theory of communicative action, english translation by Thomas McCarthy.* Boston: Beacon Press; 1984. (originally published in German in 1981).

31 Nugent M. An economy of shells: a brief history of la perouse aboriginal women's shellwork and its markets. In: Fijn N, Keen I, Lloyd C, Pickering I, editors. *Indigenous participation in australian economies: historical engagements and current enterprises. II.* Canberra, ACT: ANU Press; 2012. pp. 211–39.

32 Nugent M. Shellwork on show: colonial history, Australian aboriginal women and the display of decorative objects. *J Mater Cult.* 2014; **19**(1):75–92.

33 Scott J, Laurie R. Colonialism on display: indigenous people and artefacts at an Australian agricultural show. *Aborig His.* 2007; **31**:45–62.

34 Enright WJ. A dilly bag from the North Coast of New South Wales. *Aust J Anthropol.* 1932; **1**(6):137–8.

35 Guyula Y, Gotha K, Gurruwiwi D, Christie M. The ethics of teaching from country. *Aust Aborig Stud.* 2010; **2**:69–80.

36 Bowdler S. Hook, line, and dilly bag: an interpretation of an Australian coastal shell midden. *Aust J Anthropol.* 1976; **10**(4):248–58.

37 Smith SE. Riding the throughflow: seeking cultural humility to navigate some challenges in conducting cross-cultural research and education. In: Lian A, Kell P, Black P, Yew Lie K, editors. *Challenges in global learning: dealing with education issues from an international perspective.* Newcaslte upon Tyne: Cambridge Scholars Publishing; 2017. pp. 52–68.

38 Hickey SD, Maidment SJ, Heinemann KM, Roe YL, Kildea SV. Participatory action research opens doors: mentoring Indigenous researchers to improve midwifery in urban Australia. *Women Birth.* 2017; (in press).

39 Radford K, Mack HA, Robertson H, Draper B, Chalkley S, Daylight G, et al. The Koori Growing old well study: investigating aging and dementia in urban aboriginal Australians. *Int Psychogeriatr.* 2014; **26**(6):1033–43.

40 Hill R, Grant C, George M, Robinson CJ, Jackson S, Abel N. A typology of indigenous engagement in Australian environmental management: implications for knowledge integration and social-ecological system sustainability. *Ecol Soc.* 2012; **17**:1–17.

41 North Australian Indigenous Land and Sea Management Alliance (NAILSMA). *The NAILSMA checklist for research. Adapted from guidelines and protocols for the conduct of research.* 2007; 9. Available from: www.nailsma.org.au/sites/default/files/publications/NAILSMA_Guidelines_Jun07.pdf

42 World Health Organization. (WHO). *Indigenous peoples & participatory health research.* 2007. Available from: www.who.int/ethics/indigenous_peoples/en/print.html

43 Australian Institute of Aboriginal and Torres Strait Islander Studies, (AIATSIS). *Guidelines for ethical research in australian indigenous studies.* Canberra: AIATSIS; 2012.

25 Research methods in physical activity and health

Sexual orientation and gender identity

Damon Kendrick

Introduction

All participants in physical activity and health research should be guaranteed equality and freedom from discrimination regardless of sexual orientation and gender identity [SOGI] or because they are intersex. These are fundamental human rights that belong to all people, not only participants in research projects. Although the general principles of ethical considerations apply to all participants in research regardless of SOGI, there are further considerations to be made if the research question, research outcomes and/or hypotheses include SOGI.

Definitions and terminology

Sex: The biological differences between male and female: the visible difference in genitalia, the related difference in procreative function. An act of physical or emotional sexual arousal.

Gender: The cultural and social classification into 'masculine' and 'feminine'; the attitudes, behaviours and appearance (physical or sartorial) any given society expects from sexually mature bodies.

Sexuality: The feelings of attraction, both sexual and romantic, the emotions and the behaviours involved in intimate relationships. Common terms used to define sexuality include 'gay' (male-to-male homosexuality), 'lesbian' (female-to-female homosexuality) and 'bisexual' (sexuality involving either/both male and female).

Transgendered: Any person who identifies with a sex or gender other than the one assigned or assumed at birth.[1]

Intersex: A condition that may be a named diagnosis or be of unknown aetiology for those who are born with atypical genitalia in which it is difficult to definitively or correctly assign a sex to a new-born infant.[2]

Cisgender: Denoting or relating to a person whose sense of personal identity and gender corresponds with their birth sex.

Acronyms

The acronym most commonly used for lesbian, gay, bisexual, transgendered and/or intersex is LGBTI.[3] However, this does not cover all possibilities of sexuality or gender identity. Indeed, the City of New York recognizes 31 different terms for gender identity alone (see Table 25.1).[4]

Table 25.1 Gender identity terms accepted by New York City

Bi-Gendered, Cross-Dresser, Drag King, Drag Queen, Femme Queen, Female-to-Male,
FTM, Gender Bender, Genderqueer, Male-to-Female, MTF, Non-Op, Hijra, Pangender,
Transexual/Transsexual, Trans Person, Woman, Man, Butch, Two-Spirit, Trans, Agender,
Third Sex, Gender Fluid, Non-Binary, Transgender, Androgyne, Gender Gifted, Gender
Blender, Femme Person of Transgender Experience, Androgynous

(Adapted from NYC Commission on Human Rights, 2015)[4]

Additional terms and acronyms for expression of sexuality (in addition to lesbian, gay and bisexual) include pan-sexual [PS], asexual [AS], omni-sexual [OS], two-spirit [TS], sista-girl [SG], queer [Q] (alternatively spelled kweer), questioning [Q], bi-curious [BC], straight and cisgender ally [SCA]. Not only would utilization of all of these acronyms be difficult and unwieldy, collectively these terms may yet be regarded as not totally inclusive. Therefore, many researchers are utilizing the term "same sex attracted and gender diverse" [SSAGD] as being more inclusive and all-encompassing.[5] The term "sexual orientation and gender identity [SOGI]" is used to include all sexual orientations whether same-sex or opposite-sex attracted.

Ethical issues

All research participants are protected by the requirements of the relevant Human Research Ethics Committee [HREC] of that research institution. For most physical activity research, questions regarding SOGI are mostly irrelevant with the exception of performance or anthropometrical norms in intersex or transgendered athletes. Health research may require disclosure of sexuality only if it is directly connected with the research outcomes, research question or hypothesis. When designing a questionnaire, Information Sheet or Informed Consent Form, any questions regarding sexuality and/or gender identity must be carefully considered before inclusion. Assumption that all individuals can be classified as male or female (binary classification) will exclude many individuals. Therefore participants should be given the option of 'Other' if the question of sex is asked. The two major ethical considerations when asking SSAGD participants for disclosure of their SOGI are Justice and Confidentiality although all of the other ethical principles apply (see Table 25.2).

Legal issues

In many countries, homosexual activity has, or did have legal ramifications. To illustrate these the legal position in Australia is used here as an example, with the implications being applicable to those undertaking research in many different countries.

In Australia, homosexual activity between men was a capital offence, with the state of Victoria being the last to change from a capital offence to imprisonment in 1949. It is therefore possible that there are individuals still extant who were living when a charge of homosexuality carried the death penalty. This may have long-lasting psychological consequences and elderly SSAGD people may not disclose their sexuality or gender identity. Homosexual acts between women were never criminalized in Australia. The age of consent laws in Australia apply to all individuals regardless of sexuality or gender identity. This age is 16 in all states and territories except South Australia and Tasmania where it is 17.

Table 25.2 Ethical principles in research regarding SSAGD participants

Autonomy	Many SSAGD people have been subjected to bullying. Any pressure or persuasion required to encourage SSAGD individuals to participate in a research project may be construed as bullying. It must be impressed upon participants that they should not feel pressured in any way to participate or continue their participation if circumstances warrant an exit from the project.
Beneficence	Disclosure is only of any benefit and therefore required if the Research Question, Hypothesis or Research Outcomes is/are irrevocably connected to sexuality or gender identity.
Non-maleficence	For many SSAGD people, the process of disclosure of their SOGI (coming out) is traumatic and psychological scars may remain. Any research in the social sciences as well as any qualitative research needs to take this into consideration and the Informed Consent forms need to reflect this principle.
Justice	Despite the strides made in human rights issues for SSAGD people, inequities, inequalities and discrimination still abound and are entrenched within the legal system. Human rights and the individual rights of all research participants are incorporated within the fundamental ethical principles of research. Although discrimination based on sexuality was outlawed from 2015 in Australia, an exemption is given to religious organizations who are free to discriminate based on SOGI.
Veracity	Having faced bullying and discrimination, many SSAGD people may display a lack of trust. It is vitally important that the principle of Veracity is adhered to absolutely by every researcher in order to gain and maintain trust.
Fidelity	As many SSAGD individuals may have been discriminated against, it is important to reassure future participants that researchers will be true to their word.
Confidentiality	This principle is absolute. All information must be kept confidential according to the rules of the HREC overseeing the research project. This includes any information gathered in sex, gender, sexuality or gender identity, and all information must be de-identified. Electronic information should be kept in password-encrypted files and hard copies should be kept in a locked cabinet in a locked room.

(Adapted from Polgar and Thomas, 2008)[6]

Only in recent history, between 1975 and 1997, was male homosexuality decriminalized in all Australian states (see Table 25.3). In accordance with this the Australian Capital Territory [ACT], New South Wales [NSW], South Australia [SA] and Victoria have enacted legislation that expunges the criminal record of people who were arrested under homosexual convictions legislation.

Health and physical activity research involving SSAGD individuals may have legal, qualitative and psychological ramifications. Males who were over the age of 16 before the decriminalization of homosexuality means that they were subject to legislated discrimination. In those states which have not yet enacted legislation to pardon those offences, these people may still carry criminal convictions. They are legally regarded as sex offenders, which can therefore have legal, social and psychological ramifications for these individuals. Any qualitative, social and psychological research methods should consider the legal situation of older SSAGD participants in the methodology. These individuals may be denied work in certain sectors and be denied visas to travel to many countries.

Table 25.3 Decriminalization of homosexuality in Australia by state and territory

State	Date of decriminalization	Expungement of criminal records
Australian Capital Territory	4 November 1976	6 November 2016. *Spent Convictions (Historical Homosexual Convictions Extinguishment) Amendment Act 2015*
New South Wales	22 May 1984	24 November 2014. *Criminal Records Amendment (Historical Homosexual Offences) Bill 2014*
Northern Territory	4 October 1983	No legislation as of March 2017
South Australia	17 September 1975	South Australia. *Spent Convictions (Decriminalised Offences) Amendment Act 2013*
Tasmania	13 May 1997	No legislation as of March 2017
Queensland	29 November 1990	No legislation as of March 2017
Victoria	23 December 1980	1 September 2015. *Sentencing Amendment (Historical Homosexual Convictions Expungement Act) 2014*
Western Australia	7 December 1989	No legislation as of March 2017

On 1 August 2013, the Australian Federal Government amended the Sex Discrimination Act of 1984 to make discrimination against SSAGD people illegal (Australian Human Rights Commission: Face the Facts: Lesbian, Gay, Bisexual, Trans And Intersex People, 2014).[7] However, religious institutions were granted immunity from this law. The result is that employers who are religious organizations may legally dismiss or refuse to employ a person based on their sexuality or gender identity. Additionally, research and educational institutions who are owned and/or managed by religious institutions may insist on exercising editorial rights over research incorporating SSAGD participants. This may adversely affect the independence and validity of research performed with these institutions.

It must also be noted that five countries (Saudi Arabia, Iran, Mauritania, Sudan and Yemen) and regions of two other countries (Nigeria and Somalia) punish homosexuality with the death sentence.[8] A further 70 countries punish homosexuality by corporal punishment or imprisonment.[8] Research participants originating from these countries may not admit to SSAGD identity. This could therefore skew results if specific SSAGD information is required.

Social issues

Bullying

Homophobic and transphobic bullying has been entrenched in many sporting and social groups over the past number of years.[9] It is also entrenched in many different

countries and cultures and therefore cognizance must be made for people from culturally and linguistically diverse backgrounds [CALD] as they may be more likely to
engage in bullying behaviour. This has ramifications that will need to be considered
in qualitative and social or psychological research design. Furthermore the sporting
arena appears to be one of the last bastions of homophobia with a survey of American
professions demonstrating that professional sportspeople were more homophobic
than the US military.[10] The Out on the Fields Study (summary of data form this study-
presented in Table 25.4–25.7) conclusively demonstrated that:[9]

- 80% of all sport participants and 82% of SSAGD participants reported witnessing
  homophobia.
- 54% of gay male, 60% of bisexual males, 48% of lesbian females and 29% of
  bisexual females have personally experienced homophobia.
- 62% of gay males under 22 years of age and 53% of gay males over 22 had experienced homophobia.
- 28% of straight male participants had been personally targeted.

Table 25.4 Experience of homophobia (Denison and Kitchen, 2015)[9]

Experience of homophobia	Gay men	Lesbian women
Received verbal slurs such as faggot or dyke	84%	82%
Have been bullied	38%	18%
Have been verbally threatened	27%	16%
Have been physically assaulted	19%	9%

Table 25.5 Participants in Out on the Fields Study (Denison and Kitchen, 2015)[9]

SSAGD Status	Number of participants
Gay male	4,672
Lesbian female	1,386
Bisexual	709
Heterosexual	2,484
Other	181
Total	9,494

Table 25.6 Countries by participation in Out on the Fields Study (Denison and Kitchen, 2015)[9]

Country	Number of participants
Unites States of America	2,064
United Kingdom	1,796
Australia	3,006
Canada	1,123
Ireland	501
New Zealand	631
Other	373

Table 25.7 Participant age group (Denison and Kitchen, 2015)[9]

Participant age group	Number of participants
15–17	3%
18–21	15%
22–29	29%
30–39	24%
40–49	16%
60–59	9%
60 +	4%

Health disparities

With the exception of HIV/AIDS, there is a paucity of research into health disparities of SSAGD people compared to the heterosexual population.[11,12] In the USA, National Institutes of Health research funding SSAGD studies represented 0.1% of the total, much lower than the estimated population proportions of this population.[12] This lack of funding for research may result in health delivery inequities in this population. Important health disparities identified include adults older than 50 and who identify as SSAGD showing significantly higher prevalences of disability based on physical, mental or emotional or dependence on special equipment,[13] and the ages of SSAGD people with disabilities is younger than heterosexuals with disabilities.[13] Additionally there is a higher prevalence of substance abuse (smoking and alcohol), and poor mental health compared to heterosexuals.[13] Higher rates of excessive drinking and obesity in lesbian women compared to heterosexual women are also demonstrated.[14,15] However, bisexual women are at greater risk of mental distress and poor general health than their lesbian counterparts.[16] Gay and bisexual men generally have lower rates of obesity than heterosexual men,[16] but older gay and bisexual men display greater rates of hypertension and diabetes than heterosexual men.[17] All of these have ramifications for healthcare, housing and service delivery to SSAGD individuals, particularly as they age.

Gender issues

Gender issues include transgender, intersex conditions and biological anomalies making gender assignation at birth or later gender identity difficult. Saraswat et al.[18] found compelling evidence for a biological aetiology of gender identity in either transgendered people or those displaying gender dysphoria. Transgenderism is not a lifestyle choice, but an expression of biological reality. No biological link between transgenderism and intersex has been identified. As such these must be considered as separate conditions. The Olympic Charter states:

> Olympism seeks to create a way of life based on the joy of effort, the educational value of good example, social responsibility and respect for universal fundamental ethical principles. The practice of sport is a human right. Every individual must have the possibility of practising sport, without discrimination of any kind and in the Olympic spirit, which requires mutual understanding with a spirit of friendship, solidarity and fair play.
>
> (International Olympic Committee, in force from 2 August 2015)[19]

The transgendered athlete

The legal status of either intersex or transgendered athletes in international competition is far from clear. Although many sporting codes have clear policies regarding transgendered athletes, significantly more do not. This leaves an ethical dilemma for many sports administrators when presented with a transgendered athlete. Policies for inclusion in competition should be based on empirical evidence which is currently lacking. Research incorporating sporting performance needs to be cognizant of the possibility of transgendered athletes. Transgendered participants should be covered by any Human Research Ethics Committee (HREC) (especially regarding confidentiality). The principal issue to sports administrators is to balance the issues of fairness to other competitors with the ethical treatment of transgendered athletes. The perception is that a non-operative male-to-female athlete, who is not taking androgen antagonists will have functionally more muscle tissue and therefore have an unfair advantage over their cisgendered female competitors. Harper[20] demonstrated a reduction in running speed in seven of eight Male-to-Female (MTF) transgendered athletes. The only athlete who increased running speed after transition had an increased training load which could account for the performance improvement. However, the author noted that this study will probably not impinge on the resistance shown by cisgender women in competition against transgender women.

The United Kingdom has a legislated Gender Recognition Certificate [GRC] which is a legal document confirming the gender of that person. This is therefore used by people who have been transgendered in order to ensure that they are legally treated as that specific gender. Anyone with a GRC has the right to a new birth certificate and passport reflecting their gender according to the GRC. However, it is inappropriate to ask for either a GRC or a birth certificate in order to confirm gender.[21]

Hormone levels

Objections with respect to MTF transgendered people are often raised by fellow competitors regarding hormone levels and fairness. The perception that MTF competitors have an unfair advantage due to raised androgen levels is pervasive, and probably a contributing factor to reduced tolerance of transgendered athletes. The common scientific consensus is that the difference in testosterone between males and females accounts for the performance differences between the sexes.[22] This view however is not universally shared amongst the scientific community.[23] This is confounded by the demonstration that the prevalence of hyperandrogenism in female athletes with normal chromosomal complement (46 XX) is approximately 7 per 1,000, which is 140 times higher than the cisgendered female population.[22] Transgender women on testosterone suppression therapy show levels below that of 46 XX women.[24]

Percentage fat norms

A common component of health as well as fitness testing is the determination of body fat percentage. Most of the tests performed are indirect tests that have high degrees of correlation with the determinant of fat content by underwater weighing. Methods include various protocols of skinfold calipers, and bio-impedance techniques. Increasingly common is the utilization of dual emission X-ray absorptiometry [DEXA] testing.

Currently, there are norms for male and female but no evidence could be found for transgender or intersex norms for any of these methods. No published protocols could be found on the ethics of which norms to use with transgendered individuals. Percentage body fat and fat distribution will alter between transgendered individuals who are pre- or post-operative and whether they are prescribed hormone replacement therapy or hormone antagonist therapy. Anecdotal evidence exists on male-to-female transgendered individuals taking non-prescribed birth control pills in order to increase circulating female hormones. In the absence of invasive questioning, it is recommended that until transgendered norms are published, the norms for the identified gender should be used in all cases, i.e. if the person identifies as male, then the male norms should be used. Although this may result in anomalies in direct comparison to cisgendered individuals, any changes that may occur between pre- and post-testing should still be valid.

Performance norms

Similar to percentage body fat norms, the performance norms are for males or females, and no such norms exist for transgendered or intersex individuals.

The intersex athlete

The highly publicized case of the South African middle distance runner and 2016 Olympic Gold Medalist for the women's 800m, Caster Semenya, has highlighted

Table 25.8 Intersex conditions

Intersex Condition	Prevalence in live births
Not XX and not XY	1 in 1,666
Klinefelter (XXY)	1 in 1,000
Androgen insensitivity syndrome	1 in 13,000
Partial androgen insensitivity syndrome [PAIS]	1 in 130,000
Classical congenital adrenal hyperplasia	1 in 13,000
Late onset adrenal hyperplasia	1 in 66
Mayer-Rokitansky-Küster-Hauser syndrome [MRKH] (Mullerian agenesis; vaginal agenesis; congenital absence of vagina)	1 in 4,500
Vaginal agenesis (non MRKH)	1 in 6,000
Ovotestes (formerly called 'true hermaphroditism')	1 in 83,000
Idiopathic (no discernable medical cause)	1 in 110,000
Iatrogenic (caused by medical treatment, for example Progestin) induced virilization	Unknown
5 alpha reductase deficiency	Unknown
Mixed gonadal dysgenesis	Unknown
Complete gonadal dysgenesis	1 in 150,000
Hypospadias (urethral opening in perineum or along penile shaft)	1 in 2,000
Hypospadias (urethral opening between corona and tip of glans penis)	1 in 770
Aphallia (Talebpour Amiri 2016)	1 in 10–30 million
Clitoromegaly, micropenis, genital ambiguity	Unknown
Gonadal dysgenesis (partial and complete)	XX 1–9/100,000 XY Unknown
Mosaicism involving 'sex' chromosomes	Unknown

the need for a greater consideration of gender issues in physical activity and health research. This athlete had her confidentiality breached on several occasions after she was subject to sex testing. Had she been a participant in research, the requirements of the relevant HREC would have protected her.

The various forms of intersex conditions appear to have been ignored for many generations.[25] However the prevalence of intersex conditions is relatively common with one of the forms appearing more commonly than 1 in every 1,500 live births[2] (see Table 25.8).

Conclusion

Physical activity and health research should be cognizant of the issues surrounding the SOGI of participants that may not be covered by HREC approval. It is important that at least an 'other' option is given for sex and or gender identity. Any health research that includes psychological, social or qualitative research should consider all of the ramifications that SOGI will have on the data, particularly if the research question, hypothesis and research methodology specifically includes SSAGD participants.

References

1   Gender Education & Advocacy. *Gender variance: a primer.* 2001. Available 22/06/2007, from www.gender.org/resources/dge/gea01004.pdf.

2   Blackless M, Charuvastra A, Derryck A, Fausto-Sterling A, Lauzanne K, Lee E. How sexually dimorphic are we? Review and synthesis. *Am J Hum Biol.* 2000; **12**(2):151–66.

3   Tinney J, Dow B, Maude P, Purchase R, Whyte C, Barrett C. Mental health issues and discrimination among older LGBTI people. *Int Psychogeriatr.* 2015; **27**(9):1411–6.

4   NYC Commission on Human Rights: Gender Identity Expression. Availabe from: www1. nyc.gov/assets/cchr/downloads/pdf/publications/GenderID_Card2015.pdf

5   Symons C, O'Sullivan G, Borkoles G, Andersen MB, Polman RCJ. *The impact of homophobic bullying during sport and physical education participation on same-sex-attracted and gender-diverse young Australian's depression and anxiety levels.* Melbourne, Australia: College of Sport and Exercise Science and the Institute for Sport, Health and Active Living Victoria University; 2014.

6   Polgar S, Thomas SA. *Introduction to research in the health sciences.* 5th ed. Elsevier, Philadelphia: Churchill Livingstone; 2008.

7   Australian human rights commission: face the facts: lesbian, gay, bisexual, trans and intersex people. 2014. Available from: www.humanrights.gov.au/sites/default/files/FTFLGBTI.pdf

8   Perez GS. The protection of LGBTI rights: an uncertain outlook. *Int J Hum Rights.* 2014; **20**:143–9.

9   Denison E, Kitchen A. Out on the fields: the first international study on homophobia in sport. *Repucom, Australian Sports Commission, Federation of Gay Games.* 2015. Available from: www.outonthefields.com

10 Available from: www.pewsocialtrends.org/2013/06/13/a-survey-of-lgbt-americans/

11 Boehmer U. Twenty years of public health research: inclusion of lesbian, gay, bisexual, and transgender populations. *Am J Public Health.* 2002; **92**(7):1125–30.

12 Coulter RWS, Kenst KS, Bowen DJ, Scout. Research funded by the National Institutes of Health on the health of lesbian, gay, bisexual, and transgender populations. *Am J Public Health.* 2014; **104**(2):e105–12.

13   Fredriksen-Goldsen KI, Kim HJ, Barkan SE. Disability among lesbian, gay, and bisexual adults: disparities in prevalence and risk. *Am J Public Health*. 2012; **102**(1):e16–21.

14   Dilley JA, Simmons KW, Boysun MJ, Pizacani BA, Stark MJ. Demonstrating the importance and feasibility of including sexual orientation in public health surveys: health disparities in the Pacific Northwest. *Am J Public Health*. 2010; **100**(3):460–7.

15   Conron KJ, Mimiaga MJ, Landers SJ. A population based study of sexual orientation identity and gender differences in adult health. *Am J Public Health*. 2010; **100**(10):1953–60.

16   Fredriksen-Goldsen KI, Kim HJ, Barkan SE, Muraco A, Hoy-Ellis CP. Health disparities among lesbian, gay, and bisexual older adults: results from a population based study. *Am J Public Health*. 2013; **103**(10):1802–9.

17   Wallace SP, Cochran SD, Durazo EM, Ford CL. *The health of aging lesbian, gay and bisexual adults in California*. Los Angeles: University of California, Los Angeles Center for Health Policy Research; 2011.

18   Saraswat A, Wienand JD, Safer JD. Evidence supporting the biologic nature of gender identity. *Endocr Pract*. 2015; **12**(2):199–204.

19   International Olympic Committee. Olympic charter. Available from: https://stillmed. olympic.org/Documents/olympic_charter_en.pdf

20   Harper J. Race times for transgender athletes. *J Sport Cult Identit*. 2015; **6**(1):1–9.

21   Available from: www.icehockeyuk.co.uk/transgender-policy/

22   Bermon S, Pierre Yves Garnier PY, Hirschberg PL, Robinson N, Giraud S, Nicoli R, et al. Serum androgen levels in elite female athletes. *J Clin Endocrinol Metab*. 2014; **99**(11):4328–35.

23   Healy ML, Gibney R, Pentecost C, Wheeler MJ, Sonksen PH. Endocrine profiles in 693 elite athletes in the postcompetition setting. *Clin Endocrinol*. 2014; **81**:294–305.

24   Gooren LJ, Bunck MC. Transsexuals and competitive sports. *Eur J Endocrinol*. 2004; **151**:425–9.

25   Rosario V. The new science of intersex. *Gay Lesbian Rev*. 2009; **16**(5):21–3.

26 Conducting physical activity research within chronic disease populations

Brigid M. Lynch, Lucy Hackshaw-McGeagh and Julian Sacre

Aims of the chapter

This chapter will discuss important considerations relevant to physical activity research focused on chronic disease populations. Specifically, it aims:

- To describe ethical and practical considerations related to research involving people who have been diagnosed with chronic diseases;
- To document appropriate methods for participant recruitment, data collection, and surveillance for such studies;
- To provide a checklist for researchers intending to conduct research involving adults with chronic diseases; and
- To present case studies illustrating good practice.

Introduction

Chronic diseases (also referred to as non-communicable diseases) are the leading cause of mortality and morbidity worldwide.[1] Chronic diseases will become more prevalent in coming years, as worldwide trends in population ageing continue, and low- and middle-income countries increasingly adopt 'Western' lifestyles (see Box 26.1).

Box 26.1 Burden of disease: cancer as an example

Estimates suggest that there were 14.1 million new cancer cases diagnosed and 8.2 million cancer deaths worldwide in 2012.[2] This made cancer the second leading cause of death, behind cardiovascular disease (an estimated 17.5 million deaths globally).[3] In 2012, an estimated 32.6 million people around the world had been diagnosed with cancer within the past five years.[4] By 2020 the number of new cancer cases and cancer deaths will increase to about 17 million and 10 million, respectively.[4]

Physical activity can help prevent a range of chronic diseases, including cardiovascular disease, some cancers, type 2 diabetes, osteoporosis, anxiety and depression.[5] Emerging evidence suggests that sedentary behaviour (sitting time) may also contribute to chronic disease risk, even among physically active individuals.[6] Importantly, physical activity provides many health benefits for adults living with chronic diseases.

For example, physical activity is widely promoted to people who have been diagnosed with type 2 diabetes, as it assists with weight management, improves glycaemic control and reduces the risk of comorbid complications.[7]

Over the past few decades a large body of research has accumulated on the potential role of physical activity in the management of chronic diseases. Scientists have investigated the potential benefits of physical activity at different points across the disease trajectory, from prior to administration of primary treatments (sometimes referred to as 'prehab') through to many years after the conclusion of primary therapy (see Figure 26.1).

Box 26.2 Case study: the Colorectal Cancer and Quality of Life Study

Over a two-year period 1,996 adults diagnosed with colorectal (bowel) cancer were recruited through the Queensland Cancer Registry to take part in an observational, longitudinal study.[8] During the first data collection point (on average 4.5 months after diagnosis), participants were asked to recall their 'pre-diagnosis' phase and current physical activity. For some, current physical activity fell within the 'active treatment' phase; for others who had completed treatment, current physical activity fell within the 'survivorship' phase. A small number of participants had already moved into the 'palliative care' phase by this time. Participants of this study went on to report their physical activity annually, for five years following their diagnosis.

Ethical and practical considerations

This section focuses on ethical and practical considerations to be aware of when designing and implementing physical activity research with individuals who have chronic disease. This list is in no way comprehensive, but encompasses key considerations. Each of which will need to be included within an ethics submission for consideration by the relevant ethics committee.

Ethical considerations

Justification for carrying out the research

It is important to clearly articulate the research question to be addressed at the beginning of the research process. A sound rationale is required, supported by appropriate

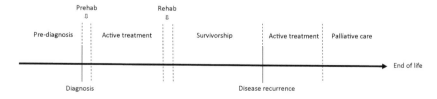

Figure 26.1 Phases across the chronic disease trajectory at which physical activity can be studied.

prior research (or lack thereof). Key questions to ask may be: Is there a clinical need? A gap in the literature? Are you trying to improve healthcare delivery? Or reduce negative health outcomes in a particular population? It is unethical to carry out research, particularly when working with vulnerable populations, without a clear purpose and research plan.

Participant deception

Most of the time, all elements of research should be transparent, including the aims and hypotheses of the study. It is unethical for a researcher to avoid disclosing information, such as how the research outcomes will be assessed, to study participants. From time to time, however, the research question may necessitate non-disclosure of information or participant deception. Note this is rare, and should only take place when no other method would suffice. In these instances, further expert guidance should be sought, and participants should be debriefed upon completion of the study.

Exclusions based on language barriers

When considering inclusion and exclusion criteria, it is preferable to be as inclusive as possible and thus improve representativeness of the study sample. One factor to consider is the potential participant's ability to speak, read or write English (or the primary language of the research team). Inclusion of non-English-speaking participants should be encouraged, however the practical limitations need to be considered. Is it feasible to have a physical activity intervention group that includes participants who have limited English skills? Does the research project have the resources to pay for a translator to attend research clinics? Do you have the means to translate all written materials into different languages? Questions such as this would need to be considered prior to compiling inclusion/exclusion criteria.

Confidentiality

Confidentiality is paramount in health and medical research. Research participants who have a chronic disease may be more sensitive to issues of confidentiality; it is likely you will be collating personal information about their health status, treatment history or physical limitations. It is therefore important to clearly communicate practices that will be followed for retaining such information securely and privately. Examples of standard confidentiality practices include: making sure all data are encrypted and stored securely; removing identifiable information from data sets; and, securely storing participant contact details in a separate location to other research data.

Participant burden

When designing research a balance must be struck between individual burden and community benefits. It may be in participants' best interest to restrict data collection to a small number of variables that are essential for addressing the research question at hand, particularly for populations with chronic disease, who may already face additional challenges in their daily lives due to their health status. However, researchers also have to be accountable for the resources utilized to undertake research, and ensure research outputs provide value for the time and resources put into the study.

Beware of assumptions and judgements

When working with chronic disease populations it is important to adopt a judgement-free approach. Beware of assumptions you may have, for example, about the physical limitations of the population or expectations that you may have formed based on previous experience. Bearing this in mind, you must equally ensure that you do consider physical limitations and contraindications during, for example, exercise testing or intervention delivery.

Informed consent

Consent to research must be fully informed and given voluntarily. Individuals must be provided with detailed information about what the research is about, and what their participation entails. This information must be provided at an appropriate level, and individuals should be given an opportunity to ask questions, and time to consider participation (see next subsection).

Whilst the decision to participate in research should be made by the individual, it is advisable that physical activity researchers consider whether medical clearance is required for their study. Participants with chronic diseases may have a number of disease- or treatment-related physical activity contraindications. The level of medical clearance required will depend upon factors such as the clinical population being recruited, the type of intervention being delivered or the physical function testing being administered. Individuals should be informed that they can withdraw their participation at any point, without providing a reason for doing so, and without it affecting their standard care (this could be an additional concern for an individual with chronic disease).

In the case where research is being conducted with a population who, by definition, are unable to provide fully informed consent, we advise you to seek expert, specific guidance. Clinician researchers should not provide medical clearance to their own patients; instead, they should refer their patients to other health professionals for review, to avoid conflict of interest.

Time to consider participation

Potential participants must be given time to consider whether they wish to participate in the research or not. They should never be rushed. They should be given time to reflect, time to read over any literature, and talk to family and friends. There is no specific guidance about how long this consideration period should be; it would depend greatly upon the nature of the research. For example, a year-long physical activity intervention trial, involving time consuming or uncomfortable procedures may take longer to consider than completing a brief, self-report questionnaire on one occasion. There may be certain situations where the consent process is subject to time limitations, such as research taking place in Accident and Emergency departments.

Ethical approval

All research, regardless of population or environment, should be reviewed and granted ethical approval from a research ethics committee. This may be an internal committee such as within a university department, or an external research ethics committee. For example, in the UK any research taking place within the National Health Service (NHS) must successfully apply for Health Research Authority approval from an NHS Research Ethics Committee (REC). Although it is the responsibility of the ethics committee to ensure the research protocol is ethically sound, it is ultimately the researcher's responsibility to ensure that all ethical guidelines and considerations are adhered to. Research involving humans must be conducted in line with the World Medical Association Declaration of Helsinki Ethical Principles for Medical Research Involving Human Subjects.[9]

Practical considerations

Identify and maintain key relationships

When undertaking research within chronic disease populations, positive working relationships are key to the success of a study. From the outset it is important to identify who the stakeholders, gatekeepers and key personnel are, and then establish and maintain relationships with the relevant individuals or groups. When working with clinical populations this could be the clinicians, research nurses, hospital administrators, primary care receptionists or, of course, representatives from the clinical population itself. Having open and honest discussions, addressing concerns or resolving misconceptions early on can generate a positive working relationship.

Patient and public involvement

It is now a general expectation that patient and public involvement (PPI) groups (sometimes referred to as consumer groups) are consulted in the development of new research protocols. This is equally important, if not more so, when working with chronic disease populations. It is therefore not only important to involve a relevant PPI group, but to ensure you act upon the feedback provided.

Maintain participant relationships

When carrying out longitudinal research, maintaining relationships with participants is an important element. In some research projects it may be possible to maintain regular contact with participants via face-to-face meetings; other studies may need to maintain contact through sending out newsletters or making telephone calls. These efforts help to make participants feel valued, and will help to reduce attrition rates.

Intervention-specific considerations

If you are developing an intervention study there may be additional considerations. For example the specific elements of the physical activity intervention may be the key factor in the success or failure of the research. When working with populations with chronic disease, in a similar way to other populations, you may wish to consider the intervention being easy to do, enjoyable, delivered by trained individuals who understand the disease and it being compatible with the individual's current routine.

Involving partners or carers in the research

You may conduct research where partners or carers are participants in their own right within the research. Alternatively, you may wish to include them, not as a participant, but by inviting them to accompany participants to their research appointments. Some participants welcome their partner or carer being involved. Involving partners or carers can facilitate shared recall during qualitative interviews. Partners can also be important stakeholders to consider when physical activity interventions are being administered; their support and encouragement can be critical to an intervention's success. However, be cognizant that some participants may not want their partners or carers involved. Participants may feel they are unable to speak freely in front a partner or carer, or wish for the research to be something that is uniquely theirs.

Allow flexibility

Disease- and treatment-related factors need to be considered when planning and delivering research projects. Issues such as participant fatigue, or their inability to participate in vigorous physical activity, need to be considered. Long interview schedules, for example, may need to be broken down into brief sections to accommodate fatigue; or, intervention protocols may need to be delayed due to complications with clinical treatment.

Systematically check data as they are collected

Data are often not collated, cleaned and analysed until the end of a research study. However it is important to systematically monitor data as they are collected to ensure that they are in the expected format. This is particularly important when using devices, such as accelerometers, to objectively measure physical activity. If errors are made, for example when initializing the devices, the data will not be collected successfully. To identify this at the end of a research study (when it is not possible to return to participants to collect the necessary data) would be highly disappointing, and compromise the entire study. Where possible, use high-quality devices that have been pilot-tested in the target population beforehand.

Methods

Recruitment

Recruitment difficulties are amongst the most common reasons for a study to be halted prematurely. With the exception of pilot/feasibility studies, the sample size required to detect a clinically meaningfully effect (whether it be change in $\dot{V}O_{2max}$, differences in rates of hospitalization/mortality, reduction in blood glucose, etc) should be calculated a priori. It is unethical to initiate a study if it is not possible to recruit the required number of participants within the timeframe afforded by available resources/funding. Thus, feasibility of recruitment should be a key consideration by investigators in the first instance, but also at ethical/governance review level.

The research question itself often defines the best method of recruitment, though in many cases a variety will be needed to achieve target sample size. It is also often overlooked that methods of recruitment can have a substantive impact on the results of a study and how generalizable these results will be to the broader population that the study sample is supposed to represent. For example, two studies of individuals with type 2 diabetes may differ markedly if one recruits primarily from a hospital diabetes clinic and the other from community-based settings (where the former generally gives rise to individuals with poorer disease control/management and more comorbidities/complications).

The following is a list of frequently used methods to recruit participants with chronic diseases; it is by no means exhaustive.

Registries

A registry is a collection of information about individuals, often focused on a specific population or disease. Some registries are coordinated by governments, and may collect data relating to notifiable diseases. For example, many countries around the world have legislation that requires health institutions (such as hospitals) to notify a registry about all cancer diagnoses and deaths. Through this process it is possible for cancer registries to achieve almost complete coverage of cancer incidence for their country/state/county, providing an accurate picture of the distribution of cancer throughout the population. Other registries are populated by voluntary reporting of data. Such registries may be sponsored by not-for-profit organizations, healthcare facilities or even private companies.

Registries usually have processes to facilitate recruitment for research. Researchers can apply to access information about individuals with registries, but requests must have ethics approval and be approved by the registry before information is provided. Recruitment through registries is ideal when study samples are required to be (approximately) representative of the chronic disease group being studied.

Patient support groups

Many formal and informal support groups, established to assist individuals with chronic diseases, exist. Sometimes groups are organized and facilitated by healthcare institutions (such as community health centres) or not-for-profit groups. Patient support groups can be excellent channels through which research participants can be recruited. It is best to contact patient support group leaders to discuss potential recruitment, as some groups will require study protocols to be formally approved by their governing committees. Patient support groups can facilitate recruitment by: directly emailing their members about the study; including information about the study in newsletters; or by distributing information about the study at group meetings.

Hospitals and clinical practices

Hospitals can be an important and even necessary source of recruitment for studies of certain patient populations, such as diseases that require frequent hospitalization (e.g. heart failure) or complex conditions managed primarily by hospital-based specialists (e.g. advanced kidney disease). For stable conditions that do not generally mandate hospitalization (e.g. obesity, diabetes), hospitals may not be a suitable recruitment avenue.

Community-based clinics tend to demonstrate patient profiles that are generally 'healthier' and more stable compared with hospitals. However, there is still significant variation in populations, depending on factors such as the geographic location or the clinic and its billing practices. For example, general practice clinics in economically deprived areas tend to have the highest proportion of patients with chronic disease. Thus, researchers pursuing clinic-based recruitment need to be strategic in deciding which clinics to direct their resources to.

Common strategies used when recruiting patients via hospitals or clinics include: placing promotional materials (posters, postcards) in waiting areas (this is a passive method of recruitment that is low cost but not typically very effective); sending letters to potentially eligible patients (this is still a passive form of recruitment that requires participants to reply, but it may be possible to follow-up non-responders with telephone calls); and, in-person approaches made to patients during clinic visits (usually the most time consuming and expensive option, but results in highest response rate).

Social and traditional media

Media can be an effective method of recruitment, particularly when studies are promoted via journalistic means (e.g. the study is mentioned in a newspaper article or television segment related to the chronic disease). Other options include paid advertisements in newspapers, magazines or on radio. Although researchers can expect a high volume of enquiries when soliciting research participants via the media, it is a non-targeted approach and may be less effective for rarer conditions. The rate of screening failures (i.e. not eligible for study) also tends to be higher. Social media represents a less expensive alternative to traditional media advertising. In pursuing these avenues, researchers need to consider the capacity for the social medium to reach their target population. Mediums such as Facebook can target paid advertisements to broad demographic categories, such as women over the age of 60, which may be sufficiently specific if your study wishes to recruit postmenopausal breast cancer survivors.

Data collection

A variety of data collection methods can be utilized to collect physical activity information from adults with chronic diseases. The best method is often determined by the research question itself. Are you interested in obtaining an accurate estimate of the duration of moderate-vigorous physical activity within a chronic disease population? Or do you wish to find out what motivates individuals with a chronic disease to exercise?

Exercise testing

Exercise capacity (broadly encompassing measures of cardiorespiratory fitness) is a powerful predictor of prognosis for many chronic diseases. It is also intrinsic to the definition of some clinical syndromes (e.g. chronic heart failure, which can mandate exercise capacity below a given % of predicted to achieve a diagnosis) and a primary target of therapy in others (e.g. individuals with peripheral artery disease and intermittent claudication, whose limited walking ability is of foremost concern). Exercise capacity may also be available as an adjunct measure to tests performed for other reasons (e.g. screening for ischaemic heart disease through exercise stress testing).

The choice of exercise testing modality will be governed by a number of factors, including: clinical context (safety/appropriateness and degree of expected exercise limitation); the number of participants relative to resources available (more accurate tests are also more resource intensive); the equipment and expertise available to the study team; and how much time is available to be spent with participants (participant burden will be a factor to consider).

Cardiopulmonary exercise testing (CPET; for peak oxygen uptake [$\dot{V}O_2$peak]) is considered the gold standard,[10] but CPET requires a significant amount of time and expertise, and specialized equipment is required. Because of this, CPET is most suited to smaller clinical studies. As a 'maximal' test (i.e. participants are instructed to attain their highest, symptom-limited workload), it is contraindicated in some patients and generally requires medical supervision. CPET is most commonly performed in conjunction with a treadmill or cycle ergometer protocol (incremental increases in workload in a ramp or stepwise manner). If CPET equipment is unavailable, the highest workload achieved by participants undertaking a treadmill or cycle ergometer protocol (maximum METs or watts) correlates well with $\dot{V}O_2$peak and still provides highly relevant information.

Functional tests, such as the six-minute walk test, may also be administered. The six-minute walk test is not an alternative to CPET but is nevertheless a useful test of aerobic/exercise capacity that has been widely applied in many chronic diseases. Although the test is simple in that it only involves measuring the distance walked by a patient within six minutes, its administration must comply with standardized methodology[11] to ensure reliability.

Self-report

Self-report measures can be self-administered as questionnaires or diaries; interviewer-administered, either in person or via telephone; and, in some cases (where participants are too ill or unable to write) proxy measures are used.[12] Self-report measures can be administered to large numbers of people at a time and are cost-efficient. However, self-report measures of physical activity have a number of limitations, particularly that they are prone to recall error, social desirability and other biases.[13] Healthy populations have been used to establish the validity and reliability of most measures used to assess the physical activity of adults with chronic diseases. It is important, where possible, to use physical activity measures for which psychometric properties have been established amongst the chronic disease population being studied.

Accelerometry

Accelerometers are small, wearable devices that accurately measure movement patterns. Accelerometers provide the opportunity to examine other elements of physical activity and sedentary behaviour, such as the time of day when these behaviours most frequently occur, and how frequently participants 'break up' their sitting time. Collecting accelerometer data remains time consuming and expensive, but it provides objective data that are not susceptible to some of the biases inherent in self-reported data.[14] An important issue to consider when using accelerometers in chronic disease populations is how to best reduce the raw, acceleration data into meaningful summary variables. Most chronic disease studies using accelerometry to date have used cut-points developed and tested in young, healthy adult populations. Thus, there is a need for more methodological work in this field to develop suitable cut-points or algorithms to reduce accelerometer data into summary variables that are reflective of the physical activity performed by older adults, including those with chronic disease.[15]

Wearable technology

Consumer wearable devices – or 'wearables' – track and promote physical activity. Wearables have been described as a potential method to overcome some of the difficulties in monitoring, assessing and promoting physical activity to adults with chronic diseases.[16] Wearables have the potential to be used across different phases of the chronic disease trajectory, and data linked to clinical data (e.g. number of hospitalizations, or falls) used to identify onset of disease complications (e.g. oedema, neuropathy). Chronic disease populations have also been reported to perceive wearables as useful and acceptable.[17] Thus, wearables may be a low-cost, feasible and accessible way for promoting physical activity to adults with chronic disease. However, this is a new field of research, and further research is needed.

For further information on the methods, technologies and issues associated with measuring physical activity, please see Chapter 18.

Box 26.3 Case study: the ACTIVATE Trial

The ACTIVATE Trial is a randomized controlled trial that will evaluate the efficacy of an intervention that combines wearable technology (the Garmin Vivofit2®) with traditional behavioural change approaches to increase physical activity and reduce sedentary behaviour performed by breast cancer survivors. Eighty-three women have been randomly assigned to the primary intervention group (Garmin Vivofit2®; behavioural feedback and goal-setting session; and, five telephone-delivered health coaching sessions) or to the wait-list control group. The primary intervention is delivered over a 12-week period.

Participants are invited to share their Garmin Vivofit2® data with the study team via the Garmin Wellness API (application programme interface). This API provides the research team with access to near real-time data, which informs the content of the telephone-delivered health coaching sessions. Participants who are non-compliant with the intervention (not using the wearable), or those who are not meeting their daily step goals, are provided with additional encouragement and strategies to overcome barriers to physical activity during the telephone call.

Checklist

Here are the key steps necessary to successfully develop and implement a physical activity research project within a chronic disease population:

- Find patient/consumer collaborators. Their involvement is critical from the outset, and they should be involved in all stages of the project.
- Define your research question clearly, and justify why the research should be undertaken.

- Select a method to appropriately address the research question.
- Develop a thorough research protocol, carefully considering the ethical and practical considerations described in this chapter.
- Secure the required human research ethics approval(s).
- Establish and maintain positive working relationships with key stakeholders and gatekeepers, keeping them informed of the study's progress.
- Recruit your sample through the most appropriate method(s).
- Carry out the research, collecting data using methods that balance the need for high-quality data with participant burden.
- Ensure you provide participants with updates on the status of the research, and feedback study results.

Conclusion

Chronic disease will become more prevalent in coming years, as worldwide trends in population ageing continue, and low- and middle-income countries increasingly adopt 'Western' lifestyles. This will generate significant economic and social burdens. Physical activity levels are low amongst adults with chronic disease, despite there being convincing epidemiologic and experimental evidence demonstrating a range of health benefits. Many questions remain regarding the most appropriate dose (frequency, intensity, duration) of physical activity to be recommended to adults with different chronic diseases. It is likely that there will be different optimal doses for different health outcomes (e.g. survival, prevention of comorbidities, health-related quality of life). Understanding how physical activity can help to manage chronic diseases more efficiently, and provide adults living with chronic disease an improved quality of life, is critical moving forward.

References

1 Moore SC, Lee IM, Weiderpass E, Campbell PT, Sampson JN, Kitahara CM, et al. Association of leisure-time physical activity with risk of 26 types of cancer in 1.44 million adults. *JAMA Intern Med.* 2016; **176**(6):816–25.
2 Ferlay J, Soerjomataram I, Dikshit R, Eser S, Mathers C, Rebelo M, et al. Cancer incidence and mortality worldwide: sources, methods and major patterns in GLOBOCAN 2012. *Int J Cancer.* 2015; **136**(5):E359–86.
3 World Health O. *Global status report on noncommunicable diseases 2014.* Geneva, Switzerland: World Health Organization Press. 2014.
4 Ferlay J, Soerjomataram I, Ervik M, Dikshit R, Eser S, Mathers C, et al. *GLOBOCAN 2012 v1.0, Cancer incidence and mortality worldwide: IARC CancerBase No. 11 Lyon.* France: International Agency for Research on Cancer; 2013.
5 Haskell WL, Lee IM, Pate RR, Powell KE, Blair SN, Franklin BA, et al. Physical activity and public health: updated recommendation for adults from the American college of sports medicine and the american heart association. *Med Sci Sports Exerc.* 2007; **39**(8):1423–34.
6 Biswas A, Oh PI, Faulkner GE, Bajaj RR, Silver MA, Mitchell MS, et al. Sedentary time and its independent risk on disease incidence, mortality and hospitalization in adults: a meta-analysis. *Ann Int Med.* 2015; **162**(2):123–32.
7 Eakin EG, Reeves MM, Marshall AL, Dunstan DW, Graves N, Healy GN, et al. Living well with diabetes: a randomized controlled trial of a telephone-delivered intervention for maintenance of weight loss, physical activity and glycaemic control in adults with type 2 diabetes. *BMC Public Health.* 2010; **10**:452.

8 Lynch BM, Cerin E, Newman B, Owen N. Physical activity, activity change, and their correlates in a population-based sample of colorectal cancer survivors. *Ann Behav Med*. 2007; **34**(2):135–43.

9 General Assembly of the World Medical Association. World medical association declaration of helsinki: ethical principles for medical research involving human subjects. *J Am Coll Dent*. 2014; **81**(3):14–8.

10 Palange P, Ward SA, Carlsen KH, Casaburi R, Gallagher CG, Gosselink R, et al. Recommendations on the use of exercise testing in clinical practice. *Eur Respir J*. 2007; **29**(1):185–209.

11 Butland RJ, Pang J, Gross ER, Woodcock AA, Geddes DM. Two-, six-, and 12-minute walking tests in respiratory disease. *Br Med J (Clin Res Ed)*. 1982; **284**(6329):1607–8.

12 Sallis JF, Saelens BE. Assessment of physical activity by self-report: status, limitations, and future directions. *Res Quar Exerc Sport*. 2000; **71**(2):S1–S14.

13 Ainsworth BE, Caspersen CJ, Matthews CE, Masse LC, Baranowski T, Zhu W. Recommendations to improve the accuracy of estimates of physical activity derived from self report. *J Phys Act Health*. 2012; **9**(1):S76–84.

14 Wijndaele K, Westgate K, Stephens SK, Blair SN, Bull FC, Chastin SF, et al. Utilization and harmonization of adult accelerometry data: review and expert consensus. *Med Sci Sports Exerc*. 2015; **47**(10):2129–39.

15 Barnett A, van den Hoek D, Barnett D, Cerin E. Measuring moderate-intensity walking in older adults using the ActiGraph accelerometer. *BMC Geriatr*. 2016; **16**(1):211.

16 Phillips SM, Cadmus-Bertram L, Rosenberg DE, Buman MP, Lynch BM. Wearable technology and physical activity in chronic disease: opportunities and challenges. *Am J Prev Med*. 2017; In press.

17 Nguyen NH, Hadgraft NT, Moore MM, Rosenberg DE, Lynch C, Reeves MM, et al. A qualitative evaluation of breast cancer survivors' acceptance of and preferences for consumer wearable technology activity trackers. *Support Care Cancer*. 2017; **25**(11):3375–84.

27 Research studies with populations with mental health issues

Andy Smith and Nathalie Noret

Aims of the chapter

The objectives of this chapter are to provide researchers with a resource which:

- Highlights a number of issues to be considered when conducting research on exercise and mental health;
- Signposts the reader to published studies which illustrate current methodological approaches; and
- Suggests future research questions and methodologies. By so doing the chapter addresses ethical issues in relation to research in populations with mental health issues.

Introduction

Research exploring relationships between exercise and mental health can be undertaken exploring exercise as a predictor of mental health, mental health as a predictor of physical activity and exercise as a mechanism for improving mental health. Undertaking research to examine these relationships and mechanisms poses ethical and methodological challenges.

Methodological issues when conducting research on exercise and mental health

Local regulatory frameworks, such as the research ethics and research integrity policies of the institution in which one works, and factors specific to the proposed study are often more important than the generic 'issues' considered here. Therefore, whilst it is necessary to consider the issues presented below it is not sufficient to consider them in isolation from the 'issues' raised by any specific research proposal.

Stigma

Sadly in some communities and societies there is a stigma surrounding mental illness. This has the following implications for researchers:

- Research should be conducted in such a way as to help break down this stigma;
- Those who feel stigmatized may feel less inclined to volunteer to be participants in studies, a recruitment factor which may bias findings; and
- There may be less funding to study mental rather than physical illness.

Poverty

Care needs to be taken not to confound mental illness with poverty. As the Joseph Rowntree Foundation concluded: *"Poverty increases the risk of mental health problems and can be both a causal factor and a consequence of mental ill health . . . "*.[1] Research into mental illness often means working with some of the most vulnerable and hard-to-reach members of our communities i.e. those who are both poor and unwell. As a result they may be homeless and struggle with reading and writing. Researchers have a profound responsibility to attempt to recruit such people to participate in research and when doing so treat them with respect and to protect and enhance their dignity. When designing methodologies in the area of mental health, researchers should familiarize themselves with the relevant literature on poverty (see for example Barr et al.,[2] Wickham et al.[3] and Lund[4]).

Conflation

Care needs to be taken not to conflate different types of mental illness into one overall category. The gradations may be subtle but crucially important. For example, when conducting research into depression care needs to be taken to define both the type and severity of the condition. Similarly different types of exercise should not be conflated. The prescribed exercise should be reported using the "Consensus on Exercise Reporting Template" (CERT).[5-7]

Comorbidity

As Wegner et al.[8] report "in a survey conducted in over sixty countries, Moussavi and colleagues found that depressive disorders have more detrimental effects on overall health status than diseases like diabetes, arthritis, or asthma" (p. 1003). This is an issue both from a safety perspective and it needs to be controlled for within study methodologies.

Pharmacology

People with mental illness are oftentimes prescribed drugs which help them manage their conditions. Researchers need to be aware of what drugs participants in their studies are taking. This is so that they can:

- Exclude those who are taking drugs which may adversely interact with exercise;
- Control for the effect of the drugs. It is important that researchers in this area get professional advice and guidance from qualified and experienced medical doctors on all drug-related matters connected to their studies. This will help keep participants safe and secure the methodological rigour of the study. When considering the impact that the drugs taken by some people may have on the methodology of research in this area, care needs to be taken to account for "*antipsychotic-induced weight gain*" (p. 547 – Alvarez-Jimenez et al., 2008).[9] If this is not accounted for the potential positive impact of exercise in enabling people on this medication to maintain a healthy weight or reduce this side-effect of the drugs may go unreported.

Neuroscience

One can argue that when designing studies it is possible to adopt a methodology from neuroscience focusing on disease of the brain (e.g. Alzheimer's) *or* a psychological/ psychiatric methodology focusing on disease of the mind (e.g. depression). As the review conducted by Kandola et al.,[10] on the effect of aerobic exercise (AE) on hippocampal plasticity states: "*AE is associated with cognitive enhancements **and** stimulates a cascade of neuroplastic mechanisms that support hippocampal functioning*" (p. 1 – emphases of the word 'and' added by the authors of this chapter).

Outcomes

An essential part of designing a research methodology, is to clearly state from the outset what potential outcome is being investigated. For example, if designing a RCT comparing an exercise intervention, is the aim of the study to:

- Investigate the effect of exercise as a treatment for a mental illness (e.g. depression)?
- Or as a therapy for a comorbidity (e.g. CHD risk factors) and will the intervention be successful if the effect is 'acute'?
- Or will only 'chronic' response(s) be judged effective?

Ideally issues such as these should be formally recorded before any data is collected. A number of journals now enable researchers to pre-register their hypothesis.

Community

Given the number of researchers working in the area of exercise and mental health and their disciplinary and geographical spread, it may be over-claiming to call them a community. The output from workers in this field is increasing in both quality and quantity. However, the literature is relatively quiet as to the long-term purpose of this endeavour. This is largely because most of the current research is not 'directed' toward a common purpose but is motivated by curiosity or the need to develop evidence to underpin practice and policy. To a large extent this 'free market' of ideas is to be celebrated and encouraged. Nonetheless, if one was to speculate as to a long-term goal, would it be to use exercise as a therapy for those with mental illness or to help the general population be happy?

Interdisciplinary

In the UK at least, calls for an interdisciplinary approach to almost every conceivable research question have become almost a cliché. Demands for interdisciplinarity have become so loud as to deafen those who might benefit from hearing the suggestion. It is then with some trepidation, for fear of being accused of stating the obvious, that we suggest that more methods designed by interdisciplinary teams are required. Our justification is that research on exercise and mental health by its very nature involves that most fundamental interface between the body (the exercise) and the mind (the mental health). We strongly suggest that every research method in this area is developed in partnership between at least an exercise scientist and a psychologist. Even such a partnership is arguably fundamentally weakened by the exclusion of a neuro-scientist, psychiatrist, exercise leader, etc. So we conclude this point with a contrac-tion of all that has gone before by stating that there is still space for the sole author buried deep in their parent discipline investigating one very specific factor.

Consent

Some people with certain types of mental illness may not be able to give informed consent and others may need help and support to understand the process. When planning research in this area, care needs to be taken to put in place appropriate mechanisms to gain consent and to allocate sufficient time to gain consent from each individual participant.

Acute or chronic response

In designing methodologies to investigate the effect of exercise on mental health the researcher needs to clearly state from the outset if they are seeking to measure acute or chronic responses. A good example of a study on the acute effect of exercise on obsessive-compulsive disorder (OCD) was conducted by Abrantes et al.[11]

Age

Research by Tao et al.,[12] which found that "*physical activity might not be the protective fac-tor for health risk behaviours and psychopathology symptoms in adolescents*" (p. 762), points to the importance of not assuming that findings in adults hold true for other age groups. An example of a methodology specifically looking at older adults, aged 50–94 can be found in the work of Strawbridge et al.,[13] whose work demonstrates what can be found when a longitudinal study is conducted.

A golden rule?

As research happens at the frontiers of knowledge and is constantly changing and morphing in nature, it is impossible to draft a golden rule that can be applied in all contexts. Perhaps the nearest one can get is to state that research should do no harm and to ask ourselves would we let a loved one participate in the studies we conduct. Undertaking research on mental health has the potential to be distressing for some participants. We should therefore endeavour to do such research ethically and sensi-tively to ensure no inadvertent resulting harm.

Given the prevalence of mental illness any large-scale study into any aspect of exercise and health is likely to 'inadvertently' recruit participants with mental health problems. This is the reverse of the comorbidity issue described earlier in this chapter. As research-ers in exercise and mental health we have a responsibility to educate our colleagues conducting, for example, research on exercise and obesity to take into account the like-lihood that participants in their studies are likely to include people with mental illness.

Research which illustrates current methodological approaches

There is some remarkable research being conducted around the world on exercise and mental health using robust, rigorous and sometimes very creative methodologies.

What follows cannot capture the scale, breadth or overall quality of this work. However, it does signpost the reader to studies which illustrate some of the methodological approaches being used.

Surveys: Cross-sectional surveys can provide an important first step in identifying an initial relationship between variables, such as between exercise and mental health.[14] Such methods provide a quick, cheap and effective method of establishing an initial relationship across variables. However, they are limited in the extent to which causality can be inferred, and research is now moving more towards a greater use of longitudinal survey designs to identify changes in relationships over time (e.g. Sagatun et al. 2007[15]) and towards examination of variables which affect the relationship between exercise and mental health, such as mediating and moderating factors.[16,17]

Randomized Controlled Trails: The literature now includes a number of high-quality RCTs.[18] The work of Sturm et al.[19] has a number of strong methodological features including:

- Working safely with a group of people with a high risk of suicide; and
- A clear statement of limitations.

Methodological Studies: The maturity of the literature on exercise and mental health is demonstrated as there are studies which investigate methodological issues in the area. Stubbs et al.[20] have published a meta-analysis and meta-regression on drop out rates in RCTs studying exercise and depression. As they state "dropouts, from RCTs pose a threat to the validity of this evidence base, with drop out rates varying across studies" (p. 457). This work makes an important contribution to our understanding of how best to conduct research in this area.

Neuroscience studies: A good example of research methods in this area is the study by Haslacher et al.,[21] entitled "physical exercise counteracts genetical susceptibility to depression" (p. 168). Their methodology included genotyping rs6265 (a variant of the brain-derived neurotropic factor linked to depression) in controls ($n = 58$) as compared to marathon runners ($n = 55$). Work such as this challenges researchers who do not come from a neuroscience background to develop the skill set and methodological competencies to contribute to work in this area.

Meta-analysis: The authors of this chapter consider the meta-analysis conducted by Schuch et al.[22] to be an essential read for those considering using this methodological approach. The study looks at the use of exercise to treat people with depression. Those who study this publication will find that the work contains an adjustment for publication bias and a fail-safe assessment (see p. 47). Meta-analysis has proved such a powerful methodology that the literature now includes at least one meta-meta-analysis conducted by Rebar et al.,[23] on physical activity and depression and anxiety.

Animal studies: Whilst animal studies must only be taken after careful consideration of the ethical issues they raise there is some such work in the literature. One such study is the work of Bjørnebekk et al.,[24] using rats to study the effect of exercise on the hippocampus.

Reviews: Arguably any new reviewer of the literature should begin their methodological reflections by visiting the Cochrane Library. The reviews contained there represent some of the best methodological practice across a range of subject areas. In 2013 a review on exercise and depression was added to this collection.[25] Both this review and a subsequent criticism by Schuch et al.[22] are worth reading to gain an insight into how to review the literature.

Readers of the literature may find it a stimulating intellectual exercise to identify and justify what they think have been the studies which have, historically, shaped our current thinking and approach to research on exercise and mental health. In 1959 Shamos did something similar in physics writing "viewed in retrospect,[26] the most significant ideas in physics stand out in simple elegance against a background shadowed by confusion" (p. v). Reflective, critical thinking on the research methodologies that have 'got us here' may provide insights to guide future research questions and methodologies.

Suggested future research questions and methodologies

With the development of systematic reviews and meta-analysis techniques, along with the advent of 'big data', it is likely that the coming decade will see even more advances in new ways of 'mining' existing data. By combining data points from hundreds of high-quality separate studies it may be that we will be able to identify factors not apparent at the level of individual studies. However, care must be taken to ensure that empirical studies remain our top priority. Empirical work should, in the view of the authors of this chapter, attract most of the research funding and be held in the highest esteem. In addition, whilst systematic reviews have arguably revolutionized how we interrogate the literature, they are not the only method for such analysis. Grant et al. (2009)[27] identified "14 review types and associated methodologies" (p. 91). Without wishing to add needlessly to this typology the authors of this chapter are currently working on a literature-based, 'evidence-based practice framework' to guide exercise prescription for people with mental illness.

Whilst population-level studies that look at mental health as a public health issue at a national level are important (see ten Have et al.,[28] Pratt et al.,[29] for good examples), future research may also benefit from the investigation of local issues. For example, in the home city of the authors, York, more people require emergency admission to hospital as a result of self-harm than the average in the UK.[30] A local study on how exercise intervention might, or might not, help tackle this problem could be justified.

With the predicted increase in the power of computing and the growth of online exercise programmes it is foreseeable that technological progress will enable the development of new methodologies and research questions. There is already work in the literature which hints at this direction of travel. See for example the RCT by Hallgren et al.,[31] comparing physical activity with an internet-based intervention and the work of Kimhy et al.[32] on the use of 'active-play video games' with people with schizophrenia.

If, as seems probable, the number of peer-reviewed publication on exercise and mental health continues to grow there will be a need to develop unified approaches. An 'early attempt' has already been made to do this.[33] More work to develop and apply suitable methodologies is needed if the many disparate studies published and underway are to be joined up. There is also a need to join up the exercise science literature with the recreation literature.

Recent evidence has demonstrated the effectiveness of exercise programmes to support an individual's suffering with stress-related symptoms such as symptoms of anxiety and post-traumatic stress disorder (PTSD), in both adults and children and adolescents.[34,35] The apparent utility of exercise in reducing mental health symptoms gives rise to the opportunity to develop evidence-based exercise interventions to ease mental health symptoms in particular populations. One such avenue is to support victims of aggressive and/or violent behaviours. Experiencing aggressive behaviours such as rape, sexual assault and bullying has been found to be related to a range of mental health symptoms.[36,37] Given the available evidence, exercise may provide a framework for intervention to buffer the impact of such negative experiences on mental health. Although limited, the emerging literature on the use of exercise to support victims of violence and aggression has demonstrated that physical activity such as yoga can increase positive coping strategies and lessen depressive symptomology in female victims of sexual assault,[38] and a dedicated women's-only fitness class was found to develop feelings of empowerment in victims of sexual assault compared to those in other more traditional physical activities.[39] Exercise is also recommended as a means to increase the social activity of children and adolescents who have been victims of bullying, the aim being to provide social contact and reduce social rejection.[40] Although the literature to date is limited, it does suggest a role for exercise in buffering the negative impact experiences of violent and aggressive behaviour.

References

1   Elliott, I. *Poverty and mental health: a review to inform the joseph rowntree foundation's anti-poverty strategy.* London: Mental Health Foundation; 2016.

2   Barr B, Kinderman P, Whitehead M. Trends in mental health inequalities in England during a period of recession, austerity and welfare reform 2004 to 2013. *Soc Sci Med.* 2015; **147**:324–31.

3   Wickham S, Anwar E, Barr B, Law C, Taylor-Robinson D. Poverty and child health in the UK: using evidence for action. *Arch Dis Child.* 2016; archdischild-2014.

4   Lund C. Poverty, inequality and mental health in low-and middle-income countries: time to expand the research and policy agendas. *Epidemiol Psychiatr Sci.* 2015; **24**(2):97.

5   Slade SC, Dionne CE, Underwood M, Buchbinder R, Beck B, Bennell K, Holland A. Consensus on Exercise Reporting Template (CERT): modified delphi study. *Phys Ther.* 2016; **96**(10):1514–24.

6   Kent P, O'Sullivan PB, Keating J, Slade SC. Evidence-based exercise prescription is facilitated by the Consensus on Exercise Reporting Template (CERT). *Br J Sports Med.* 2018; **52**; 147–8.

7   Slade SC, Keating JL. Exercise prescription: a case for standardised reporting. *Br J Exerc Med.* 2012; **46**(16):1110–13.

8   Wegner M, Helmich I, Machado S, Nardi AE, Arias-Carrion O, Budde H. Effects of exercise on anxiety and depression disorders: review of meta-analyses and neurobiological mechanisms. *CNS Neurol Disord Dr Targets.* 2014; **13**(6):1002–14.

9   Alvarez-Jimenez M, Gonzalez-Blanch C, Crespo-Facorro B, Hetrick S, Rodriguez-Sanchez JM, Perez-Iglesias R, Vazquez-Barquero JL. Antipsychotic-induced weight gain in chronic and first-episode psychotic disorders; a systematic critical reappraisal. *CNS Drugs.* 2008; **22**(7):547–62.

10   Kandola A, Hendrikse J, Lucassen PJ, Yucel M. Aerobic exercise as a tool to improve hippocampal plasticity and function in humans: practical implications for mental health treatment. *Front Hum Neurosci.* 2016; **10**:373.

11   Abrantes AM, Strong DR, Cohn A, Cameron AY, Greenberg BD, Mancebo MC, Brown RA. Acute changes in obsessions and compulsions following moderate-intensity aerobic exercise among patients with obsessive-compulsive disorder. *J Anxiety Disord.* 2009; **23**:923–7.

12 Tao FB, Xu ML, Kim SD, Sun Y, Su PY, Huang K. Physical activity might not be the protective factor for health risk behaviours and psychopathological symptoms in adolescents. *J Paediatr Child Health.* 2007; **43**(11):762–7.

13 Strawbridge WJ, Deleger S, Roberts RE, Kaplan GA. Physical activity reduces the risk of subsequent depression for older adults. *Am J Epidemiol.* 2002; **156**(4):328–34.

14 Monshouwer J, ten Have M, van Poppel M, Kemper H, Vollebergh W. Possible mechanisms explaining the association between physical activity and mental health: findings from the 2001 Dutch health behaviour in school-aged children survey. *Clin Psychol Sci.* 2013; **1**(1):67–74. DOI: 10.1177/2167702612450485

15 Sagatun A, Søgaard AJ, Bjertness E, Selmer R, Heyerdahl S. The association between weekly hours of physical activity and mental health: a three-year follow-up study of 15–16-year-old students in the city of Oslo, Norway. *BMC Public Health.* 2007; **7**(1):155.

16 Scarapicchia TMF, Sabiston CM, O'Loughlin E, Brunet J, Chaiton M, O'Loughlin JL. Physical activity motivation mediates the association between depression symptoms and moderate to-vigorous physical activity. *Prev Med.* 2014; **66**:45–48. DOI: 10.1016/j.ypmed.2014.05.017

17 Horman KJ, Tylka TL. Appearance-based exercise motivation moderates the relationship between exercise frequency and positive body image. *Body Image.* 2014; **11**(2):101–8. DOI: 10.1016/j.bodyim.2014.01.003

18 Stubbs B, Vancampfort D, Rosenbaum S, Ward, PB, Richards J, Ussher M, Schuch FB. Challenges establishing the efficacy of exercise as an antidepressant treatment: a systematic review and meta-analysis of control group responses in exercise randomised controlled trials. *Sports Med.* 2016, **46**(5):699–713.

19 Sturm J, Plöderl M, Fartacek C, Kralovec K, Neunhäuserer D, Niederseer D, Fartacek R. Physical exercise through mountain hiking in high-risk suicide patients. A randomized crossover trial. *Acta Psychiatr Scand.* 2012; **126**(6):467–75.

20 Stubbs B, Vancampfort D, Rosenbaum S, Ward PB, Richards J, Soundy A, Schuch FB. Drop-out from exercise randomized controlled trials among people with depression: a meta-analysis and meta regression. *J Affect Disord.* 2016; **190**:457–66.

21 Haslacher H, Michlmayr M, Batmyagmar D, Perkmann T, Ponocny-Seliger E, Scheichenberger V, Wagner O. Physical exercise counteracts genetic susceptibility to depression. *Neuropsychobiology.* 2015; **71**(3):168–75.

22 Schuch FB, Vancampfort D, Richards J, Rosenbaum S, Ward PB, Stubbs B. Exercise as a treatment for depression: a meta-analysis adjusting for publication bias. *J Psychiatr Res.* 2016; **77**:42–51.

23 Rebar AL, Stanton R, Geard D, Short C, Duncan MJ, Vandelanotte C. A meta-meta- analysis of the effect of physical activity on depression and anxiety in non-clinical adult populations. *Health Psychol Rev.* 2015; **9**(3):366 78.

24 Bjørnebekk A, Mathé AA, Brené S. The antidepressant effect of running is associated with increased hippocampal cell proliferation. *Int J Neuropsychoph.* 2005; **8**(3):357–68.

25 Cooney GM, Dwan K, Greig CA, Lawlor DA, Rimer J, Waugh FR, Mead GE. Exercise for depression. *Cochrane Database of Syst Rev.* 2013; **9**, Art. No.: CD004366.

26 Shamos MH. *Great experiments in physics: firsthand accounts from galileo to einstein.* New York: Holt, Rinehart and Winston; 1959.

27 Grant MJ, Booth A. A typology of reviews: an analysis of 14 review types and associated methodologies. *Health Inf Libr J.* 2009; **26**(2):91–108.

28 ten Have M, de Graaf R, Monshouwer K. Physical exercise in adults and mental health status: findings from the Netherlands mental health survey and incidence study (NEMESIS). *J Psychosom Res.* 2011; **71**(5):342–8.

29 Pratt LA, Druss BG, Manderscheid RW, Walker ER. Excess mortality due to depression and anxiety in the United States: results from a nationally representative survey. *Gen Hosp Psychiat.* 2016; **39**:39–45.

30 City of York Council. Self-harm: local identification of needs. Available 14/03/2018, from: http://democracy.york.gov.uk/documents/s107984/Annex%20B%20-%20Summary%20 Self%20Harm%20Needs%20Asesssment%20-%20FINAL%2003.08.16.pdf

31 Hallgren M, Kraepelien M, Öjehagen A, Lindefors N, Zeebari Z, Kaldo V, Forsell Y. Physical exercise and internet-based cognitive – behavioural therapy in the treatment of depression: randomised controlled trial. *Br J Psychiat.* 2015; **207**(3):227–34.

32 Kimhy D, Khan S, Ayanrouh L, Chang RW, Hansen MC, Lister A, et al. Use of active-play video games to enhance aerobic fitness in schizophrenia: feasibility, safety, and adherence. *Psychiatr Serv.* 2015; **67**(2):240–3.

33 Salmon P. Effects of physical exercise on anxiety, depression, and sensitivity to stress: a unifying theory. *Clin Psychol Rev.* 2001; **21**(1):33–61.

34 Newman CL, Motta RW. The effect of aerobic exercise on childhood PTSD, anxiety, and depression. *Int J Emerg Ment Health.* 2007; **9**(2):133–58.

35 Rosenbaum S, Vancampfort D, Steel Z, Newby J, Ward PB, Stubbs B. Physical activity in the treatment of Post-traumatic stress disorder: a systematic review and meta-analysis. *Psychiat Res.* 2015; **230**(2):130–6. DOI: 10.1016/j.psychres.2015.10.017

36 Ttofi MM, Farrington DP, Lösel F, Loeber R. Do the victims of school bullies tend to become depressed later in life? A systematic review and meta-analysis of longitudinal studies. *J Aggress Confl Peace Res.* 2011; **3**(2):63–73. DOI: 10.1108/17596591111132873

37 Chen LP, Murad MH, Paras ML, Colbenson KM, Sattler AL, Goranson EN, Zirakzadeh A. Sexual abuse and lifetime diagnosis of psychiatric disorders: systematic review and meta-analysis. *Mayo Clin Proc.* 2010; **85**(7):618–29.

38 Crews DA, Stolz-Newton M, Grant NS. The use of yoga to build self-compassion as a healing method for survivors of sexual violence. *J Religion Spiritual Soc Work Soc Thought.* 2016; **35**(3):39–156. DOI: 10.1080/15426432.2015.1067583

39 Cole AN, Ullrich-French S. Exploring empowerment for sexual assault victims in women's only group fitness. *Women Exerc Phys Act J.* 2017; **25**(2):96–104.

40 Crothers LM, Kolbert JB. Tackling a problematic behavior management issue: teachers' intervention in childhood bullying problems. *Interv Sch Clin.* 2008; **43**(3):132–9.

28 Research studies in populations with physical disabilities

Christof A. Leicht, Barry Mason and Jan W. van der Scheer

Chapter aims

The aims of this chapter are to introduce readers to the issues associated with doing research with people who have a physical disability. We cover the following themes: population-specific physical activity guidelines; assessment of physiological and anatomical parameters; risks and considerations when undertaking exercise assessments or prescribing exercise; and specialized or modified equipment used when researching with this group.

Physical activity guidelines for people with disabilities

Many people with physical disabilities face specific physical, psychosocial and environmental barriers to physical activity (PA).[1] As such, they are often less active and more physically deconditioned than people from the general population.[2,3] This, in turn, further increases their risk of secondary health conditions such as cardiovascular disease, diabetes and mental health problems.[4] There is no clear-cut solution for people with disabilities to engage in a more physically active lifestyle, which is further complicated by differences in age and health condition. Effective strategies require collaboration between rehabilitation and community settings and should give people with disabilities the possibility to find PA opportunities that fit their needs and preferences.[5,6]

A first step towards using PA to improve a population's fitness and health is formulating and implementing evidence-based PA guidelines.[7] PA guidelines are systematically developed, evidence-based statements that provide age and ability specific information on what is required to maintain or improve fitness, performance and health.[7] Such guidelines describe types of PA that are effective and advise on the frequency, intensity and duration of the required PA.

Over the past decade, international and national agencies have used systematic literature reviews and expert panel discussions to develop PA guidelines for the general population. For instance, the World Health Organization and the UK Chief Medical Officer recommend at least 150 min/week of moderate-intensity aerobic activity or 75 min/week of vigorous-intensity activity, in addition to muscle-strengthening activity twice per week.[8,9] However, these guidelines were not specifically meant to be applicable to people with physical disabilities.[8] Their unique characteristics and barriers to PA warrant the need for disability-specific PA guidelines that take into consideration the benefits, risks, values and preferences of the people who will use the guidelines.[10]

Recently, groups consisting of researchers, clinicians and people with disabilities have addressed this gap, leading to evidence-based PA guidelines for people with spinal cord injury and those with multiple sclerosis.[11,12] The evidence underpinning these guidelines, as well as the guidelines themselves, can be an important starting point when designing research studies on PA and disability. They provide information on what we know or do not yet know, highlight the risks when people with disabilities engage in PA, indicate what is feasible for a specific disability population, and outline their preferences when engaging in PA. This information should be based on evidence and developed through a rigorous, systematic and transparent process that adheres to internationally accepted standards for formulating PA guidelines.[10,13]

Part of the PA guideline development processes is describing research gaps that limited the development of the guidelines (e.g. lack of evidence for a specific exercise type or specific health outcome).[11,12] Addressing these gaps will not only advance research in this field, but also give people with disabilities more opportunities to improve their fitness, performance and health – on the basis of evidence rather than assumptions.

In the sections below, we outline some of the unique caveats and challenges facing researchers when working with people with physical disabilities. The aims are to increase awareness of these matters and in so doing, to facilitate the collection of high quality scientific data and thereby to reach meaningful conclusions. We further provide an overview how research can be conducted, focusing on exercise testing related and disability-specific issues.

Assessment of physiological and anatomical parameters

Physical capacity is a determinant of many health-related outcomes and a key concept frequently assessed in exercise and health research. As such its accurate determination is of central importance. Disabilities often lead to a reduction of physical capacity resulting from a reduced active muscle mass, missing limbs or impaired function. In laboratory settings, peak variables (such as peak oxygen uptake) can be determined in graded exercise tests to exhaustion. Adjusting the start load and load increment relative to the severity of the impairment is therefore central to achieving exhaustion in an optimal timeframe,[14] i.e. not too short to result in excessive loading of the working muscles, but not too long to result in exercise duration dependent fatigue. For example, start loads and load increments are reduced by ~50% in athletes with high-level spinal cord injuries (resulting in tetraplegia) when compared with athletes with low-level spinal cord injuries.[15] A reduced peak heart rate and the lack of a linear response between heart rate and work rate can be found in disabilities related to neurological dysfunction such as high-level spinal cord injuries. Subsequently, in these populations there is limited use for heart rate as a monitoring tool during exercise, and alternatives such as subjective rating of exercise intensity have been explored. There is promise in the use of ratings of perceived exertion for exercise prescription,[16,17] but also to give the researcher an indication of the relative strain of exercise.

Disabilities may further alter the anatomy of an individual, examples being altered or missing limbs, burn scars or altered location of blood vessels. Some flexibility in study protocols may be required to deal with such problems, e.g. application of surface markers or performing venepuncture at the contralateral, unimpaired side.

Exercise risks and contraindications

Disabilities may lead to changes that make investigations related to exercise a potential hazard to study participants. Impairment of autonomic function (e.g. because of neural damage) can lead to autonomic dysreflexia, a condition accompanied by potentially life-threatening spikes in blood pressure. Autonomic dysreflexia can be triggered by a full bladder or compression of the area affected by neural damage.[18] It is therefore crucial to check for potential pressure points (either on seating surface, or on contact points with prostheses) and to void the bladder before any testing.

Where muscular function is impaired, limb or core stability may be compromised. Applying strapping to the participant can increase stability (e.g. strapping of the upper body to a wheelchair), whilst hand rails or a harness decrease the risk of falls in ambulatory studies. Impaired muscular function is often associated with reduced bone mineral density, which may prove an issue in studies investigating impactful movements, with fractures as a worst-case scenario. Sensitivity to temperature may also be altered, and thermoregulation can be impaired for disabilities affecting the autonomic nervous system. Objective monitoring of body temperature in hot environments or during physical strain represents an important tool for conducting research that is safe.[19]

Equipment and technology

In populations with disabilities, mobility performance is not only dependent on the physical capacity of the individual, but also their equipment (e.g. wheelchair, prostheses) and the interaction between the two. For wheelchair users, the wheelchair and how it is configured/maintained can have a significant bearing upon many aspects of performance, such as manoeuvrability, acceleration, efficiency and stability.[20] Specific wheelchair selections (e.g. smaller wheels, increased camber) and maintenance issues (e.g. reduced tyre pressure, worn castor bearings) can increase the rolling resistance, which increase the physical strain imposed on the user.[21] Subsequently, researchers should pay close attention to the individuals' equipment and any changes they have made to it over time, especially if longitudinal monitoring is an objective of the research. Researchers should take as many steps as possible to standardize the users' equipment (e.g. tyre pressure etc.) given its effect on performance. This helps to determine whether any changes in performance are the result of changes to the individual rather than confounding variables owing to equipment.

Equipment and modalities for testing disabled populations often require innovation, either from the researcher or via assistive technology. To maximize ecological validity, over-ground propulsion studies in a field-based environment are generally favourable. However, if physiological or biomechanical outcome parameters are of interest it may not be possible to assess those in the field even with recent developments in technology (e.g. portable gas analysis systems, wearable technology for real-time 3D motion capture). Subsequently, laboratory-based testing can be considered a good, although sometimes expensive, alternative. Bespoke treadmills, wide enough to accommodate cambered sports chairs or the increased hip circumduction of above-knee amputees are often required with specific adaptations needed to ensure health and safety (Figure 28.1). Roller ergometer systems also enable wheelchair users to be tested in their own wheelchairs. An advantage of these systems is that they enable the user to determine the speed of propulsion, which means that sprinting performance can be assessed, which is not possible on most treadmills. In addition, dual-roller ergometers can independently assess the force applied on both sides, allowing researchers to explore propulsion asymmetries in greater detail (Figure 28.2). However, the mass of the rollers and difficulties associated with attaching wheelchairs can often inflate the rolling resistance experienced to values beyond those experienced

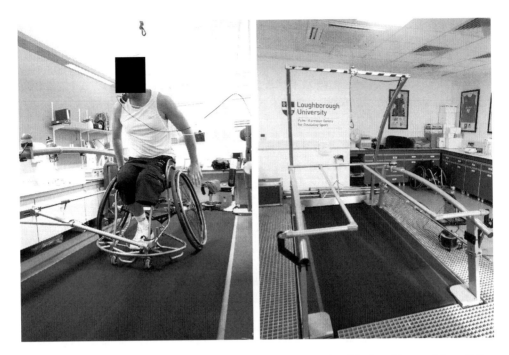

Figure 28.1 Bespoke treadmill developed to accommodate wheelchair athletes with a sliding
safety rail (left) and an attachable handrail for ambulant runners or cyclists (right).

during over-ground propulsion,[22] as well as causing issues with reproducibility. To
more accurately reflect the conditions experienced during over-ground propulsion
(e.g. resistance, physiological and biomechanical responses) treadmill-based propulsion at a gradient between 0.7% and 1.0% has been recommended.[22]

Upper-body exercise performance can further be assessed using arm crank ergometry (Figure 28.3). Arm cranking can be performed in a standardized chair. This elim-
inates the contribution of the individuals' equipment and their interaction with the
equipment, which may be of interest for some research questions. Importantly, arm
crank ergometry does not involve the synchronous activities of wheelchair propulsion
or handcycling that are more commonly performed in sport and leisure activities. Due
to the asynchronous action, rotational movements are performed, requiring greater
core stability.[23] Therefore, arm crank ergometry may not be suitable for individuals
with heavily impaired trunk function. One major advantage of arm crank ergometry,
however, is that an arm crank ergometer is not such a specialist and expensive piece
of equipment as the wheelchair treadmills or ergometers. This makes it more readily available and of potential use in rehabilitation or fitness settings to help promote
physical activity in populations with disabilities.

Conclusion

This chapter describes approaches taken to outline evidence-based physical activity
guidelines that are specific to populations with disabilities. Whilst large steps have

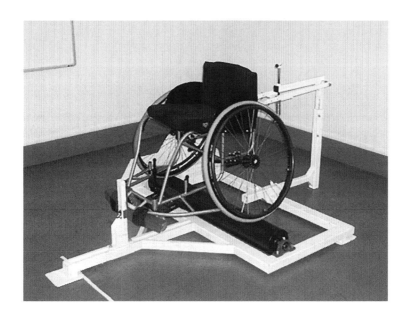

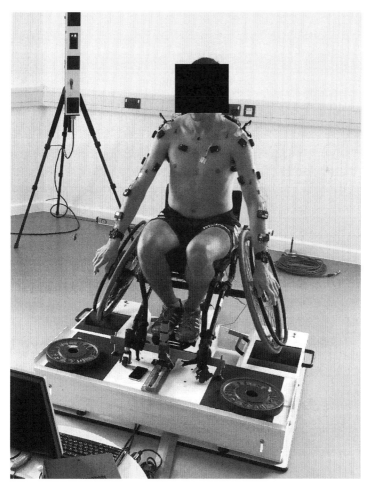

Figure 28.2 A single (top) and dual-roller (bottom) ergometer which enable sprinting performance to be assessed in individuals' own wheelchairs.

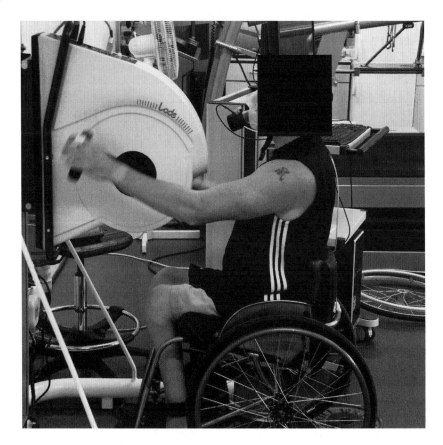

Figure 28.3 A manual wheelchair user performing exercise on an arm crank ergometer.

been taken in recent years to produce disability-specific guidelines based on peer-reviewed research, no guidelines exist for a large number of the many disability subgroups, making this an objective for future research. We further highlight some considerations when conducting research with individuals with disabilities. Awareness of disability-specific issues should allow the researcher to account and prepare for them and enable them to put procedures into place to minimize risk and safeguard the study participants' health and wellbeing.

References

1   Martin Ginis KA, Ma JK, Latimer-Cheung AE, Rimmer JH. A systematic review of review articles addressing factors related to physical activity participation among children and adults with physical disabilities. *Health Psychol Rev.* 2016; **10**:478–94. DOI: 10.1080/17437199.2016.1198240

2   Haisma JA, van der Woude LH, Stam HJ, et al. Physical capacity in wheelchair-dependent persons with a spinal cord injury: a critical review of the literature. *Spinal Cord.* 2006; **44**:642–52. DOI: 10.1038/sj.sc.3101915

3   van den Berg-Emons RJ, Bussmann JB, Stam HJ. Accelerometry-based activity spectrum in persons with chronic physical conditions. *Arch Phys Med Rehabil.* 2010; **91**:1856–61. DOI: 10.1016/j.apmr.2010.08.018

4   Rimmer JH, Schiller W, Chen MD. Effects of disability-associated low energy expenditure deconditioning syndrome. *Exerc Sport Sci Rev.* 2012; **40**:22–9. DOI: 10.1097/JES.0b013e31823b8b82

5   Alingh RA, Hoekstra F, van der Schans CP, et al. Protocol of a longitudinal cohort study on physical activity behaviour in physically disabled patients participating in a rehabilitation counselling programme: ReSpAct. *BMJ Open.* 2015; **5**:e007591. DOI: 10.1136/bmjopen-2015-007591

6   Rimmer J, Lai B. Framing new pathways in transformative exercise for individuals with existing and newly acquired disability. *Disabil Rehab.* 2017; **39**:173–80. DOI: 10.3109/09638288.2015.1047967

7   Tremblay MS, Shephard RJ, Brawley LR. Research that informs Canada's physical activity guides: an introduction. *Can J Public Health.* 2007; **98**(Suppl 2):S1–8.

8   WHO. *WHO | Global recommendations on physical activity for health.* WHO; 2010. Available 26/03/2018, from: www.who.int/dietphysicalactivity/factsheet_recommendations/en/

9   Gov.uk. Start active, stay active: a report on physical activity from the four home countries' Chief Medical Officers. 2011. Available 26/03/2018, from: www.gov.uk/government/publications/start-active-stay-active-a-report-on-physical-activity-from-the-four-home-countries-chief-medical-officers

10 Brouwers MC, Kho ME, Browman GP, et al. AGREE II: advancing guideline development, reporting and evaluation in health care. *Can Med Assoc J.* 2010; **182**:E839–E842. DOI: 10.1503/cmaj.090449

11 Martin Ginis KA, van der Scheer JW, Latimer-Cheung AE, et al. Evidence-based scientific exercise guidelines for adults with spinal cord injury: an update and a new guideline. *Spinal Cord.* 2018; **56**:308–21. DOI: 10.1038/s41393-017-0017-3

12 Latimer-Cheung AE, Martin Ginis KA, Hicks AL, et al. Development of evidence-informed physical activity guidelines for adults with multiple sclerosis. *Arch Phys Med Rehab.* 2013; **94**:1829–36.e7. DOI: 10.1016/j.apmr.2013.05.015

13 Martin Ginis KA, van der Scheer JW, Latimer-Cheung AE, et al. Response to correspondence from the ESSA Statement authors. *Spinal Cord.* 2018; **56**:409–11. DOI: 10.1038/s41393-017-0051-1

14 Yoon BK, Kravitz L, Robergs R. V̇O₂max, protocol duration, and the V̇O₂ plateau. *Med Sci Sports Exerc.* 2007; **39**:1186–92. DOI: 10.1249/mss.0b13e318054e304

15 Leicht CA, Tolfrey K, Lenton JP, et al. The verification phase and reliability of physiological parameters in peak testing of elite wheelchair athletes. *Eur J Appl Physiol.* 2013; **113**:337–45. DOI: 10.1007/s00421-012-2441-6

16 Au JS, Totosy DE Zepetnek JO, Macdonald MJ. Modeling perceived exertion during graded arm cycling exercise in spinal cord injury. *Med Sci Sports Exerc.* 2017; **49**:1190–96. DOI: 10.1249/MSS.0000000000001203

17 van der Scheer JW, Hutchinson MJ, Paulson T, Martin Ginis KA, Goosey-Tolfrey VL. Reliability and Validity of Subjective Measures of Aerobic Intensity in Adults With Spinal Cord Injury: A Systematic Review. *PM R* 2018; **10**:194–207. DOI: 10.1016/j.pmrj.2017.08.440

18 Krassioukov A. Autonomic function following cervical spinal cord injury. *Respir Physiol Neurobiol.* 2009; **169**:157–64. DOI: 10.1016/j.resp.2009.08.003

19 Griggs KE, Leicht CA, Price MJ, Goosey-Tolfrey VL. Thermoregulation during intermittent exercise in athletes with a spinal-cord injury. *Int J Sports Physiol Perform.* 2015; **10**:469–75. DOI: 10.1123/ijspp.2014-0361

20 Mason BS, van der Woude LHV, Goosey-Tolfrey VL. The ergonomics of wheelchair configuration for optimal performance in the wheelchair court sports. *Sport Med.* 2013; **43**:23–38. DOI: 10.1007/s40279-012-0005-x

21 van der Woude LH, Veeger HE, Dallmeijer AJ, et al. Biomechanics and physiology in active manual wheelchair propulsion. *Med Eng Phys.* 2001; **23**:713–33.

22 Mason B, Lenton J, Leicht C, Goosey-Tolfrey V. A physiological and biomechanical comparison of over-ground, treadmill and ergometer wheelchair propulsion. *J Sports Sci.* 2014; **32**:78–91. DOI: 10.1080/02640414.2013.807350

23 Faupin A, Gorce P, Meyer C. Effects of type and mode of propulsion on hand-cycling biomechanics in nondisabled subjects. *J Rehabil Res Dev.* 2011; **48**:1049–60.

29 Using health equity to guide future physical activity research involving people living with serious mental illness

Paul Gorczynski, Shanaya Rathod and Kass Gibson

Introduction

Serious mental illness can be defined as a mental, behavioural or emotional disorder that is currently diagnosable or was diagnosed within the past year, of sufficient duration to meet the statistical diagnostic criteria in the Diagnostic and Statistical Manual of Mental Disorders classification (*DSM-V*), and which results in severe functional impairment that impedes or limits major life activities.[1] As a result of these severe functional impairments, people living with serious mental illness are considered vulnerable individuals. A major area of research interest in this population has been the use of physical activity to promote physical, mental and social health. This chapter will provide an overview of the importance of physical activity to the overall health and wellbeing of people living with serious mental illness and how social determinants of health need to be first addressed in this population in order to afford them the opportunity to become active and healthy. First the health benefits of physical activity as well as the consequences of physical inactivity in serious mental illness are reviewed, followed by a discussion of a lack of physical activity programming within clinical care in this population. Then, the broader social determinants of health that influence physical activity in this population are highlighted and how their neglect has affected not only physical activity, but the overall health of individuals living with serious mental illness. Finally, the chapter concludes with suggestions for future research, including ethical considerations, as well as the political engagement necessary to improve the physical activity and health of people living with serious mental illness.

Physical activity and serious mental illness

There are many physical, psychological and social health benefits to regular physical activity.[2–4] Despite these health benefits, many people living with serious mental illness are insufficiently active. In their comparative systematic review and meta-analysis examining activity levels between individuals living with and without serious mental illness, Stubbs and colleagues found individuals living with serious mental illness engaged in roughly the same amount of light physical activity as those living with no serious mental illness.[5] However, people living with serious mental illness engaged in significantly less moderate and vigorous physical activity (MVPA), only approximately 48 minutes per week, far below global recommendations of 150 minutes.[6] Such low levels of MVPA contribute to the poor cardiorespiratory fitness of people living with serious mental illness and exacerbates many morbidities often found in this population,[7] including high incidence of chronic conditions like metabolic syndrome,[8] type 2 diabetes[9] and cardiovascular disease.[10] Furthermore, results from Stubbs et al.'s work also found that individuals living with serious mental illness residing within inpatient psychiatric facilities were less active than those who lived in the community,[5] illustrating that those living with greater psychiatric disability were even further disadvantaged.

Inaction on inactivity

Despite much literature showing the benefits of regular activity in this population, tailored physical activity interventions for those living with serious mental illness have been sparse. There is a long history of recommending daily physical activity to people living with serious mental illness as part of their overall treatment.[11] In 1968, as part of the orthomolecular approach embedded within the medical model used in the US, some individuals living with schizophrenia and their families were provided with information about the psychotic illness and told about the clinical importance of daily physical activity.[11,12] More recently, Richardson and colleagues called for the complete integration of physical activity into mental health services for people living with serious mental illness.[13] They noted that physical activity could be delivered in group settings, composed of simple activities that were easy to organize and execute, like walking groups. They further noted that physical activity was often well received amongst individuals living with serious mental illness and that adherence to such programmes was similar to those living with no serious mental illness. Unfortunately, despite such calls for action, little has been done. Although there is sufficient evidence that physical activity improves health and wellbeing in people living with serious mental illness, there has been a complete failure at using such evidence to inform the design of sustainable interventions or produce meaningful change in clinical practice.[14] Put simply: our collective knowledge around the area of physical activity and serious mental illness has not led to the overall improvement of health of this population.

Unfortunately, people living with serious mental illness experience a disproportionately high level of poor physical health when compared to those living with no serious mental illness. Ultimately, people with serious mental illness have a decreased life expectancy of approximately 10 to 20 years.[15] While insufficient levels of MVPA undoubtedly are contributory factors, understanding unhealthy behaviours (e.g. inactivity, unhealthful eating, smoking) as causes of ill-health is insufficient. Therefore, those researching physical activity for people with serious mental illnesses should shift attention to the 'causes of the causes' of inactivity[16] or as Williams and Gibson (2017, p. 5) ask: "what *causes* people to behave in ways that *causes* ill-health?"[17]

The approach of researchers seeking to increase physical activity levels generally, and in mental health research specifically, has been to frame physical activity as a cost-effective treatment modality with minimum side-effects. As such, the strategy relies on robust evidence compelling people to active. Such an approach stresses choice but often overlooks opportunities for activity and factors that limit the ability for people to be active. For instance, qualitative research that has involved individuals living with serious mental illness residing both within and outside psychiatric facilities in Canada found that physical activity programmes often were not available or difficult to access.[18,19] Individual and environmental barriers such as low motivation and dealing with isolation caused by mental illness–related stigma resulted in many individuals living with serious mental illness becoming completely sedentary and resigned to a "culture of sitting".[19] Given such neglect, it is unsurprising that serious mental illness has been described as an 'abandoned illness' and that the complete neglect of the poor physical and social health of these individuals has resulted in what some call a "civil rights issue".[20] The results of the Schizophrenia Commission, conducted in the UK in 2011 to systematically evaluate provisions of care for people living with schizophrenia, called for strategies to prevent, rather than wait for, poor physical and social health to develop in people living with serious mental illness. Specifically, with respect to physical activity, the Schizophrenia Commission called for systematic implementation of exercise prescription schemes, complete with tailored exercise programmes, at the outset of treatment. Therefore, we maintain that less research effort should be expended on demonstrating efficacy of physical activity and more effort focusing on developing sustainable programmes that meet the needs, beyond physical health, for people with serious mental illness.

Physical activity interventions do not operate in isolation from other areas of support for people living with serious mental illness. In addition to addressing aspects of care related to physical activity for people living with serious mental illness, the Schizophrenia Commission called for interventions to address issues of health equity to achieve overall wellbeing.

What is health equity?

Health involves a state of complete physical, mental and social wellbeing and not just the absence of disease or disability.[21] Equity can be defined as fairness, an ethical principle rooted in distributive justice.[22] Health equity can be defined as the absence of systematic disparities in health and social determinants of health between groups with differing levels of social advantages and disadvantages.[23] Social determinants of health are conditions people are born into and live with and are largely based on distributions of money, power and resources, both regionally and internationally.[24] Social determinants of health can include levels of housing stability, early age experiences, employment, food security, access to healthcare services, access to education, education attainment, income and levels of social exclusion and isolation.[25] Additionally, racial, ethnic, gender and sexual identities compound health disparities.[26] A great deal of research shows that individuals living with serious mental illness are more likely to experience deprivation in relation to the social determinants of health than those living with no serious mental illness.[26] From unstable housing situations to food insecurity to poor access to healthcare, the social determinants of health are good predictors of disease burden – with physical, mental and social health consequences – in people living with serious mental illness.

A growing evidence base reveals an inverse relationship between adherence to health behaviours and socioeconomic status.[27,28] Additionally, evidence shows that regardless of how socioeconomic status is conceptualized and operationalized, individuals of low socioeconomic status, which disproportionately includes individuals with serious mental illness, are less physically active recreationally than those with higher socioeconomic status.[29–31] Furthermore, Buck and Frosini's review of health behaviours highlighted focusing on increasing awareness does not sufficiently increase opportunity.[32] A health equity perspective demonstrates improving health and wellbeing for people with severe mental illnesses requires addressing inactivity and inequality.[17]

How can health equity guide future physical activity research in serious mental illness?

Faulkner and Gorcyznski[2] have recommended that physical activity research within serious mental illness adopt a behavioural epidemiological framework to enhance practice.[33] Their recommendations included the:

- Establishment of the relationship between physical activity and physical and mental health;
- Development of valid and reliable methods to measure physical activity;
- Identification of factors that determine physical activity;
- Evaluation of interventions that promote physical activity;
- Translation of research into clinical practice.

In serious mental illness, translation of physical activity research into meaningful clinical practice has consistently failed because it has neglected to acknowledge the diverse social determinants of health. Research that has examined the correlates of physical activity in serious mental illness has found that the social determinants of health have been consistently positively associated with physical activity as well as overall improvements in physical and mental health outcomes.[2,34,35] For instance, individuals living with serious mental illness who are employed, have higher socioeconomic statuses, higher educational attainments, eat healthier diets and are not socially isolated, tend to be more physically active and experience better overall health. This research illustrates that addressing the social determinants of health may help establish a set of optimal conditions to allow individuals living with serious mental illness to become active and to improve their health.

Although calls have been made for multi-disciplinary approaches to increase physical activity amongst individuals living with serious mental illness,[36] few attempts have been made to actually address the social determinants of health to help establish optimal conditions for physical activity for individuals in this population. With respect to future physical activity research, we need to embrace individual-level factors, such as psychological, cognitive, emotional and behavioural factors, but also address broader socio-ecological factors such as employment, income, education, food security and social isolation.[2,35] This approach means three things for physical activity researchers working in serious mental illness:

- To recognize and acknowledge that people living with serious mental illness need to have their social determinants of health addressed in order to be active and healthy;
- To design physical activity interventions that currently work within the constraints of poor social determinants of health; and
- To advocate for policy changes at community, local and national levels to improve the social determinants of health.[25]

Along with mental health professionals, researchers can use their expertise to advocate for policy changes to establish programmes to address broader social determinants of health. Researchers can also become actively involved in local and federal politics, advocating for policies that address social determinants of health as well as helping to shape legislation and policy interventions that will improve the lives of people living with serious mental illness. As the Schizophrenia Commission points out,[20] advocating for legislation to address employment provisions within clinical care, income assistance, secure housing and support for those with greatest psychiatric disability is key to the long-term improvement of health for people living with serious mental illness. Researchers of physical activity in serious mental illness cannot ignore the evidence that clearly shows how physical activity behaviours will be influenced by broader social factors. In a sense, physical activity researchers must play a role in helping shape the social conditions where physical activity behaviours can thrive and people with serious mental illness can lead healthier lives.

Ethical challenges and considerations

The World Medical Association Declaration of Helsinki states that "Medical research involving an underprivileged or vulnerable population or community is only justified if the research is responsive to the health needs and priorities of that population or community and if there is a reasonable likelihood that this population or community stands to benefit from the results of the research".[37] This means that there is an ethical imperative for researchers to not only conduct physical activity research to ensure a robust evidence base to guide physical activity practice, but more importantly, to ensure that the wider community can benefit. From our perspective, this creates an ethical imperative for researchers to ensure that their research endeavours are at least sensitive to, if not directly address, social determinants of health.

In being sensitive to social determinants of health, researchers should give serious consideration to post-trial access to interventions for those participating in the trials. Post-trial access is more usually associated with drug trials. However, if researchers do truly consider physical activity to be medicine then plans must be in place to manage participant access to physical activity programmes and schemes after the research has concluded. Indeed, according to the Declaration of Helsinki: "At the conclusion of the study, patients entered into the study are entitled to be informed about the outcome of the study and to share any benefits that result from it, for example, access to interventions identified as beneficial in the study or to other appropriate care or benefits". Naturally, there are a number of practical considerations and pressures facing researchers. Nonetheless, careful consideration to post-trial access to physical activity initiatives should be considered early in research design and clearly communicated to both potential participants and other stakeholders, such as gatekeepers, in the research.

References

1 2015. Available from: www.nimh.nih.gov/health/statistics/prevalence/serious-mental-ill ness-smi-among-us-adults.shtml
2 Faulkner G, Gorczynski P. Evidence of impact of physical activity on schizophrenia. In: Clow A, Edmunds S, editors. *Physical activity and mental health*. Champaign, IL: Human Kinetics Publishers; 2013. pp. 215–35.

3 Firth J, Cotter J, Elliott R, French P, Yung AR. A systematic review and meta-analysis of exercise interventions in schizophrenia patients. *Psychol Med.* 2015; **45**:1343–61. DOI: 10.1017/S0033291714003110

4 Rosenbaum S, Tiedemann A, Sherrington C, Curtis J, Ward P B. Physical activity interventions for people with mental illness: a systematic review and meta-analysis. *J Clin Psychiat.* 2014; **75**:964–74. DOI: 10.4088/JCP.13r08765

5 Stubbs B, Firth J, Berry A, Schuch FB, Rosenbaum S, Gaughran F, Vancampfort D. How much physical activity do people with schizophrenia engage in? A systematic review, comparative meta-analysis and meta-regression. *Schizophr Res.* 2016; **176**:431–40. DOI: 10.1016/j.schres.2016.05.017

6 World Health Organization. Global recommendations on physical activity for health. 2010. Available from: http://apps.who.int/iris/bitstream/10665/44399/1/9789241599979_eng.pdf

7 Vancampfort D, Rosenbaum S, Ward PB, Stubbs B. Exercise improves cardiorespiratory fitness in people with schizophrenia: a systematic review and meta-analysis. *Schizophr Res.* 2015; **169**:453–7. DOI: 10.1016/j.schres.2015.09.029

8 Vancampfort D, Stubbs B, Mitchell AJ, De Hert M, Wampers M, Ward PB, Correll CU. Risk of metabolic syndrome and its components in people with schizophrenia and related psychotic disorders, bipolar disorder and major depressive disorder: a systematic review and meta-analysis. *World Psychiat.* 2015; **14**:339–47. DOI: 10.1002/wps.20252

9 Stubbs B, Vancampfort, D, De Hert M, Mitchell AJ. The prevalence and predictors of type two diabetes mellitus in people with schizophrenia: a systematic review and comparative meta-analysis. *Acta Psychiat Scand.* 2015; **132**:144–57. DOI: 10.1111/acps.12439

10 Gardner-Sood P, Lally J, Smith S, Atakan Z, Ismail K, Greenwood KE, IMPaCT team. Cardiovascular risk factors and metabolic syndrome in people with established psychotic illnesses: baseline data from the IMPaCT randomized controlled trial. *Psychol Med.* 2015; **45**:2619–29. DOI: 10.1017/S0033291715000562

11 Hawkins DR. Treatment of schizophrenia based on the medical model. *J Schizophr.*1968; **2**:3–10.

12 Pauling L. Orthomolecular psychiatry. Varying the concentrations of substances normally present in the human body may control mental disease. *Science.* 1968; **160**: 265–71.

13 Richardson CR, Faulkner G, McDevitt J, Skrinar GS, Hutchinson DS, Piette JD. Integrating physical activity into mental health services for persons with serious mental illness. *Psychiatr Serv.* 2005; **56**:324–31. DOI: 10.1176/appi.ps.56.3.324

14 Gorczynski P, Stitch M, Faulkner G. Examining methods, messengers, and behavioural theories to disseminate physical activity information to individuals with a diagnosis of schizophrenia: a scoping review. *J Ment Health.* (In Press). DOI: 10.1080/09638237.2016.1276535

15 Walker ER, McGee RE, Druss BG. Mortality in mental disorders and global disease burden implications: a systematic review and meta-analysis. *JAMA Psychiat.* 2015; **72**: 334–41. DOI: 10.1001/jamapsychiatry.2014.2502

16 Marmot, M. Social determinants of health inequalities. *Lancet.* 2005; **365**:1099–104.

17 Williams O, Gibson K. Exercise as a poisoned elixir: inactivity, inequality and intervention. *Qual Res Sport Exerc Health.* 2017; Online First. DOI: 10.1080/2159676X.2017.1346698

18 Faulkner G, Gorczynski P, Cohn T. Psychiatric illness and obesity: recognizing the "obesogenic" nature of an inpatient psychiatric setting. *Psychiatr Serv.* 2009; **60**:538–41.

19 Gorczynski P, Faulkner G, Cohn T. Dissecting the 'obesogenic' environment of a psychiatric setting: client perspectives. *Can J Community Ment Health.* 2013; **32**:65–82.

20 The Schizophrenia Commission. The abandoned illness: a report from the schizophrenia commission. 2012. Available from: www.rethink.org/media/514093/TSC_main_report_14_nov.pdf

21 World Health Organization. Constitution of the world health organization. 1948. Available from: http://apps.who.int/gb/bd/PDF/bd47/EN/constitution-en.pdf?ua=1

22 Braveman P, Gruskin S. Defining equity in health. *J Epidemiol Community Health.* 2003; **57**:254–8.

23 Whitehead M. The concepts and principles of equity in health. *Int J Health Serv Plan Adm Eval.* 1992; **22**: 429–45.

24 Blas E, Sivasankara Kurup A. *Equity, social determinants and public health programmes.* Geneva, Switzerland: World Health Organization Press; 2010.

25 Shim R, Koplan C, Langheim FJP, Manseau MW, Powers RA, Compton MT. The social determinants of mental health: an overview and call to action. *Psychiatr Ann.* 2014; **44**:22–6.

26 Swinson Evans T, Berkman N, Brown C, Gaynes B, Palmieri Weber R. *Disparities within serious mental illness. Technical brief No. 25.* Rockville, MD: Agency for Healthcare Research and Quality; 2016.

27 Stringhini S, Dugravot A, Shipley M, Goldberg M, Zins M, Kivimäki M, et al. Health behaviours, socioeconomic status, and mortality: further analyses of the British Whitehall II and the French GAZEL prospective cohorts. *PLoS Med.* 2011: **8**:e1000419.

28 Pampel FC, Krueger PM, Denney JT. Socioeconomic disparities in health behaviors. *Ann Rev Soc.* 2010; **36**:349–70.

29 Beenackers MA, Kamphuis CB, Giskes K, Brug J, Kunst AE, Burdorf A, van Lenthe FJ. Socioeconomic inequalities in occupational, leisure-time, and transport related physical activity among European adults: a systematic review. *Int J Behav Nutr Phys Act.* 2012; **9**:116.

30 Elhakeem A, Hardy R, Bann D, Caleyachetty R, Cosco TD, Hayhoe RP, Muthuri SG, Wilson R, Cooper R. Intergenerational social mobility and leisure-time physical activity in adulthood: a systematic review. *J Epidemiol Community Health.* 2017; **71**: 673–80.

31 Farrell J, Hollingsworth B, Propper C, Shields MA. The socioeconomic gradient in physical inactivity: evidence from one million adults in England. *Soc Sci Med.* 2014; **123**:55–63.

32 Buck D, Frosini F. *Clustering of unhealthy behaviours over time: implications for policy and practice.* London: The King's Fund; 2012.

33 Sallis J, Owen N. *Physical activity and behavioral medicine.* Thousand Oaks, CA: Sage; 1999.

34 Shor R, Shalev A.Barriers to involvement in physical activities of persons with mental illness. *Health Promot Int.* 2016; **31**:116–23. DOI: 10.1093/heapro/dau078

35 Vancampfort D, Knapen, J, Probst M, Scheewe T, Remans S, De Hert M. A systematic review of correlates of physical activity in patients with schizophrenia. *Acta Psychiatr Scand.* 2012; **125**:352–62. DOI: 10.1111/j.1600-0447.2011.01814.x

36 Vancampfort D, Faulkner G. Physical activity and serious mental illness: a multidisciplinary call to action. *Ment Health Phys Act.* 2014; **7**:153–4. DOI: 10.1016/j.mhpa.2014.11.001.

37 World Medical Association. WMA declaration of helsinki – ethical principles for medical research involving human subjects. 2013. Available from: www.wma.net/policies-post/wma-declaration-of-helsinki-ethical-principles-for-medical-research-involving-human-subjects/

30 Disseminating the research findings

Ashleigh Moreland and Joshua Denham

Introduction and aims

By definition, disseminate means to 'spread widely'. In the context of physical activity and health research, it is critical to consider all stakeholders when it comes to sharing our important findings. After all, the only way to create meaningful change and develop knowledge and best practice in the wider community is by sharing scientific evidence in a way that is understandable to appropriate audiences. This chapter will provide a brief overview of considerations for disseminating research findings, including publishing in scientific journals, presenting at national and international conferences, and more informal sharing of information via social media and other means.

Publishing in scientific journals

Having your work published in reputable scientific journals is currently the gold standard for research dissemination, and also ensures the quality and robustness of experimental designs and study findings. However, the peer-review process is complex and can take lengthy periods of time (e.g. typically 3–6 months, or more). The first complexity of publishing is selecting a target journal. With this task, one must consider not only the content matter and target audience, but also whether to choose a traditional journal or an open access journal, and further, the journal's impact, as determined by an ever-growing list of metrics. An additional complexity of publishing relates to authorship – who goes on the paper, and where are they positioned in the list of authors?

Who is your target audience?

One sensible approach to selecting a journal is by asking the question, 'who cares?' If a particular type of researcher or end-user of your results is for whom your findings are likely to be most relevant, the ideal journal may be one that is a 'niche' journal. For example, the *Journal of Strength and Conditioning Research* has a target audience primarily of strength and conditioning coaches, it thus includes a 'practical applications' section that is geared towards translating scientific findings to practice. This may be an ideal journal for your findings if they have a practical application rather than submitting to a physiology journal, such as *Physiological Genomics*, which focuses on publishing articles describing mechanisms underpinning physiological responses at the molecular level, which would be of interest to a different readership. Likewise, if you are aspiring towards a career as an academic in applied exercise science, the former could also be a better choice as it is the most relevant to your chosen field.

Traditional or open access publication?

In addition to considering your target audience, you may find yourself weighing up the pros and cons of selecting a traditional journal versus an open access journal. Prior to the internet era, journals were hardcopy publications that scientists would subscribe to in order to remain up-to-date with the most recent evidence in their field, and to also identify collaborative opportunities. They or their institution's library would then receive a hard copy of the journal at designated intervals, such as monthly or quarterly. It is quite possible, though, that scholars working in the 21st century never lay their hands on a hardcopy scientific journal, as technological advancements provide us with access to publications through digital devices. Along with this has emerged the concept of open access journals. In short, open access journals are an alternative business model, offering faster publication speeds and higher acceptance rates, but shift the expense of research dissemination to the researcher, rather than the consumer. That is, traditional publications usually charge little to no fees to authors, but are prohibitive to end-users due to subscription fees that are typically paid by institutions; whereas open access journals shift the financial responsibility to the authors by charging hundreds or thousands of dollars in article processing and publication charges (e.g. US $1,595 per PLoS One manuscript in 2018), in return for enhanced accessibility and visibility of research findings. This allows almost anyone with an internet connection to access the article, usually at no cost to the reader. Björk[1] discusses the benefits and challenges of open access publishing. However, whilst it is clear that open access journals offer advantages over traditional journals, be cautious of predatory publishers, who often send soliciting emails 'inviting' you to submit papers to them, and who present with a façade of a scholarly journal, but don't employ adequate or ANY peer-review processes and will publish virtually anything, provided the fee is paid.[2] Publishing in these journals may adversely affect the reputation of academics trying to establish a publication record, and has been a driving force in emphasizing the 'quality' of publications, rather than merely the quantity. As a consequence, researchers need to be aware of the status of journals they are contemplating submitting their research to, and to assist with this there are a number of reputable metrics that relate to journals as well as researchers.

What are 'metrics', and what do they tell us about the quality of research?

With the emphasis being placed on quality research outputs, journal metrics and researcher metrics are evolving as a way for researchers and readers to assess the calibre of the journal that the work is published in, and also to demonstrate a research track record for job opportunities, grant applications and promotions. According to Elsevier,[3,4] these metrics include CiteScore, Source Normalized Impact per Paper (SNIP), SCImago Journal Rank (SJR), H-index, Impact Factor (annual or five-year), Immediacy Index, and the Eigenfactor and Article Influence. For a summary of each of these metrics, see Table 30.1. Publications in high-impact journals are, no doubt, goals of most scientists, as they tend to lead to career opportunities and promotions – though they are not requisites. Another useful fact to consider when deciding where to submit your research, is where the journal is ranked in the list of journals relevant to your field. Sites such as Scimago (https://www.scimagojr.com/) rank journals for each field and then indicate in which quartile the journal is ranked (Q1–Q4). Publishing in a Q1 journal is therefore likely to be deemed more prestigious and potentially have greater benefit than publishing in a journal ranked in one of the lower

Table 30.1 Definitions of publication metrics

Metric	Explanation
Researcher metrics	
H-index*	Calculated by identifying the number of articles a researcher has published and determining whether that number of articles has generated at least the same amount of citations each (e.g. 9 articles, each cited at least 9 times equates to an H-index of 9).
i10-index*	The number of published articles that have been cited at least 10 times.
Journal metrics	
SCImago Journal Rank (SJR)	SJR is calculated by the mean weighted citations generated over a given year by the articles published in the particular journal over the previous three years.
CiteScore	The average citation count of all papers published in a particular journal over the previous three years.
Source Normalized Impact per Paper (SNIP)	SNIP is the ratio of a source's average citation count per paper and the citations potential of its subject field (Elsevier 2018).
Immediacy index	The number of times a paper is cited in the year it is published.
Eigenfactor score	A measure of a journal's total importance to the scientific community. It is calculated based on the number of citations within the reporting year of articles published in a given journal within the last five years.

Note: Number of documents (overall and over *x*-amount of years) and citations are also important researcher metrics.

* Typically calculated over a researcher's career and also over a five-year period in an attempt to quantify past and more recent research productivity.

quartiles. This ranking within fields also has the benefit of overcoming some of the problems with other metrics, where for example in a relatively small field it would be difficult for a publication to get as many citations as one in a much larger field, and hence the magnitude of journal impact factors are affected by the size of the field.

What are the considerations for authorship?

Authorship can be a sensitive issue, as career progression and research grant success can be highly dependent upon publications. Whilst there are several variations as to what constitutes authorship, the International Committee of Medical Journal Editors (ICMJE) recommends that an author is someone who:

- Substantially contributes to the conception or design of the work; or the acquisition, analysis, or interpretation of data for the work; AND
- Drafts the work or revises it critically for important intellectual content; AND
- Approves the final version to be published; AND
- Agrees to be accountable for all aspects of the work in ensuring that questions related to the accuracy or integrity of any part of the work are appropriately investigated and resolved.

(International Committee of Medical Journal Editors 2018)[5]

Typically, in medical and most science journals, the 'prime real-estate' is that of first author and last author, whereby the first author is often the person who has primarily conducted most of the research and written the paper, and the last author is the most senior person overseeing the project. Middle authors are those who meet the authorship guidelines, but are seen as having had a more secondary role, thus these positions tend to hold less weight when establishing a research track record. Interestingly, the number of authors on papers has significantly increased over the past few decades, with many regular research papers having six or more authors.[6] This is possibly an outcome of improved collaborative opportunities provided by web-based platforms. Indeed, a larger proportion of middle authors who may have had a significant contribution to the work may now not be receiving appropriate recognition for their efforts. This has created a relatively new phenomena calling for equal attribution recognition for papers with 'multiple first authors', or 'multiple last authors'.[7] This needs further development in the field of physical activity and health research, but allows fairness and equality in an environment that is promoting cross-discipline research by recognizing the significant contributions of experts from their respective fields. Regardless, though, it is imperative that conversations regarding authorship expectations occur early to prevent disputes when it is time to publish. One way to prevent authorship disputes is by establishing formal authorship agreements that outline the roles and responsibilities of all parties. Authorship agreements should be developed early in the project, and be updated when necessary as the project progresses.

Presenting at scientific conferences or seminars

Conferences and seminars are great opportunities to bring together research and industry. Often, practitioners, coaches or other industry stakeholders will attend conferences for professional development purposes, and other scientists will attend and present either poster or oral presentations for the purpose of not only dissemination of their own work, but also for immediate networking and collaborative opportunities. The process for selecting a conference to attend is very similar to that of selecting a journal, and requires consideration of the target audience or relevance of the content, costs of attendance and likely benefits of attendance. There are convenient web-collections of conference listings, such as Conference Management Software,[8] which you may wish to browse to determine whether your work fits the theme and would add value to conference proceedings.

Presenting findings to participants

An important consideration that is often overlooked during the research process is disseminating the overall study findings and relevant individual results back to research participants. Providing a summary of the study findings and implications in easy-to-understand language (lay terminology) is a great way to show gratitude to participants, whilst improving community engagement and rewarding participants for their dedication to the study (i.e. time, physical and mental efforts). Results from outcome measures of interest, such as anthropometric variables, cognitive data, physical performance or other variables can be presented relative to population normative data. This can help to educate participants on their current health status, and by knowing what the study findings mean and how they can incorporate them into their own physical activity behaviours, they may benefit their own health. This can be achieved with an on-the-spot discussion of results after a testing session, emails with graphs displaying their personal data relative to normative data (which dot they are on the scatterplot and what it indicates), or a presentation delivered face to face or online. In some situations, group presentations are also possible, sometimes in the form of evening celebrations upon completion of the research, but on these occasions, researchers need to be mindful of maintaining individual privacy and anonymity when presenting any results.

Informal dissemination of research findings

As eluded to previously, the rise of web-based platforms has created an insatiable hunger for information. Social media outlets like Facebook, Twitter, Yammer, Instagram and even Snapchat contain never-ending feeds of information, and an enormous audience to broadcast snippets of your research highs and lows. Hashtags are used to follow live updates at conferences, 'Facebook lives' are used to interview researchers, and TED talks and YouTube channels are powerful vehicles to achieve the ultimate goal of widespread exposure of your research. Although social media and other media outlets (e.g. television, radio, newspapers and magazines) are great methods of disseminating research findings, they also have their challenges. For instance, the key research finding/s or take-home message/s can be presented in a palatable form either graphically or in a few sentences (150 characters) via social media – an effective dissemination outlet, especially if the audience re-posts the findings to their 'followers' or 'friends'. However, unlike journal articles with lengthy discussions and limitations sections, many social media–related research posts fail to acknowledge the shortfalls of research, which can lead to heated online discussions. At times, conclusions from research are at risk of misinterpretation or dilution, which can result in the evolution of 'anecdata'. Therefore, one must be conservative when interpreting the research findings, acknowledge limitations and use language that is comprehensive to a layperson. There are also researcher profile platforms such as ResearchGate and LinkedIn that enable you to connect with other researchers and freely share your projects and key findings. Finally, a relatively new initiative, 'Science Matters', is attempting to give formal recognition of research observations in an informal setting and without the narrative required in full publications.[9]

Conclusion

It is clear that the landscape of research dissemination has, and will continue to, change, particularly in the realms of open access publishing, equal attribution of authors and the widespread use of social media. It has also been established that there is no one best approach to disseminating your findings; rather you should ask yourself a series of questions to determine the best option for your work on a case-by-case basis. However, regardless of how you choose to disseminate your research, you should aim to remain authentic in your purpose of creating and sharing knowledge for the growth of science and humanity.

References

1 Björk BC. Open access to scientific articles: a review of benefits and challenges. *Int Emerg Med.* 2017; **12**(2):247–53.
2 Shen C, Björk BC. Predatory' open access: a longitudinal study of article volumes and market characteristics. *BMC Med.* 2015; **13**(1):230.
3 Elsevier. Measuring a journal's impact. Available 29/06/2018, from www.elsevier.com/authors/journal-authors/measuring-a-journals-impact
4 Elsevier. How is SNIP (Source Normalized Impact per Paper) used in Scopus? Available 04/06/2018, from https://service.elsevier.com/app/answers/detail/a_id/14884/c/10547/supporthub/scopus/related/1/session/L2F2LzEvdGltZS8xNTMwNjYyMTA4L3NpZC9mVUd6eXB5V2RXQmFrcHBBWTVRtSFRZRlBBBc0N3dmQ1MTh2cFR3OHNYS3djZmQzWWIBeFJCOW1CcHE0d1JYUzVEYlAwNzhCb2lhQ3MxdzNxazZJOG5jRFdJdjVGcmRRuT0p1WXh3UTMyX1hydVpCVHRGNVJMXzJDWEElMjElMjE%3D/
5 International Committee of Medical Journal Editors. Defining the role of authors and contributors. Available 29/06/2018, from www.icmje.org/recommendations/browse/roles-and-responsibilities/defining-the-role-of-authors-and-contributors.html
6 Zetterström R. The number of authors of scientific publications. *Acta Paediatr.* 2004; **93**(5):581–2.
7 Akhabue E, Lautenbach E. Equal contributions and credit: an emerging trend in the characterization of authorship. *Ann Epidemiol.* 2010; **20**(11):868–71.
8 Conference Management Software. Conferences and meetings on sport and exercise medicine, physical therapy. Available 29/06/2018, from: www.conference-service.com/conferences/sports-medicine.html
9 Science Matters. *The next-generation science publishing platform.* Available 28/06/2018, from www.sciencematters.io/

31 Translating research findings into community interventions. Considerations for design and implementation

A case-based approach

Andrew D. Williams, Lucy K. Byrne, Lindsey B. Strieter, Greig Watson, and Ross Arena

Aims of the chapter

The aims of this chapter are to illustrate how research can contribute to informing better practice and attaining better health outcomes.

Introduction

Despite extensive evidence that there are numerous physical and psychological benefits of physical activity across the human lifespan,[1,2] worldwide 31.1% of adults are classified as inactive.[3] Indeed, the World Health Organisation (WHO) identifies physical inactivity as a major risk factor across the globe for morbidity and premature mortality,[4] yet it is estimated that approximately 5.3 million deaths per year could be avoided if all inactive people became moderately active.[5] In addition to its effects on the health and wellbeing of individuals, physical inactivity has a considerable negative impact on the economy. The economic costs of physical inactivity through increased mortality and disease burden is immense with reported conservative estimates of the global direct health costs of physical inactivity to be INT$53.8 billion in 2013 with an additional $13.7 billion in lost productivity associated with physical inactivity–related deaths.[6] Recognition of the importance of physical activity to health through wider policy initiatives designed to increase global physical activity levels therefore is of paramount importance. However, increasing the physical activity levels of millions of people is not an easy task, indeed, just increasing the physical activity levels of a small community can be fraught with complexities.

This chapter presents challenges involved in getting people to become more active, profiles several initiatives designed to increase physical activity and improve health risk factors across a range of population groups, and examines some of the issues related to delivery and ongoing sustainability of physical activity programmes. Finally, some recommendations for their future delivery are made.

Factors affecting participation in physical activity?

A number of interrelated factors or elements can influence the decision for an individual to participate in physical activity. These elements, which in combination constitute the ecological framework of active living, include intra- and interpersonal factors,[7, 8] organizational, policy, and community or environmental factors that work in isolation or together and potentially across the complete ecological framework resulting in a culmination of their effects. To illustrate this, Evenson and Aytur provide an example "where a person who does not know how to swim lacks skills (intrapersonal),[9] but this may have been influenced by having siblings who did not swim (interpersonal), living in a town without a public pool (community/environmental), or not having affordable swimming lessons (policy)". All of these factors 'add up' to create barriers to physical activity and to successfully encourage increases in physical activity through policy all these factors need to be considered and addressed where relevant.[9] Thus, despite the large and indisputable health benefits for physical activity, translating adherence to physical activity in daily life is far more complicated, and adherence to physical activity routines over time remains a major challenge.[10] This has remained the situation despite widespread reporting of the benefits of physical activity to health within the media and growing awareness of this in the general population.

Physical activity population interventions

To be truly effective, population physical activity interventions need to increase physical activity in not only the short term, but must also lead to long-term increases in physical activity in the target population. Research indicates that to optimize success particularly at the community-wide level, interventions must address all decisions made by members of the target community that influence their physical activity – in other words, optimal interventions act across all relevant levels of the ecological framework.[11] However, while interventions to improve health outcomes through the delivery of physical activity or exercise interventions are common, historically much of the research has focused on the impact of structured programmes that target small groups of individuals with specific illness.[12] This may be at least in part due to the complexities involved in implementing community-wide initiatives,[13] because community- or population-based strategies to increase physical activity are difficult to implement and where they have occurred and have been evaluated, the effect sizes are often small.[11,14] A recent Cochrane Review,[11] for example, reports that the failure to demonstrate improvements may be due to narrow engagement strategies that fail to reach the target population, and limitations in the research methods utilized in the reviewed studies including selection bias, lack of control communities and lack of analysis against equity markers such as socioeconomic status.

To reiterate, population-based physical activity initiatives that adopt multiple strategies to promote the benefits of physical activity and engage communities in higher rates of participation may have the best chance of increasing physical activity levels in the general community and improving health outcomes.[11] The strategies most likely to contribute to population-level change in physical activity participation include supportive environments, mass media and educational programmes, community interventions, broad population engagement, professional guidance and ongoing care.[15,16]

Case studies

The following section describes three case studies of community physical activity programmes which demonstrate how strategies listed above have been implemented to promote increased physical activity across a range of populations. The discussion of these cases covers the context, overview and outcomes (where available) from each project and a summary of key learnings coming from the case studies then follows.

University of Illinois at Chicago Health and Wellness Academy case study

Substantial growth in school- and community-based health-intervention programmes has occurred over the last 15 years in the United States, which, if implemented effectively, can have a positive impact on important health issues such as childhood obesity (currently 17%).[17] In fact, many 'focused-based', or youth intervention programmes focus on the prevention of a chronic disease diagnosis (e.g. cardiovascular disease, diabetes, etc.). Focused-based programmes commonly facilitate physical activity and healthy eating practices;[18–20] primary outcomes/objectives include body weight/fat loss or weight maintenance[21–23] and enhanced cardiorespiratory fitness.[24] However, it is important to differentiate between an 'obesity prevention programme' and "school-based wellness programmes" (SBWP). SBWPs are comprehensive, multilevel approaches that may include components focused on disease prevention, but with the primary goal of facilitating health-promoting change in the school environment, as well as changes in the lifestyles of children, family groups and ultimately the broader community. Current evidence suggests SBWPs can positively impact health behaviours, including physical activity patterns.[18,25–27]

Through a partnership fostered between an academic medical centre and urban public school system, the Department of Physical Therapy in the College of Applied Health Sciences (CAHS) at the University of Illinois at Chicago (UIC) created a SBWP, focusing on two key components of healthy living – physical activity and nutrition. The UIC SBWP incorporated evidence-based approaches from the literature in conjunction with established educational models.[18,25–28] The primary intention of this SBWP is to empower participants, children between the age of 8 and 11, to make choices that build a positive relationship with physical movement and nutrition, thus promoting healthy living practices and motivating them to sustain such practices. The SBWP began as a summer health camp in 2016 for grade school children who lived in the immediate neighbourhood. The health camp incorporated healthy living practices utilizing students from departments in the CAHS, including nutrition and kinesiology, and physical therapy. The camp was held on the UIC's campus, and in doing so, the children not only learned information about healthy lifestyle choices, but were also given the opportunity to see the university and engage with its students. From this camp, the Health and Wellness Academy (HWA) evolved the following spring of 2017 as a three-credit community outreach experiential learning course (PT 592: The Health and Wellness Academy).

The HWA was structured in a way that children, teachers and school administrators serve as vital stakeholders. As such, their input, support and participation were crucial for optimal efficacy of the SWBP. In this context, by utilizing trained educators to develop, deliver and disseminate curriculum specifically tailored to the health needs of each student in their classroom the HWA is designed in a way that puts education of youth at the forefront for health promotion efforts to be sustainable, have long-term impact potential and produce and maintain educational efficacy. A UIC faculty member housed within the Department of Physical Therapy, who was a former

Chicago Public Schools classroom teacher, currently serves as the Education Director (ED) of the HWA. The HWA was tested as a 1.5-hour after-school session held twice per week, delivered to approximately 40 elementary students (ES – third through fifth grade). In conjunction with the HWA, the parallel spring semester course (PT 592) provided training to 14 college students (CS) from the departments of kinesiology and nutrition and physical therapy. Course content included didactic learning, open-discussions (1 time per week) and community outreach experiential learning sessions (twice per week) at the Chicago elementary school.

Once the interdisciplinary team of CS was compiled, the ED conducted participant interviews in order to familiarize themselves with the learners/population. From there, areas of strength and growth were identified, and learning objectives were created. The ED with the CS planned, created and implemented learning activities that were tailored to the needs and interests of the ES, so that ES could achieve mastery of the content. Bringing the various disciplines together in one course created multi-tiered mentorships. The planning and collaboration occurred in the 2-hour didactic discussion session each week. The after-school programme at the elementary school then served as their community outreach experiential learning. During each session with the ES there were both movement and nutrition activities. During the movement component, CS engaged ES into creative physical activity games in order to facilitate movement. By the end of the programme, ES had shown that they were able to know the content, apply the content and then teach the content, by presenting their mastery of knowledge and skills in an event shared with the surrounding community. Additionally, CS gained valuable insight into multi-disciplinary problem-solving and increased their awareness of social, political and cultural factors that influence the surrounding community.

Lastly, a research-focused faculty member, also from the UIC Department of Physical Therapy, with expertise in community-based health and wellness interventions, is establishing a HWA research agenda. The main goal of this research programme will be to *inform the HWA*; findings will be used on an ongoing basis to make adjustments to the programme that will ideally enhance efficacy and long-term outcomes.

Limitations of HWA, like many other SBWPs, can be found in the resource management between academic institutions and elementary schools. HWA's strengths can be found in its interdisciplinary and innovative approach that is reproducible and has the potential to bring about positive environmental change and improve health outcomes for children and their families.

Strength 2 Strength case study

Strength 2 Strength (S2S) was a 12-week supervised exercise programme targeted at elderly, frail and aged individuals, Indigenous Australians and those with or at high risk of developing chronic medical conditions. Participants were able to self-refer or were referred by their general practitioner or other health professionals. The programme ran in Tasmania between June 2013 and June 2016. This programme was funded by the Australian government as part of the Tasmanian Health Assistance Package with money allocated across a number of projects aimed to address inequities in the Australian and Tasmanian health systems. Projects funded as part of this scheme addressed primary and secondary preventive health outcomes as well as issues with high elective surgery waiting lists.

S2S involved the delivery of evidence-based individualized exercise programmes to participants within a group setting by Accredited Exercise Physiologists over a 12-week period and was accompanied by home-based exercise programmes for clients to complete in their own time.[29,30] Participants were also provided with the opportunity to attend optional additional sessions focused on improving their health and wellbeing and assisting self-management (e.g. the benefits of physical activity, diet and nutrition, management or prevention of chronic conditions and falls prevention). Over the life of the project at least 1,573 individuals enrolled and received exercise prescription and more than 1,115 completed the S2S programme although data quality issues from those enrolled in regional locations prevents exact numbers being available.

Multiple outcomes related to physical activity adherence and health risk factors were assessed as part of the Strength 2 Strength programme [unpublished data]. Improvements in physical activity participation were observed by participants during the 12-week intervention and a limited evaluation of the outcomes that was performed revealed mean improvements in shuttle and six-minute walk test distance, in functional strength measures and reductions in waist circumference and resting blood pressure in those with higher levels on entry into the programme suggesting reduced risk of comorbidities. The proportion of participants continuing to undertake their home-based programme following completion of the S2S programme was 65% at 3 months, 56% at 6 months and 52% at 12 months indicating that the approach was successful in educating and motivating many participants to be more physically active. A comprehensive health economics assessment of the programme was not performed as part of the analysis of the programme due to timeframes required for the delivery of the report and issues associated with participant identifiers.

Active Launceston case study

The Active Launceston health promotion initiative involved a partnership between the Tasmanian State Government, Launceston City Council, University of Tasmania, as well as local businesses, community groups and not-for-profit organizations. An outline of the project direction and its preliminary outcomes have been described elsewhere.[31] Briefly, Active Launceston was underpinned by the Ottawa Charter for Health Promotion focusing primarily on the fifth action area which was to reorient (health) services towards a prevention focus.[32] It ran in the city of Launceston, a city of approximately 100,000 residents, between 2008 and 2015 and aimed to fill an identified gap in lack of coordination in the community for physical activities.[33] The initiative included a suite of physical activity programmes designed to accommodate people of all ages, interests and abilities, an extensive marketing campaign, input from health and industry professionals, and advocacy for environmental and policy change. The Active Launceston programme adopted a community-engagement, population-based approach with a goal to mobilize community members to increase their voluntary participation in physical activity by:[34] filling gaps in provision, reducing barriers and targeting those with the highest need. A stated aim was to fill identified gaps in physical activity provision in the community and to develop capacity within the community to ensure sustainable participation in physical activity.

Over its lifespan Active Launceston programmes attracted 11,887 attendees who attended a total of 30,342 sessions amounting to over 38,000 hours of physical activity. Semi-regular evaluations of both process and impact of the intervention using mixed methods design (combination of qualitative and quantitative evaluation) were performed in 2008, 2012 and again in 2015. The process evaluation was conducted through use of focus group, stakeholder interviews and a cross-sectional serial online survey. It identified that participants believed the programmes provided personal benefits through improved health, personal development and social connectedness. Facilitators of participation included free and accessible programmes as well as catering for people with different abilities and specific needs in non-threatening environments. The impact evaluation involved assessments of community-wide engagement in physical activity measured using telephone surveys of approximately 900 residents of Launceston in 2008, 2012 and again in 2015. Results of the surveys indicated gradual increases in the proportion of the population who achieved sufficient activity for health (defined as 150 min or more per week) over the years, with a significantly higher proportion achieving sufficient activity levels in 2015 compared to 2008 ($p < 0.01$). Awareness of the Active Launceston programme almost doubled from 31.9% to 61.5% over the same timeframe and the proportion of those interviewed who were sufficiently active for health was higher in those aware of Active Launceston (57.5%) than those who were not (44%) in the 2015 survey.

A retrospective cost-benefit analysis on the programme conducted by the Menzies Institute for Medical Research at the University of Tasmania [unpublished data] estimated a good return on investment. Using an estimated return on investment of 1.61 (based on a meta-analysis of 51 studies[35]) and a total investment of $1.9 million from 2008 to 2015, the cost to deliver Active Launceston was $160 per participant, and the estimated economic benefit and return of Active Launceston was $416 and $257 per participant respectively. The outcomes of this project indicate that inter-sectoral partnerships to increase population-wide physical activity levels using multi-strategy and wide-scale interventions can be effective in encouraging individuals to increase physical activity levels and may then lead to improved health outcomes and generate a positive return on investment for funding bodies.

Key learnings

Multiple important learnings are revealed through the implementation and evaluation of physical activity interventions that operate in community settings, including those summarized above. Importantly these programmes can successfully increase physical activity levels of participants and reduce health risk factors during the intervention period,[11] and potentially for many years following the cessation of the intervention,[36] although further evaluation of a range of programme types and foci are required to confirm these results. These programmes can also provide less tangible or measurable benefits through increasing social capital and health literacy for participants.[31]

Often there is an assumption that because benefits of an intervention such as exercise have been shown in rigorously controlled laboratory-based studies, these benefits will transfer to community- or population-based interventions. However as the scale of any study is increased, the complexities involved in designing, implementing and evaluating the intervention also increase.[37] The randomized controlled trial is considered the pinnacle of study design.[38] However, it is often not possible to evaluate community physical activity programmes with this type of design given the diversity of settings and complexity of interventions. Alternative designs don't provide the same evidence of programme effectiveness but are more feasible in many situations,[38] where balancing of the optimal evaluation design against what is achievable in practice is required. None of the case studies in this chapter used a randomized controlled intervention, as this was not feasible at the time. However their success can possibly be attributed to considering multiple aspects of the ecological framework,[7,8] adopting numerous strategies to increase physical activity, developing partnerships and incorporating specific evaluation as part of the design process.

Despite their successes, the two Tasmanian case studies described in this chapter relied on substantial public and philanthropic funding for their development and operation, which while significant, was not sufficient to fund randomized controlled trials or to fully evaluate outcomes. The failure to fully evaluate these programmes represents a missed opportunity given the limited funding available for these types of initiatives. A problem with preventive health initiatives is that the investment required for the initiative may precede the return on that investment by many years.[39] The benefits can often be quite difficult to quantify as they may result not only in reduced or delayed acute healthcare and disability costs, but also increased work productivity and the building of social capital. A world-class study conducted by researchers at the University of Queensland and Deakin University in Australia used economic modelling to quantify the benefits of 150 different health interventions, of which 123 were preventive.[40] The study found that if the Australian government were to implement the top 20 health interventions it would cost Australia $4.6 billion over 30 years. However, this expense would be offset by predicted cost savings of $11 billion over the same timeframe due to reduced acute care costs and increased productivity. Such a programme which included interventions across taxation, regulation, health promotion and clinical intervention was predicted to pay for itself within 10 years and result in 1 million additional years of healthy life across the Australian population.[40]

The sustainability of initiatives is important as health and productivity benefits from community initiatives require time to become apparent. A weakness in the implementation of both the S2S and Active Launceston initiatives was to achieve sustainability of the programmes. As follow-up assessments were not planned, it is unclear whether participants of the programmes continue to maintain improvements in activity and health measures independent of the programme. Although in its early stages, the Health and Wellness Academy initiative has taken an approach likely to lead to ongoing sustainability through training future teachers how to deliver the programme. This approach ensures that subject to time being available within the curriculum the programme can be delivered in schools by these mentors independent of the ongoing status of HWA.

Educating communities and participants should be a key element of community health programmes as this education helps to empower individuals to increase responsibility for their own health.[41] Methods of providing this education can vary and while widely distributed messages through advertising or social media can initiate awareness and interest in health, more targeted/individualized education, as is delivered in both the HWA and S2S programmes, delivered to smaller groups of participants or individuals are likely to have longer-term benefits in empowering those who receive it. Initiatives that do not overtly plan to achieve project sustainability in their target population or are dependent on the resources such as staffing, volunteers, facilities, equipment and materials they provide are less likely to lead to sustainable outcomes in the long term. To assist with exercise adherence and therefore sustainability of outcomes S2S implemented home-based exercise programmes and low-cost resources such as elastic bands to enable participants to exercise independently.

The long-term sustainability of community interventions may also be influenced by involving a range of stakeholders in partnership. Active Launceston effectively utilized partnerships to sustain the initiative for nine years. During this time ongoing funding was received from a number of partners including federal, state and local government as well as the university sector and industry. Changes to government policy in 2016 resulted in state government funding being withdrawn which caused the initiative to reduce its offerings. Although a retrospective cost-benefit analysis was performed, prospective analyses of the potential economic benefits were considered but not implemented. Due to the weaknesses of retrospective compared to prospective economic analyses it is more difficult to ascertain the true economic benefits arising from Active Launceston than if prospective economic analyses were performed. A higher degree of certainty of reported economic benefits would have helped to justify the expenditure of public funding as an ongoing expense. As part of the S2S initiative, a limited economic evaluation, that compared the cost of setting up and delivering the programme with the estimated savings from a reduction in falls causing injury within 12 months of programme completion, was conducted. The analysis projected a small positive monetary saving of ~AU$70,000 from the programme. Given the benefits observed in a range of health risk factors and the ongoing compliance with home-based exercise by half of participants it is possible that these savings would continue into the future.

Conclusion

Physical inactivity is an increasing problem globally. However overcoming the increasing problem of physical inactivity is complicated due to the numerous issues involved in getting people to be more physically active. Initiatives involving multiple strategies to encourage increased activity levels and empower participants are more likely to be effective. Planning and incorporating evaluation strategies into initiatives is essential to inform wider policy. To maximize likelihood of positive outcomes and inform stakeholders, future community-based physical activity initiatives should:

- Investigate opportunities to share knowledge and resources between stakeholders.
- Address all relevant aspects of the ecological framework to the target population in the design of the initiative.
- Adopt multiple strategies to encourage participation within the target community and to educate and empower participants to sustain habitual physical activity.
- Embed evaluation processes including cost-benefit assessments into the initiative (see Nutbeam and Bauman,[38] for planning evaluations).

References

1 Lear SA, Hu W, Rangarajan S, Gasevic D, Leong D, et al. The effect of physical activity on mortality and cardiovascular disease in 130000 people from 17 high-income, middle-income, and low-income countries: the PURE study. *Lancet.* 2017; **390**(10113):2643–54.
2 Tucker SJ, Carr LJ. Translating physical activity evidence to hospital settings: a call for culture change. *Clin Nurse Spec.* 2016; **30**(4):208–15.
3 Hallal PC, Andersen LB, Bull FC, Guthold R, Haskell W, Ekelund U. Global physical activity levels: surveillance progress, pitfalls, and prospects. *Lancet.* 2012; **380**(9838):247–57.
4 World Health Organization. *Physical inactivity: a global public health problem.* 2014. Available from: www.who.int/dietphysicalactivity/factsheet_inactivity/en/index.html.

5 Lee IM, Shiroma EJ, Lobelo F, Puska P, Blair SN, Katzmarzyk PT. Effect of physical inactivity on major non-communicable diseases worldwide: an analysis of burden of disease and life expectancy. *Lancet.* 2012; **380**(9838):219–29.

6 Ding D, Lawson KD, Kolbe-Alexander TL, Finkelstein EA, Katzmarzyk PT, et al. The economic burden of physical inactivity: a global analysis of major non-communicable diseases. *Lancet.* 2016; **388**(10051):1311–24.

7 Ainsworth BE, Macera CA. *Physical activity and public health practice.* Boca Raton: CRC Press; 2012.

8 Sallis J, Owen N, Fisher E. Ecological models of health behavior. In: Glanz K, Viswanath K, editors. *Health behavior and health education: theory, research and practice.* San Francisco: Jossey-Bass; 2008. pp. 465–82.

9 Evenson K, Aytur S. Policy for physical activity promotion. In: Ainsworth BE, Macera CA, editors. *Physical activity and public health practice.* New South Wales: CRC Press; 2012.

10 Reiner M, Niermann C, Jekauc D, Woll A. Long-term health benefits of physical activity – a systematic review of longitudinal studies. *BMC Public Health.* 2013; **13**:813.

11 Baker PR, Francis DP, Soares J, Weightman AL, Foster C. Community wide interventions for increasing physical activity. *Cochrane Database Syst Rev.* 2015; **1**:CD008366.

12 Bazzano AT, Zeldin AS, Diab IR, Garro NM, Allevato NA, Lehrer D; WRC Project Oversight Team. The healthy lifestyle change program: a pilot of a community-based health promotion intervention for adults with developmental disabilities. *Am J Prev Med.* 2009; **37**(6 Suppl 1):S201–8.

13 O'Hara BJ, Phongsavan P, Eakin EG, Develin E, Smith J, Greenaway M, Bauman AE. Effectiveness of Australia's get healthy information and coaching service(R): translational research with population wide impact. *Prev Med.* 2012; **55**(4):292–8.

14 Bauman AE, Reis RS, Sallis JF, Wells JC, Loos RJ, Martin BW; Lancet Physical Activity Series Working Group. Correlates of physical activity: why are some people physically active and others not? *Lancet.* 2012; **380**(9838):258–71.

15 Bauman A, Finegood DT, Matsudo V. International perspectives on the physical inactivity crisis – structural solutions over evidence generation? *Prev Med.* 2009; **49**(4):309–12.

16 Hillsdon M, Foster C, Thorogood M. Interventions for promoting physical activity. *Cochrane Database Syst Rev.* 2005; (1):CD003180.

17 Ogden CL, Carroll MD, Kit BK, Flegal KM. Prevalence of childhood and adult obesity in the United States, 2011–2012. *JAMA.* 2014; **311**(8):806–14.

18 Dobbins M, Husson H, DeCorby K, LaRocca RL. School-based physical activity programs for promoting physical activity and fitness in children and adolescents aged 6 to 18. *Cochrane Database Syst Rev.* 2013; (2):CD007651.

19 Gortmaker SL, Peterson K, Wiecha J, Sobol AM, Dixit S, Fox MK, Laird N. Reducing obesity via a school-based interdisciplinary intervention among youth: planet health. *Arch Pediatr Adolesc Med.* 1999; **153**(4):409–18.

20 Sallis JF, McKenzie TL, Conway TL, Elder JP, et al., Environmental interventions for eating and physical activity: a randomized controlled trial in middle schools. *Am J Prev Med.* 2003; **24**(3):209–17.

21 Caballero B, Clay T, Davis SM, Ethelbah B, Rock BH, et al. Pathways: a school-based, randomized controlled trial for the prevention of obesity in American Indian schoolchildren. *Am J Clin Nutr.* 2003; **78**(5):1030–8.

22 Hoelscher DM, Springer AE, Ranjit N, Perry CL, Evans AE, et al. Reductions in child obesity among disadvantaged school children with community involvement: the Travis County CATCH Trial. *Obesity* (Silver Spring). 2010; **18**(Suppl 1):S36–44.

23 Fitzgibbon ML, Tussing-Humphreys LM, Porter JS, Martin IK, Odoms-Young A, Sharp LK. Weight loss and African-American women: a systematic review of the behavioural weight loss intervention literature. *Obes Rev.* 2012; **13**(3):193–213.

24 Ross R, Blair SN, Arena R, Church TS, Després JP, et al. Importance of assessing cardiorespiratory fitness in clinical practice: a case for fitness as a clinical vital sign: a scientific statement from the American heart association. *Circulation.* 2016; **134**(24):e653–e699.

25   Barrett-Williams SL, Franks P, Kay C, Meyer A, Cornett K, Mosier B. Bridging public health and education: results of a school-based physical activity program to increase student fitness. *Public Health Rep.* 2017; **132**(Suppl 2):81S–7S.

26   Braun HA, Kay CM, Cheung P, Weiss PS, Gazmararian JA. Impact of an elementary school-based intervention on physical activity time and aerobic capacity, georgia, 2013–2014. *Public Health Rep.* 2017; **132**(Suppl 2):24S–32S.

27   Burke RM, Meyer A, Kay C, Allensworth D, Gazmararian JA. A holistic school-based intervention for improving health-related knowledge, body composition, and fitness in elementary school students: an evaluation of the HealthMPowers program. *Int J Behav Nutr Phys Act.* 2014; **11**:78.

28   Santos RG, Durksen A, Rabbanni R, Chanoine JP, Lamboo Miln A, et al. Effectiveness of peer-based healthy living lesson plans on anthropometric measures and physical activity in elementary school students: a cluster randomized trial. *JAMA Pediatr.* 2014; **168**(4):330–7.

29   Al-Jundi W, Madbak K, Beard JD, Nawaz S, Tew GA. Systematic review of home-based exercise programmes for individuals with intermittent claudication. *Eur J Vasc Endovasc Surg.* 2013; **46**(6):690–706.

30   Clegg AP, Barber SE, Young JB, Forster A, Iliffe SJ. Do home-based exercise interventions improve outcomes for frail older people? Findings from a systematic review. *Rev Clin Gerontol.* 2012; **22**(1):68–78.

31   Byrne L, Ogden K, Auckland S. The active launceston health promotion initiative. In: Bartkowiak-Theron I, Anderseon K, editors. *Knowledge in action. University community engagement in Australia.* Newcastle: Cambridge Scholars; 2014. pp. 33–52.

32   World Health Organisation. *The ottawa charter for health promotion.* 2014. Available from: www.who.int/healthpromotion/conferences/previous/ottawa/en/

33   Australian Bureau of Statistics. *2016 Census Quickstats.* Australian Bureau of Statistics; 2017. Available from: http://www.abs.gov.au/websitedbs/censushome.nsf/home/quickstats?op endocument&navpos=220

34   Mittelmark MB, Hunt MK, Heath GW, Schmid TL. Realistic outcomes: lessons from community-based research and demonstration programs for the prevention of cardiovascular diseases. *J Public Health Policy.* 1993; **14**(4):437–62.

35   Baxter S, Sanderson K, Venn AJ, Blizzard CL, Palmer AJ. The relationship between return on investment and quality of study methodology in workplace health promotion programs. *Am J Health Promot.* 2014; **28**(6):347–63.

36   Li G, Zhang P, Wang J, Gregg EW, Yang W, et al. The long-term effect of lifestyle interventions to prevent diabetes in the China Da Qing Diabetes Prevention Study: a 20-year follow-up study. *Lancet.* 2008; **371**(9626):1783–9.

37   Deakin University. *Identifying effective strategies to increase recruitment and retention in community-based health promotion programs.* Melbourne: Deakin University; 2012. p. 54.

38   Nutbeam D, Bauman A. *Evaluation in a nutshell. A practical guide to the evaluation of health promotion programs.* North Ryde, NSW: McGraw-Hill; 2006.

39   Sassi F. *Obesity and the economics of prevention: fit not fat.* Paris: OECD; 2010.

40   Vos T, Carter R, Barendregt J, Mihalopoulos C, Veerman L, et al. *Assessing Cost-Effectiveness in Prevention (ACE-Prevention): Final Report.* Melbourne: University of Queensland, Brisbane and Deakin University; 2010.

41   Nutbeam D. Health literacy as a public health goal: a challenge for contemporary health education and communication strategies into the 21st century. *Health Promot Int.* 2000; **15**(3):259–67.

Index

informed consent: children, work with, and 239–40; chronic disease and 291; mental illness and 303; overview 60; questionnaires and 98

Integrated Research Application System (IRAS) 60

intensity of exercise: older people and 258–9; standardizing 223–5, *225*

inter-class correlation 173, 176

interdisciplinary approaches 302–3

internal validity 160, 179–80

International Physical Activity Questionnaire (IPAQ) 255

International Society for the Advancement of Kinanthropometry 158

interquartile range 170, **171**

inter-rater reliability 114

intersex 278, **285**

intersex athletes 284–6

interval data 169

intervention study: control group for *121*, 125–6; defined 118; designing 119–20; recruitment for 122–3

interviews: case study of project using 87–90; conducting 85–6; defined 80–1; designing 83–4, **84**; preparation for 84–5; in qualitative research 111; quality criteria for 86–7; uses of 81, **82**, 83

INVOLVE 49, 243

journals, publishing in 324–7

knowledge, Indigenous 267, **267**

knowledge-based questions 97

Kolmogorov-Smirnov test 170

language barriers 290

legal issues: illegal and banned activities, research on 68–9, 233–5; negative impacts of exercise research 232; SOGI and 279–81

liability insurance 67

life history approach 89

Life in Motion (LIM) programme 260–1

LIFE-P study 260

light physical activity (LPA) 147

Likert-type scales 96

limitations: on generalizability 131; of meta-analysis 182; of proposed study 47–8; of qualitative research 111

literature review of exercise and mental illness 304–5; *see also* systematic literature review

longitudinal observational studies 74–8

loss to follow-up bias 141

Male-to-Female transgendered athletes 284

malpractice, deliberate scientific 59

matching groups 126

mean 170, **171**

measurement: accuracy of 185–6; of affective responses to exercise 217–20; of clinical health 194–8; of physical behaviours 138, 186–91, *188*, 255–8; repeating 128–9; of sedentary behaviour 148–50; of strength and functional capacity 198–201

media: dissemination of findings via 328; misinformation from 11; negative impacts of exercise and 233; recruitment via 295

median 170, **171**

Medical Subject Headings (MeSH) 35, *35–6*

Medline 31, *37*

memory distortion 111

mental health population, research with: examples of 303–5; future directions for 305–6; methodological issues and 300–3; overview 300; *see also* serious mental illness, people with

meta-analysis 40, 181–3, *183*, 304

meta-bias 41

metabolic equivalent tasks (METs) 147, 185, 258–9

metabolic measurement 186

meta-synthesis 41

methodological practices, entrenched 211–12, 214–15

methods of proposed study 47, 51–2

metrics, publication 325–6, **326**

misconduct, reporting 59

mode 170, **171**

moderate-to-vigorous physical activity (MVPA) 147, 184, 317

monitoring physical activity of children and adolescents 243, *244*, 245

mood, defined 219

multichotomuous variable 138

muscle strength measurement 198–9

NAILSMA (North Australian Indigenous Land and Sea Management Alliance) checklist **273**, 275

narrative literature review 28–9

narrative synthesis 40

'nature' vs. 'nurture' 21–5

nayri kata model 269

negative impacts of exercise: ethical and legal issues and 232; importance of study of 230–1; as 'looking for trouble' 231–2; media and 233; outliers and 232–3; research questions on 235–6; scenarios for 233–5

neuroscience 302

nominal data 168

nominal variable 138

non-differential misclassification 139

non-random sampling 105